The National Medical Series for Independent Study

5th edition

review for USMLE

United States Medical Licensing Examination

Step **1**

John S. Lazo, Ph.D.

Chairman, Department of Pharmacology
Allegheny Foundation Professor of Pharmacology
University of Pittsburgh
*   School of Medicine*
Pittsburgh, Pennsylvania

Bruce R. Pitt, Ph.D.

Vice Chairman, Department of Pharmacology
Professor of Pharmacology
*   and Anesthesiology*
University of Pittsburgh
*   School of Medicine*
Pittsburgh, Pennsylvania

Joseph C. Glorioso, III, Ph.D.

Chairman, Department of Molecular
*   Genetics and Biochemistry*
William S. McEllroy Professor of
*   Biochemistry*
University of Pittsburgh
*   School of Medicine*
Pittsburgh, Pennsylvania

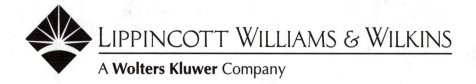

LIPPINCOTT WILLIAMS & WILKINS
A **Wolters Kluwer** Company

Editor: Elizabeth A. Nieginski
Senior Managing Editor: Amy G. Dinkel
Marketing Manager: Jennifer Conrad

Copyright © 1999 Lippincott Williams & Wilkins

351 West Camden Street
Baltimore, Maryland 21201-2436 USA

Rose Tree Corporate Center
1400 North Providence Road
Building II, Suite 5025
Media, Pennsylvania 19063-2043 USA

Printed in the United States of America

Library of Congress Cataloging-in-Publication Data

Lazo, John S.
   Review for USMLE: United States medical licensing examination,
step 1 / John S. Lazo, Bruce R. Pitt, Joseph C. Glorioso, III.—
5th ed.
     p. cm.—(The National medical series for independent study)
   ISBN 0-683-30490-9 (pbk.)
   1. Medicine—Examinations, questions, etc. I. Pitt, Bruce R.
II. Glorioso, Joseph C. III. Title. IV. Series.
  [DNLM: 1. Medicine examination questions. W 18.2L431r 1998]
R834.5.L393 1998
610'.76—dc21
DNLM/DLC
for Library of Congress   98-33988
                                               CIP

To purchase additional copies of this book, call our customer service department at **(800) 638-0672** or fax orders to **(800) 447-8438.** For other book services, including chapter reprints and large quantity sales, ask for the Special Sales department.

Canadian customers should call **(800) 665-1148,** or fax **(800) 665-0103.** For all other calls originating outside of the United States, please call **(410) 528-4223** or fax us at **(410) 528-8550.**

Visit Williams & Wilkins on the Internet: http://www.wwilkins.com or contact our customer service department at **custserv@wwilkins.com.** Williams & Wilkins customer service representatives are available from 8:30 am to 6:00 pm, EST, Monday through Friday, for telephone access.

98 99 00
1 2 3 4 5 6 7 8 9 10

5th edition

review for USMLE

United States
Medical Licensing
Examination

Step 1

Dedication

To Jacqui, Shayna, and Stacy

Permissions

Test I:

Figure 33 has been reprinted with permission from Harrison: *Principles of Internal Medicine,* 12th edition, New York, McGraw-Hill, 1991

Figure 50 has been reprinted with permission from Berne RM, Levy MN: *Human Physiology,* 3rd edition, St. Louis, CV Mosby, 1993

Figure 56 has been reprinted with permission from Murray J: *The Normal Lung,* Philadelphia, WB Saunders, 1976

Figure 60 has been reprinted with permission from Gilman AG, Rall TW, Nies AS, et al: Goodman and Gilman's: *The Pharmacologic Basis of Therapeutics,* 8th edition, Elmsford, NY, Pergamon Press, 1990

Figures 70–74 and 114–118 have been reprinted with permission from Hoffman BF, Cranefield PF: *Electrophysiology of the Heart,* New York, McGraw-Hill, 1960

Test III:

Figure 20–22 has been reprinted with permission from Robbins, St.: *Pathologic Basis of Disease,* 3rd edition, Philadelphia, WB Saunders, 1989

Figure 61–65 has been reprinted with permission from Bates DV, Macklem PT, Christie RV: *Respiratory Function in Disease,* 2nd edition, Philadelphia, WB Saunders, 1971

Figure 79 has been reprinted with permission from Wilson, Braunwald, Isselbacher: *Principles of Internal Medicine,* 12th edition, New York, McGraw-Hill, 1991

Test IV:

Figures 23 and 103 have been reprinted with permission from Guyton AC: *Textbook of Medical Physiology,* 8th edition, Philadelphia, WB Saunders, 1991

Test VI:

Figure 31–33 has been reprinted with permission from Sokolow M: *Clinical Cardiology,* 5th edition, East Norwalk, CT, Appleton & Lange, 1990

Contents

Preface

There are major changes currently occurring in the approach to medical education in the United States. There have been rapid advances in our understanding of the molecular basis of diseases; an enormous increase in the data that can be presented to medical students; and a consolidation of experimental methodologies in the basic sciences. As a result, there is now a general consensus that a greater emphasis should be placed on an integrated presentation of information during the first 2 years of medical school.

With the advent of the new USMLE Step 1 that de-emphasizes the traditional basic science disciplines and stresses the integrated approach, we believe it is especially important to provide students with a series of questions that will prepare them for this new format. Since the first edition, the *Review for USMLE Step 1* has undergone several iterations, reflecting the thoughtful comments of both students and faculty. In the most recent edition, we have substantially increased the patient-based questions that we hope will test your ability to integrate key basic science concepts with relevant clinical problems.

The National Board of Medical Examiners (NBME) will implement computer-based administration of the USMLE Step 1 in April of 1999. According to the NBME, the purpose and fundamental content of the exam will not change with the implementation of computer administration. This book provides question types that are now used on the USMLE and will continue to be used when the exam converts from paper-and-pencil format to the new computerized format. We hope you will find this book useful, and we, as well as the publisher, welcome any comments you may have.

John S. Lazo
Bruce R. Pitt
Joseph C. Glorioso, III

Acknowledgments

The writing of this book could not have been accomplished without the assistance of many individuals in the Departments of Pharmacology, Molecular Genetics and Biochemistry, Human Genetics, Psychiatry, and Pathology who helped with the first four editions. We are particularly grateful to Ronald J. Bernardi and Robert Rice, M.D./Ph.D. students at the University of Pittsburgh School of Medicine, who formulated many of the questions in the fifth edition. Thanks are also extended to Drs. Jeff Towers, Laura Finn, and Sam Yousem for supplying photomicrographs.

QUESTIONS

DIRECTIONS: *Single best answer questions* consist of numbered items or incomplete statements followed by answers or by completions of the statement. Select the ONE lettered answer or completion that is BEST in each case.

Matching questions consist of a list of four to twenty-six lettered options (some of which may be in figures) followed by several numbered items. For each numbered item, select the ONE lettered option that is most closely associated with it. Each lettered option may be selected once, more than once, or not at all.

Questions 1–5

The schematic drawing of a cholinergic synapse in the figure below should be used to answer the following questions.

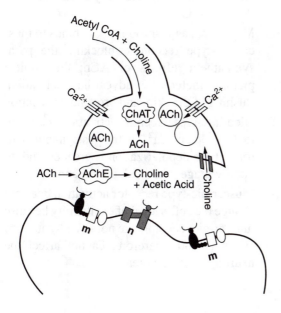

1. All of the following statements about neurons are correct EXCEPT

(A) presynaptic neurons usually do not have receptors for the neurotransmitter that they release

(B) neurons that release acetylcholine (ACh) are found in both the parasympathetic and the sympathetic branches of the autonomic nervous system

(C) cholinergic neurons in the basal nucleus of Meynert selectively degenerate in the brains of patients with confirmed Alzheimer's dementia

(D) the toxin produced by the bacterium *Clostridium tetanae* blocks inhibitory signals to cholinergic motor neurons in the anterior horn

(E) neurons releasing ACh make connections with cell types other than neurons, including cells found in glands, muscles, and blood vessels

2. All of the following statements about the proteins labeled *m* (i.e., muscarinic) and *n* (i.e., nicotinic) in the diagram are true EXCEPT

(A) muscarinic receptors have been found to carry signals via closely associated G proteins

(B) nicotinic receptors activate the inositol triphosphate (IP_3) pathway leading to the release of stored calcium (Ca^{2+})

(C) drugs that act at muscarinic sites are important in blocking the undesirable side effect of salivation during the administration of inhaled anesthetics

(D) drugs that act at nicotinic sites are important for temporarily paralyzing patients before tracheal intubation

(E) both receptor types bind the endogenous ligand ACh with high affinity

3. With respect to the postsynaptic neuron in the preceding diagram, which one of the following statements best describes signal transduction following the binding of ACh to the postsynaptic membrane?

(A) Nicotinic-type receptor activation leads to rapid influx of potassium (K^+), which causes hyperpolarization and decreased excitability in the postsynaptic neuron

(B) Muscarinic-type receptor activation may be inhibitory or excitatory, because the muscarinic receptors are a class of ligand-gated ion channels that allow the entry of chloride ions (Cl^-) and Ca^{2+}

(C) Muscarine, a mushroom toxin, binds to muscarinic-type receptors, blocking the parasympathetic effects of ACh; the clinical picture includes bradycardia, salivation, flushing of the skin, and bronchoconstriction

(D) Nicotinic-type receptor activation may lead to the influx of Ca^{2+} in the postsynaptic neurons, if the depolarization is great enough to open voltage-gated calcium channels

(E) Muscarinic-type receptor activation does not change the cell's level of excitability because muscarinic receptors are not ligand-gated ion channels and, therefore, cannot affect the neuron's resting potential

4. Which of the following statements about ACh release and deactivation is true?

(A) ACh release is blocked by the toxin associated with *Clostridium tetanae*
(B) Uptake of ACh into the presynaptic receptor is the most important mechanism in terminating the ACh signal
(C) Acetylcholinesterase (AChE) inhibitors, such as physostigmine, are not effective in the treatment of myasthenia gravis, because patients with myasthenia have no cholinergic nerve terminals to release ACh
(D) The influx of Ca^{2+} into the depolarized axon terminal is a prerequisite for the release of stored ACh
(E) Inhibitors of the enzyme monoamine oxidase (MAO) are important in the treatment of depression because they inhibit the breakdown of ACh into its constituents, acetic acid and choline

5. All of the following statements about the protein choline acetyltransferase (ChAT) in the preceding diagram are true EXCEPT

(A) ChAT is an enzyme that is synthesized on ribosomes located in the nerve terminal of the presynaptic neuron
(B) ChAT synthesizes ACh from the substrates acetyl coenzyme A (acetyl CoA) and choline
(C) ChAT exists in nerve terminals of both the central and peripheral nervous systems
(D) ChAT is responsible for synthesizing the neurotransmitter ACh before vesicular storage
(E) ChAT levels are decreased in the cerebral cortices of Alzheimer's patients whose brains have been analyzed postmortem

6. All of the following are anaerobes that can be found in the normal (disease-free) human body EXCEPT

(A) propionibacter organisms
(B) bacteroides
(C) pseudomonads
(D) fusobacterium organisms
(E) clostridia

7. A 60-year-old man has an abscess for which his physician prescribes a 7-day course of clindamycin. Before completion of the course the patient returns to the office with cramps, diarrhea, and a fever of 102.2°F. The patient is admitted to the hospital for sigmoidoscopy. Results demonstrate yellowish-white patchy areas on the wall of the colon. All of the following are true EXCEPT

(A) a Gram stain from the pseudomembrane would yield dark purple rods
(B) the pseudomembranous infection can be fatal if not treated
(C) clindamycin should be discontinued, and an aminoglycoside should be used until the pseudomembranes resolve
(D) the causative agent of the pseudomembranes is anaerobic
(E) the causative agent of the pseudomembranes produces toxins that act as monoglucosyltransferases specific for mammalian Rho protein

8. A young child has a low-grade fever, malaise, and unwillingness to eat. On physical examination, enlarged cervical lymph nodes and a gray membrane covering the tonsils and throat are found. A throat speciman shows gram-positive rods shaped like clubs that grew in "Chinese letter" forms. All of the following statements are true EXCEPT

(A) an adequate dose of penicillin will lead to complete recovery
(B) this illness could have been prevented by vaccination
(C) the causative organism expresses its toxin only in low-iron environments
(D) the gene for the toxin that is present in this disease is carried on a bacteriophage
(E) the causative organism's only host is the human body

9. A 55-year-old white man states that he has been having occasional episodes of chest pain for the past several months, but that the discomfort usually goes away after a few minutes. Three days ago, the patient had an episode of chest pain that lasted for over 20 minutes. Which one of the following statements is most likely correct?

(A) The patient's creatine kinase (CK-MB) levels are normal; therefore, he could not have had a myocardial infarction
(B) The patient's electrocardiogram (ECG) shows ST-segment elevation in leads II, III, and aVF; therefore, he had a myocardial infarction in the anterior wall of the heart
(C) The patient's lactate dehydrogenase (LDH$_1$) levels are normal; however, if he had a myocardial infarction 3 days ago, they could have been elevated earlier but returned to normal by now
(D) Based on the history alone, it is clear that the patient did not have a myocardial infarction
(E) ECG changes seen in leads I, V$_5$, and V$_6$ indicate that the left circumflex coronary artery was likely involved
(F) A decrease in serum myoglobin is detected

10. A 21-year-old man dies suddenly during his track workout. The man had a history of occasional fainting, as does his brother. On autopsy, his heart showed a hypertrophic interventricular septum out of proportion with the rest of the heart. Which one of the following is the most likely diagnosis?

(A) Sarcoidosis
(B) Amyloidosis
(C) Idiopathic hypertrophic cardiomyopathy
(D) Hemochromatosis
(E) Hypertensive heart disease
(F) Acute respiratory distress syndrome

11. All of the following statements about mitral valve prolapse are correct EXCEPT

(A) diagnosis of mitral valve prolapse rarely can be made before symptoms occur
(B) mitral valve prolapse is seen in approximately 7% of the population
(C) mitral valve prolapse usually causes a mid-systolic click
(D) Ehlers-Danlos syndrome and other connective tissue diseases are associated with mitral valve prolapse
(E) infective endocarditis is an infrequent, yet possible, complication of mitral valve prolapse

12. All of the following statements about rheumatic heart disease are correct EXCEPT

(A) it usually follows pharyngitis due to group A β-hemolytic streptococci

(B) all three layers of the heart—endocardium, myocardium, and pericardium—may be affected

(C) rheumatic heart disease cannot be distinguished from other forms of carditis on the basis of microscopic analysis of biopsies alone

(D) the five major criteria for diagnosis of acute rheumatic fever are carditis, polyarthritis, chorea, erythema marginatum, and subcutaneous nodules

(E) the mitral valve is the most commonly affected valve in chronic rheumatic heart disease

13. A correct description of the individual curves depicted in the log–dose response relationship below includes which of the following?

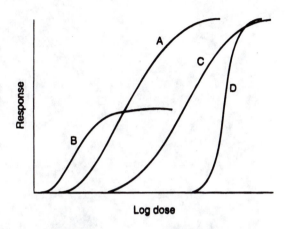

(A) Curves A and D: a full agonist (drug A) and a partial agonist (drug D)

(B) Curves B and C: an agonist in the absence of a noncompetitive inhibitor (curve B) and in the presence of one (curve C)

(C) Curves A, C, and D: three agonists with similar efficacy but different potency

(D) Curves A and C: an agonist in the absence of a competitive inhibitor (curve C) and in the presence of one (curve A)

(E) Curves A and C: drug A is less potent than drug C

14. The most common type of Ehlers-Danlos syndrome (i.e., type VI) is inherited in an autosomal recessive fashion. Which one of the following extracellular matrix molecules is affected?

(A) Laminin, which is the most abundant glycoprotein in all basement membranes

(B) Type II collagen, which is an important component of cartilage and the vitreous humor

(C) Types I and III collagen, which together have wide distributions in the skin, blood vessels, tendons, and bone

(D) Proteoglycans, which regulate connective tissue structure and permeability

(E) Fibronectin, which is an essential macromolecule secreted by endothelial cells and fibroblasts

15. A 34-year-old woman presented with pelvic pain, and ultrasound revealed a cystic ovarian mass. The multiloculated cyst pictured here was removed. The tumor can best be described as

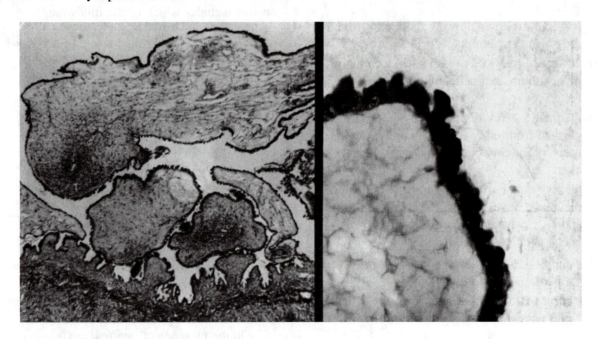

(A) being associated with elevated production of the beta subunit of human chorionic gonadotropin (hCG)

(B) a germ cell tumor requiring interventional chemotherapy

(C) being rare outside of the elderly female population

(D) being an indolent low-grade neoplasm

16. Which of the following pathophysiologic changes may be most useful in documenting, within less than 6 hours, that a patient had a myocardial infarction?

(A) Inverted or biphasic T wave on an electrocardiogram
(B) Elevated serum levels of creatine kinase
(C) Elevated serum levels of myocardial lactate dehydrogenase
(D) Maximal indices of coagulative necrosis
(E) Peak tissue infiltration of neutrophils

17. The incubation period for hepatitis A is

(A) less than 15 days
(B) 15–40 days
(C) 40–60 days
(D) 60–160 days
(E) more than 160 days

18. A healthy person is flying in an airplane that has been pressurized to 10,000 feet (523 mm Hg). Which of the following statements concerning the effects of this barometric pressure is true? It

(A) will not affect alveolar Po_2 because inspired oxygen remains at 0.21
(B) will be associated with significant desaturation of arterial hemoglobin
(C) will shift the subject's oxyhemoglobin dissociation curve to the left
(D) will decrease the vapor pressure of water in the airways
(E) will cause a modest reduction in arterial Po_2

19. The tuberculin test is used to determine if a patient has ever been exposed to *Mycobacterium tuberculosis*. If the patient has been exposed to the organism, the site where *M. tuberculosis* proteins were injected will trigger a type IV hypersensitivity response that causes the site to become red and swollen because of

(A) specific T cells recognizing the processed antigen and releasing inflammatory cytokines that increase blood vessel permeability to other immune effector cells and fluid
(B) antibodies binding the proteins and triggering neutrophils to release inflammatory cytokines that increase blood vessel permeability to other immune effector cells and fluid
(C) proteins binding to antibodies on mast cells and triggering mast cell degranulation
(D) unbound antibodies binding the proteins and the immune complex then depositing protein in the tissue, which triggers a cell-mediated response
(E) cytotoxic CD8+ T cells recognizing the processed protein and releasing inflammatory cytokines as well as causing the antigen presenting cells to undergo apoptosis

20. Cyclosporin A and FK-506 are often used in the treatment of transplant recipients. Both drugs interfere with the synthesis of the cytokine interleukin-2 (IL-2). These drugs are used to

(A) decrease plasma levels of IL-2 so that it will not bind to the foreign cells of the transplanted organ and cause rejection
(B) inhibit the IL-2 stimulus for proliferation of T cells and prevent organ rejection
(C) prevent the activation of macrophages by IL-2 and prevent organ rejection
(D) decrease the IL-2 stimulation of immunoglobulin E (IgE)-producing plasma cells and therefore hinder the recipient's allergic response to the foreign cells of the transplanted organ
(E) inhibit the suppression of T cells by IL-2 and prevent organ rejection

21. Peripheral lymphoid tissues are the sites that antigen-specific lymphocytes migrate to after developing in central lymphoid tissues. Which one of the following statements concerning lymphoid tissue is correct?

(A) The gastrointestinal system contains peripheral lymphoid tissue called gut-associated lymphoid tissue that is the site of collection of food antigens
(B) T cells develop in the bone marrow and then migrate to the thyroid for maturation
(C) The spleen is the primary site plasma cells migrate to after being activated by antigen recognition; most antibodies are released into the blood from this peripheral lymphoid tissue
(D) B cells develop in the thymus and migrate to the bone marrow for maturation
(E) Lymph nodes contain germinal centers, which are sites of massive T-cell proliferation during an infection

22. Antibodies play multiple roles in the host immune response. All of the following actions of antibodies are correct EXCEPT

(A) antibodies can serve as antigen receptors on the surface of B lymphocytes
(B) the opsonization of bacteria by antibodies enhances ingestion by macrophages
(C) the process of antibody-dependent, cell-mediated cytotoxicity relies on neutrophil recognition of antibodies bound to a target cell's Fc receptor
(D) the Fc portions of cross-linked antibodies can trigger the complement cascade and lead to the destruction of bacteria that the antibodies have bound
(E) the ability to bind toxins before they can interact with the body's cells enables antibodies to protect cells from damage

Questions 23–25

A 50-year-old man with a history of hemochromatosis presents to the emergency room coughing up bright red blood. He had his most recent phlebotomy yesterday. His blood pressure is 110/85, his pulse 115; his face is flushed, and he is diaphoretic. During the physical examination splenomegaly and a venous pattern on his chest and abdomen are noted. He seems somewhat drowsy and confused but has no focal neurologic signs.

23. What is the most likely cause of this patient's bleeding?

(A) Portal hypertension
(B) Hemoglobin deficiency
(C) Eroded gastric ulcer
(D) Bronchogenic carcinoma
(E) Protein C deficiency

24. What is the probable source of this patient's confusion?

(A) Parkinson's disease
(B) Hepatic encephalopathy
(C) Subarachnoid hemorrhage
(D) Vitamin B_{12} deficiency
(E) Shy-Drager syndrome

25. Which of the following statements concerning the etiology and pathology of hemochromatosis is true?

(A) The excess iron accumulates primarily in cells of the mononuclear phagocyte system
(B) The most severe form of the disease is found in patients with thalassemia and sideroblastic anemia
(C) The iron accumulates due to a failure of renal excretion
(D) Approximately two thirds of patients with hemochromatosis share a common human leukocyte antigen
(E) The organ damage resulting from hemochromatosis is characteristically confined to the liver

26. Which one of the following factors differentiates viruses from *Chlamydia*?

(A) Obligate intracellular parasitism
(B) The need for arthropod vectors
(C) Dependency on the host cell for energy
(D) The presence of a single type of nucleic acid

27. The probability of hepatitis B $[P(D+)]$ in a certain patient population is known to be .20 [conversely, $P(D-) = .80$]. In a study of a new diagnostic test for hepatitis B, the probability of a positive test result among patients known to have hepatitis, $P(T+|D+)$, is shown to be .90, whereas the probability that a healthy patient will have a negative result, $P(T-|D-)$, is shown to be .95. What is the probability that a new patient with a negative test result is truly healthy?

(A) .95

(B) $\dfrac{(.95)(.80)}{(.95)(.80) + (.10)(.20)}$

(C) $\dfrac{(.90)(.20)}{(.90)(.20) + (.05)(.80)}$

(D) $\dfrac{(.95)(.80)}{(.95)(.80) + (.90)(.20)}$

(E) None of the above

Questions 28–29

The following data were obtained from an arterial blood sample drawn from a hospitalized patient:

$$pH = 7.55$$
$$P_{CO_2} = 25 \text{ mm Hg}$$
$$[HCO_3^-] = 22.5 \text{ mEq/L}$$

Recall that $CO_2 = 0.03 \times P_{CO_2}$ (in mmol/L).

28. This patient's arterial blood findings are consistent with a diagnosis of

(A) metabolic alkalosis
(B) respiratory alkalosis
(C) metabolic acidosis
(D) respiratory acidosis

29. These findings indicate that the ratio of $[HCO_3^-]$ to dissolved CO_2 is

(A) 5:1
(B) 10:1
(C) 20:1
(D) 30:1

30. A 63-year-old man has experienced episodes of angina, syncope, and dyspnea on exertion for "quite some time." On auscultation, his physician notices a late-peaking systolic ejection murmur that increases in intensity with longer cardiac cycle lengths, a gallop in the fourth heart sound (S_4), and a soft aortic valve component in the second heart sound (A_2). An electrocardiogram (ECG) shows abnormally high R waves in lead aVL. Which one of the following is the most likely diagnosis?

(A) Mitral stenosis caused by rheumatic fever
(B) Aortic stenosis caused by a congenital bicuspid aortic valve
(C) Mitral regurgitation caused by infective endocarditis
(D) Aortic regurgitation caused by aortic root dilation

31. All of the following descriptions of cardiac conduction abnormalities are correct EXCEPT

(A) complete heart block—no relationship between P waves and QRS complexes
(B) first-degree atrioventricular (AV) block—prolonged PR interval, but normal QRS complex
(C) high-grade AV block—PR interval is prolonged when a beat occurs, and there is a wide QRS complex
(D) left bundle branch block—long QRS complex with a tall R wave in V_6 and a deep S wave in V_1
(E) second-degree AV block, Mobitz type I—PR interval increases with each successive beat, until a P wave is blocked at the AV node; QRS complexes are normal

Questions 32–36

A 75-year-old woman is admitted to the hospital after suffering a cerebrovascular accident. Her computed tomography (CT) scan shows a focal nonhemorrhagic infarction in the right hemisphere. During the physical examination, no muscular weakness is noted; however, the patient is not responding to any visual, auditory, or tactile stimuli on the left side of her body. The woman also has a deficit involving only the inferior portion of her left visual field in both eyes.

32. Which lobe of the brain has been principally affected by this stroke?

(A) Parietal
(B) Frontal
(C) Occipital
(D) Temporal

33. Which of the sites in the picture below best describes the location of the woman's optic tract lesion?

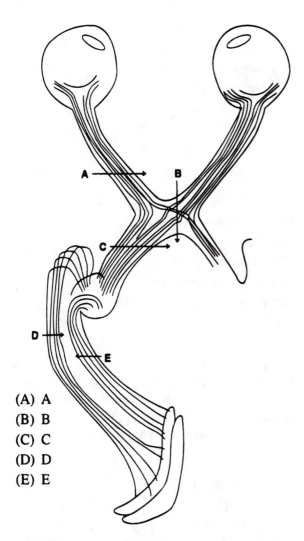

(A) A
(B) B
(C) C
(D) D
(E) E

34. Angiography later showed complete occlusion in a small branch of the middle cerebral artery with no other significant findings. Which one of the following diagnoses best explains the cause of the woman's cerebrovascular accident?

(A) Berry aneurysm
(B) Deep venous thrombosis
(C) Atrial fibrillation with mural thrombus
(D) Congestive heart failure
(E) Arteriovenous malformation

35. All of the following statements concerning the mechanism of clot formation are correct EXCEPT

(A) activation of thrombin by factor V is the final common pathway in converting soluble fibrinogen to insoluble fibrin
(B) the extrinsic pathway is activated by a lipoprotein called tissue factor, whereas the intrinsic pathway is activated by contact with foreign surfaces
(C) thrombin and several other cascade proteins are serine proteases that activate the next molecule in the pathway
(D) antithrombin III is an important regulator of the clotting cascade and acts by covalently cross-linking fibrin monomers into large meshworks in which platelets become lodged
(E) vitamin K is involved in the liver's synthesis of the factors that are calcium chelators

36. Which of the following statements correctly pairs a commonly used anticoagulant with its mechanism of action?

(A) Heparin acts to cleave the covalent linkage between fibrin monomers
(B) Tissue plasminogen activator acts by irreversibly inhibiting thrombin
(C) Dicumarol (warfarin) is a natural product which competitively inhibits the vitamin K–dependent γ-carboxylation of several cascade proteins
(D) Aspirin irreversibly binds fibrinogen, which decreases the pool of available fibrin monomers that can participate in clot formation
(E) Streptokinase is a bacterial product that causes platelet lysis, therefore inhibiting platelet aggregation

Questions 37–38

Five percent of individuals comprising a particular population are known to carry a recessive gene for poliodystrophy, an inherited disorder characterized by the onset of recurrent seizures and dementia in early childhood. A 32-year-old healthy woman, who had a brother with this disorder, seeks genetic counseling. The patient's husband, an only child, does not know if his family has a history of the disorder

37. What is the probability that the patient is a carrier of poliodystrophy?

(A) 1/20
(B) 1/10
(C) 3/8
(D) 2/3
(E) 3/4

38. What is the probability that both the patient and her husband are carriers?

(A) 1/30
(B) 1/20
(C) 3/8
(D) 2/3
(E) 3/4

Questions 39–42

A 68-year-old woman who is a volunteer at a church-sponsored kindergarten suddenly develops a fever of 38.2°C and a severe headache one evening. The following morning she also experiences a stiff neck and uncharacteristic drowsiness. At the emergency room, her temperature is 38.8°C, and there are pain and resistance on flexion of her neck. The patient is noted to be mentally competent although lethargic. A cerebrospinal fluid (CSF) sample is obtained by lumbar puncture.

39. On the basis of the history and physical examination of this patient, what is the most probable diagnosis?

(A) Viral meningitis
(B) Fungal meningitis
(C) Bacterial meningitis
(D) Viral encephalitis
(E) Brain abscess

40. On the basis of the patient's age, the probable etiologic agent is

(A) *Staphylococcus aureus*
(B) *Haemophilus influenzae*
(C) *Actinomyces israelii*
(D) *Neisseria meningitidis*
(E) *Streptococcus pneumoniae*

41. Opening pressure on lumbar puncture was slightly elevated, and the diagnosis was acute bacterial meningitis based upon the finding of gram-positive cocci in pairs in the CSF. The cell count was elevated. The prominent cell type most likely was

(A) mononuclear cells
(B) neutrophils
(C) lymphocytes
(D) red cells
(E) segmented neutrophils

42. Protein and glucose concentrations in the CSF probably were

(A) both elevated
(B) elevated and low, respectively
(C) low and elevated, respectively
(D) both low
(E) unaffected

Questions 43–44

The figure below depicts log concentration–time curves for three drugs (X, Y, and Z) after identical amounts of each drug were administered as a bolus at time zero.

43. Which of the following statements regarding these drugs is correct?

(A) Volume of distribution (V_d) of $X = Z < Y$
(B) Half-time of elimination ($t_{1/2}$) of $X = Y > Z$
(C) Clearance of X (CL_X) $= CL_Y$
(D) $CL_Z > CL_X$
(E) Elimination rate constant (k) of $X < $ (k) of Y

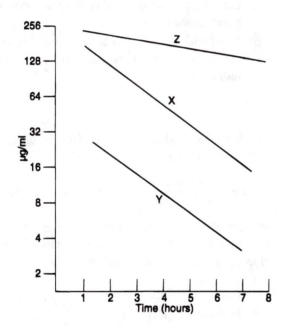

44. If drugs X, Y, and Z were independently infused in equal amounts at a constant rate, then based on the data from the figure above, which of the following statements is most accurate?

(A) At steady state, [X] > [Z]
(B) At steady state, [X] = [Y]
(C) Z would require more time to reach a steady state than either X or Y
(D) X would reach a steady state faster than Y

45. Which one of the following statements concerning infectious hepatitis is correct?

(A) Hepatitis C infection requires hepatitis B infection
(B) Diagnosis with hepatitis B carries a grave prognosis: Many people die from fulminant hepatitis, and nearly 25% of infected patients progress to hepatocellular carcinoma
(C) Hepatitis B surface antigen (HBsAg) indicates active hepatitis infection
(D) The carrier state is common in patients infected with hepatitis A
(E) Hepatitis A infection accounts for approximately 25% of all hepatitis cases in the United States

46. Of the following cell types, which would contain many mitochondria in the apical portion of the cell?

(A) Smooth muscle cells
(B) Ciliated epithelium cells
(C) Steroid-secreting cells
(D) Liver parenchymal cells
(E) Skeletal muscle cells

47. A 29-year-old man whose father died of Huntington's chorea when he was an infant is obsessively worried about developing the disease, symptoms of which appear in one's 30s or 40s. Although he knows little about the genetic disorder, he is aware that there is a 50% likelihood that he has the dominant Huntington's gene. One day, he impulsively rushes to a testing center and demands to initiate presymptomatic testing, making no attempt to hide his intention to commit suicide if he receives positive results. It would be ethically defensible for the testing center staff to

(A) refuse to initiate testing
(B) educate him about the disease and initiate testing
(C) initiate counseling to alleviate his anxieties, educate him about the disease, and defer testing until he is more stable
(D) test him and report negative results regardless of the actual results
(E) test him for other diseases

48. A 57-year-old man complains of having episodes of chest pain. His blood pressure is 160/100 mm Hg, he has been smoking 1 pack of cigarettes every day for the past 40 years, and both his legs are amputated at the knee. Which one of the following actions are most appropriate?

(A) Because of the patient's amputations, a coronary angiogram should be performed in lieu of an exercise test.
(B) The patient does not need an exercise test because his potential coronary artery disease can easily be assessed at rest
(C) The patient should immediately be rushed to the operating room for emergent bypass surgery
(D) Administration of dipyramidole should be used as a substitute for exercise in assessing the extent of the patient's potential coronary artery disease
(E) The patient is advised to quit smoking and to take one aspirin per day; he can safely return to work

49. In the general format of the Henderson-Hasselbalch equation:

$$\log \left(\frac{[\text{protonated form}]}{[\text{unprotonated form}]} \right) + pK'_a = pH$$

Phenobarbital is a weak acid. In an emergency situation, a useful maneuver to hasten its elimination in an intoxicated person might be

(A) inhalation of CO_2
(B) infusion of $NaHCO_3$
(C) infusion of NH_4Cl
(D) induction of P_{450} enzymes with a separate barbiturate
(E) infusion of dextrose

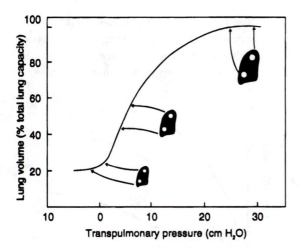

50. Which one of the following statements accurately describes pressure–volume relationships, as shown in the above figure, in the lungs of a healthy individual?

(A) At lung volumes close to functional residual capacity (FRC), alveoli at the base of the lung are smaller than alveoli at the top

(B) At lung volumes close to vital capacity (VC), alveoli at the top of the lung are smaller than alveoli at the base

(C) Alveoli in the base of the lung begin filling first during inspiration from residual volume

(D) Alveoli in the apex receive greater ventilation during inspiration from volumes near FRC

(E) Alveoli in the base of the lung close at volumes near VC

51. Which of the following statements most accurately describes specific features of neuromuscular transmission?

(A) Each muscle fiber contains multiple axon terminals

(B) The end-plate is highly enriched in electrically excitable gates

(C) Enzymatic degradation of the transmitter can terminate transmission

(D) Acetylcholine (ACh) causes chloride channels to open as a result of membrane depolarization

52. Which one of the following statements concerning expiration is correct?

(A) At lung volumes close to vital capacity (VC), expiratory air flow is independent of expiratory effort

(B) At lung volumes close to VC, airway resistance is at its peak

(C) At lung volumes close to VC, expiratory air flow increases with increasing pleural pressures

(D) At 50% of VC, increased expiratory effort results in decreased airway resistance

(E) At lung volumes close to residual volume, the elastic recoil of the chest wall is directed inward

53. A man acquires a "cold sore" from his girl-friend through ordinary kissing. Assuming that this man will exhibit recurrent infections, which nerve axon might this disease traverse during re-infection?

(A) Cranial nerve (CN) VII (upper and lower buccal branches)
(B) CN V and the marginal mandibular branch of CN VII
(C) CN V_2 and CN V_3
(D) CN V_1 only

54. Which one of the following statements about the hormonal regulation of pregnancy is correct?

(A) Human chorionic gonadotropin (hCG) is secreted by the placenta and can first be detected 4 weeks after conception
(B) hCG stimulates the corpus luteum to secrete high levels of estrogen and progesterone
(C) The β subunits of luteinizing hormone (LH), follicle stimulating hormone (FSH), and hCG are identical to one another whereas the α subunits are responsible for their different receptor affinities
(D) Maternal serum hCG levels continue to increase throughout pregnancy
(E) hCG stimulates the pituitary to maintain high LH and FSH levels to keep the corpus luteum functional

55. The process of DNA replication can be best described by which of the following statements? DNA replication

(A) initiates at random sites on the chromosome
(B) of the *Escherichia coli* chromosome begins at multiple origins
(C) is unidirectional for all DNAs
(D) is not dependent on the synthesis of RNA primers
(E) occurs during the S phase of the cell cycle

56. In the figure below, volume–pressure curves from three subjects of the same age, sex, and body size are shown. If subject B is normal, which one of the following statements is most accurate?

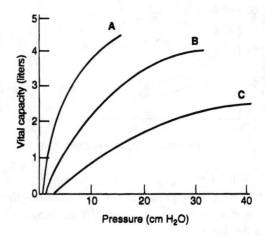

(A) Subject A has a stiff lung (fibrosis)
(B) Subject A has a flabby lung (emphysema)
(C) Subject A has a higher elastic recoil pressure than the other subjects
(D) Subject C is likely to have a higher functional residual capacity
(E) Subject C has the lowest elastic recoil pressure of the three

57. A 20-year-old man has a penile lesion that is crateriform, moist, and indurated. The patient revealed that this lesion has been present for about 20 days and is not painful. Which one of the following groups of tests is most appropriate?

(A) Gram stain, Venereal Disease Research Laboratory (VDRL) test, and culture of the lesion for *Treponema pallidum*
(B) Gram stain and culture of the lesion for *T. pallidum*
(C) VDRL and dark-field examination
(D) Fluorescent treponemal antibody absorption (FTA-ABS) test

58. Which one of the following techniques would be the best way to study a new kind of growth factor that induces proliferation of certain cell types?

(A) Measure uptake of radiolabeled methionine into cells after addition of the growth factor
(B) Measure uptake of radiolabeled thymidine into cells after addition of the growth factor
(C) Measure uptake of radiolabeled uracil into cells after addition of the growth factor
(D) Trypan blue exclusion

Questions 59–60

A 70-year-old woman is brought to the emergency room by her daughter, who noticed that her mother is not as energetic as she previously was. In the emergency room, the patient relates a history of increasing fatigability and shortness of breath over the past several months. On examination, the patient has elevated neck veins, rales in the back, and a third heart sound (S_3 gallop rhythm). Chest x-ray reveals an enlarged cardiac silhouette and increased vascular markings. The patient has a heart rate of 90 and a blood pressure of 150/100.

59. Based on the above history and physical examination, the patient is most likely to have

(A) atrial fibrillation
(B) ventricular paroxysmal tachycardia
(C) congestive heart failure
(D) adult respiratory distress syndrome
(E) rebound hypertensive crisis

60. A hypothetical series of pressure–volume loops of the left ventricle of a control subject and the patient before and after digitalis is shown below. Based on these data, which one of the following groupings is correct?

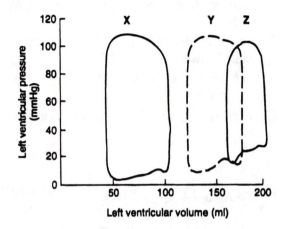

(A) X: control; Y: before digitalis; Z: after digitalis
(B) X: control; Z: before digitalis; Y: after digitalis
(C) Z: control; X: before digitalis; Y: after digitalis
(D) Z: control; Y: before digitalis; X: after digitalis

61. Which of the following areas of the central nervous system (CNS) contains structures that are considered to be phylogenically the oldest parts of the brain?

(A) Frontal lobe
(B) Limbic system
(C) Cerebellum
(D) Visual cortex

62. RNA processing can be best described by which of the following statements? It

(A) occurs in the cytoplasm
(B) results in the addition of nucleotides to the primary transcript of ribosomal RNA (rRNA)
(C) results in the formation of new covalent bonds between RNA and DNA
(D) includes the addition of a tail of polyadenylic acid at the 5′ end
(E) includes the methylation of nucleotides in RNA

Questions 63–64

A 10-year-old girl is seen by her pediatrician for flu-like symptoms that were followed (weeks later) by a peculiar expanding skin rash (erythema chronicum migrans) and monoauricular arthritis (months later). Clinical laboratory findings include a positive titer against *Borrelia burgdorferi*.

63. A likely diagnosis for this child includes which one of the following diseases?

(A) Leptospirosis
(B) Lyme disease
(C) Rocky Mountain spotted fever
(D) Relapsing fever
(E) Yaws

64. Assuming a spirochete is the causative agent in this child's syndrome, appropriate pharmacotherapy may include which one of the following drugs?

(A) Rifampin
(B) Penicillin
(C) Chloroquine
(D) Pentamidine
(E) Praziquantel

65. The following sequence is a part of a globular protein. Which of the following statements best describes this peptide?

Ser-Val-Asp-Asp-Val-Phe-Ser-Glu-Val-Cys-His-Met-Arg

(A) At pH 7.4, the peptide has a net negative charge
(B) It has only one sulfur-containing amino acid
(C) The hydrophobic amino acid content exceeds the hydrophilic content
(D) Treatment with chymotrypsin would generate four smaller fragments
(E) Only three of the side chains are capable of forming hydrogen bonds

66. A rational approach for the treatment of ventricular tachycardia associated with myocardial ischemia in a hospitalized patient includes

(A) digitalis
(B) diltiazem
(C) lidocaine
(D) propranolol
(E) verapamil

67. What color would this tumor of the kidney (pictured) be?

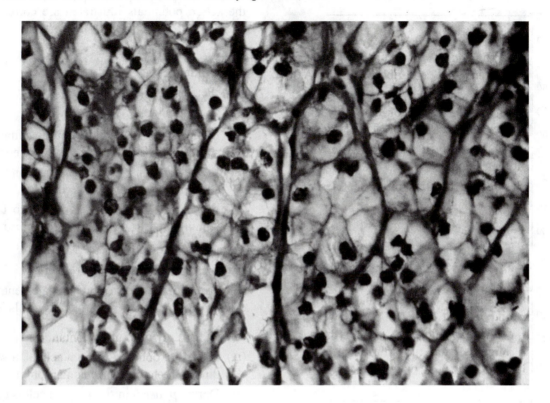

(A) Gray

(B) Translucent, with a pink hue

(C) White

(D) Yellow

68. If an individual has a genetic defect in the enzyme that produces N-acetylglutamate, the most likely clinical finding would be hyperammonemia with

(A) elevated levels of argininosuccinate (the condensation product of citrulline and aspartate)

(B) no detectable citrulline

(C) elevated levels of arginine

(D) elevated levels of urea

(E) no detectable ornithine

69. Which one of the following clinical procedures best demonstrates damage to the cerebellum?

(A) Testing for voluntary weakness by having the patient grasp the examiner's fingers and squeeze as hard as possible

(B) Tapping the patellar tendon and observing the reflex response

(C) Having the patient flex the neck, touching the chin to the sternum, to determine if this action elicits pain

(D) Passively moving the patient's limbs to elicit an increased resistance to motion

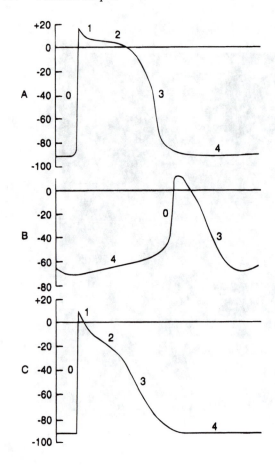

Questions 70–71

Refer to the above traces of action potentials from cardiac cells to answer the following questions.

70. All of the following statements concerning the action potentials illustrated are correct EXCEPT

(A) *trace A* represents the action potential from a myocardial cell in the left ventricle

(B) *trace B* represents the action potential from a cell in the sinoatrial (SA) node

(C) *trace C* represents the action potential from a cell in the atrioventricular (AV) node

(D) in *trace A*, contraction of the cells in the left ventricle correlates with *phase 2*

(E) in *trace A*, the cell is refractory to further stimulation during a portion of *phase 3*

71. Which one of the following statements concerning ionic currents in myocardial cells is correct?

(A) In *phase 0* of the SA node potential, inwardly directed calcium currents predominate

(B) During *phase 0* in *trace A*, the cell is rapidly depolarized by the influx of potassium

(C) During *phase 3* in *trace B*, the cell is gradually repolarized by an increase in the sodium current

(D) During *phase 3* in *trace A*, calcium-activated sodium currents are important in repolarization

(E) The ionic currents in *phase 3* of the SA node's action potential are the basis for SA node automaticity

72. A 39-year-old man presents for his regularly scheduled physical examination. During the cardiac portion of the examination, a palpable pre-systolic apical impulse is noted, and an S_4 is heard on auscultation. Which one of the following statements is most likely correct?

(A) The patient may have hypertrophic left ventricle secondary to aortic stenosis
(B) The patient likely has some form of underlying heart disease (e.g., myocardial infarction, mitral regurgitation)
(C) The patient has increased ventricular compliance
(D) The patient has aggravated hypotension
(E) The patient is undergoing atrial fibrillation

73. The upstroke of the ventricular action potential is primarily due to which one of the following actions?

(A) An inward flux of Ca^{2+}
(B) An inward K^+ current
(C) An outward K^+ current
(D) An outward Na^+ current
(E) An inward Na^+ current

74. Which one of the following statements best describes the regulation of vascular smooth muscle during exercise?

(A) There is vasoconstriction in all vessels due to the increased sympathetic outflow that occurs during exercise
(B) Increased circulating levels of metabolic products such as H^+, CO_2, and adenosine cause vasodilation in all vessels
(C) Increased blood flow during exercise causes a cascade of events leading to release of nitric oxide and vasoconstriction
(D) Local metabolic vasodilator signals in the vessels of active skeletal muscle can overcome the vasoconstrictor signals of increased sympathetic outflow and cause a net vasodilation and increased perfusion of those muscles
(E) The ability of muscles to extract a higher percentage of the delivered oxygen makes it unnecessary for any changes in vascular smooth muscle activity to occur

Questions 75–79

A 42-year-old white woman comes to the emergency room with acute onset of severe abdominal pain following a routine dinner. During a physical examination, the physician notes that she is mildly obese, and her abdominal pain is confined principally to the right upper quadrant. The physician suspects that she may have gallstones.

75. Which of the following symptoms is most specific for cholelithiasis?

(A) Excessive flatulence following a meal
(B) Hemoccult-positive stool
(C) Severe right upper quadrant pain that comes in waves over a period of hours
(D) Rigid abdominal wall with diffuse rebound tenderness
(E) Epigastric pain and nausea following a meal

76. The patient has a fever of 39.4°C and an elevated serum white cell count (12,400/mm^3). All of the following organisms are likely pathogens in acute cholecystitis EXCEPT

(A) group D streptococci (enterococci)
(B) *Escherichia coli*
(C) *Klebsiella* species
(D) *Neisseria* species
(E) *Clostridium* species

77. Which of the following statements best characterizes the prevalence of asymptomatic gallstones in western countries?

(A) The prevalence of gallstones in men over 40 years is greater than 60%
(B) The prevalence of gallstones in men over 40 years is between 20% and 60%
(C) The prevalence of gallstones in men over 40 years is less than 3%
(D) The prevalence of gallstones in women over 40 years is greater than 60%
(E) The prevalence of gallstones in women over 40 years is between 20% and 60%

78. All of the following are known predisposing factors for cholesterol and mixed stone formation EXCEPT

(A) diabetes mellitus
(B) alcoholic cirrhosis
(C) obesity
(D) ileal resection
(E) oral contraceptives

79. All of the following statements correctly characterize important contributors to the pathogenesis of cholelithiasis EXCEPT

(A) decreased hydroxymethylglutaryl coenzyme A (HMG CoA) reductase activity and increased secretion of bile acids can markedly increase the stone-forming potential of bile
(B) gallbladder hypomotility leads to the accumulation of biliary sludge, an important precursor to stone formation
(C) excess unconjugated bilirubin associated with chronic hemolysis leads to the formation of pigmented stones
(D) chronic infection of the biliary tree leads to pigment stone formation
(E) decreased lecithin or bile acid synthesis results in a decreased capacity for solubilizing biliary cholesterol

Questions 80–84

A 32-year-old white woman visits her physician because of agitation, weight loss, and the inability to sleep. When questioned further, she reveals an increased appetite and an increased frequency of bowel movements. Previously, she had regular menstrual periods, but now they are less frequent and irregular. During the physical examination, the physician notes that her skin is warm and moist and that she has a fine tremor of the fingers, hyperreflexia, and lid lag. The woman has moderately severe exophthalmos, and her upward gaze seems weak and uncoordinated.

80. Which one of the following disease processes is most likely manifesting itself?

(A) A thyroid adenoma that is secreting thyroxine
(B) Inappropriate hypothalamic secretion of thyrotropin-releasing hormone (TRH)
(C) Graves' disease
(D) Hashimoto's disease
(E) Sick euthyroid syndrome

81. Which other finding would most likely be expected on further physical examination?

(A) Sparse, dry hair that easily falls out
(B) Pericardial effusion
(C) Jaundice
(D) Dermopathy over the dorsum of the leg
(E) Diffuse hyperpigmentation of the skin

82. All of the following laboratory test results are consistent with the clinical picture EXCEPT

(A) decreased triiodothyronine resin uptake (T_3RU)
(B) decreased serum thyroid-stimulating hormone (TSH) response to a TRH challenge
(C) decreased serum TSH concentration
(D) increased serum thyroxine (T_4) concentration
(E) positive test for circulating antibodies against the TSH receptor

83. A thyroid radioactive iodine uptake scintiscan is performed and reveals uniform uptake across the gland. Which of the following conditions best describes the histopathology of this woman's thyroid gland?

(A) Multinodular goiter
(B) Multiple adenomas
(C) Single carcinoma
(D) Lymphocytic infiltration (especially plasma cells) with atrophic follicles
(E) Diffuse hyperplasia and hypertrophy

84. All of the following statements correctly pair a useful medication with its mechanism of action EXCEPT

(A) propylthiouracil blocks the coupling reaction in T_4 synthesis
(B) methimazole reduces peripheral conversion of T_4 to T_3
(C) radioactive iodine destroys follicular cells in the thyroid
(D) propranolol blocks the sympathetic components of thyrotoxicosis
(E) prednisone may relieve the mechanical exophthalmos and ophthalmoplegia by reducing inflammation

Questions 85–89

A 64-year-old man with a 40-year history of smoking 1.5 packs of cigarettes per day visits his physician's office complaining of an unproductive cough of 6 months' duration. When questioned further, the patient discloses hoarseness and generalized muscle weakness. Previously active sexually, he says that he has ''lost interest'' lately. During a physical examination, the physician notes muscle wasting, an unusual pattern of weight gain in the face and back, and abdominal stria. His serum glucose is 180 mg/dl.

85. Which single set of laboratory tests is best suited to establish a tentative diagnosis?

(A) Serum thyroxine, triiodothyronine resin uptake, and cervical ultrasound
(B) Urinary glucocorticoids, abdominal computed tomography (CT), and chest x-ray
(C) Dexamethasone suppression test and chest x-ray
(D) In-patient hospitalization with water restriction, CT of the head, and chest x-ray
(E) Glucose tolerance, urinary ketones, abdominal ultrasound, and chest x-ray

86. The test results return positive, confirming the suspicion of an endocrine abnormality secondary to a bronchogenic carcinoma. Which of the following hormone or hormone-like substances is the tumor most likely secreting?

(A) Parathyroid or parathyroid-like hormone
(B) Thyroxine
(C) Corticosteroids
(D) Adrenocorticotropic hormone (ACTH) or ACTH-like hormone
(E) Insulin or insulin-like hormone

87. Additional radiology studies to confirm the source of the endocrine abnormalities are desired. Based on the short history presented, which of the following features is most likely expected?

(A) Bilateral hypertrophy of the adrenal gland
(B) Focal enlargement in the thyroid gland
(C) Hypertrophy of a subset of cells in the pituitary gland
(D) Carcinoid tumor
(E) Hypertrophy of a subset of cells in the pancreas

88. Each of the following pieces of evidence relates cigarette smoking to bronchogenic carcinomas EXCEPT

(A) heavy smokers (more than 1 pack/day) have a 20-fold greater lifetime risk of developing bronchogenic cancer
(B) cessation of cigarette smoking for 10 years reduces cancer risk to that of nonsmokers
(C) the bronchial epithelium in more than 10% of cigarette smokers shows atypical or hyperplastic changes on autopsy
(D) tumor-initiating substances (e.g., polycyclic aromatic hydrocarbons), which have caused cancer in mice, are found in cigarette smoke
(E) lung cancer runs in families in which cigarette smoking is common

89. Each of the following is a potential paraneoplastic syndrome associated with bronchogenic tumors EXCEPT

(A) syndrome of inappropriate antidiuretic hormone (SIADH)
(B) hyperaldosteronism
(C) hypercalcemia of malignancy
(D) dermatomyositis
(E) hypertrophic osteoarthropathy

90. Of the following types of proteins, all exhibit a protein structure common for physiologic receptors or components of cellular signal transduction systems EXCEPT

(A) ion channels
(B) protein kinases
(C) guanylate cyclases
(D) guanosine triphosphate (GTP)–binding proteins (G proteins)
(E) metallothioneins

91. All of the following statements describe the genetic code EXCEPT

(A) it is nearly identical for all organisms
(B) it is composed of nucleotides containing three nucleotide code letters
(C) it represents all of the nucleotide sequence information within a transcription unit
(D) it contains transcription start and stop sequences
(E) it contains more than one codon for each amino acid

92. All of the following statements about γ-aminobutyric acid (GABA) are true EXCEPT

(A) its receptor is coupled to a benzodiazepine receptor
(B) it is a widely distributed inhibitory neurotransmitter
(C) its activity is increased in hepatic encephalopathy
(D) its activity is increased with antispasticity drugs
(E) its activity is decreased with antiseizure drugs

93. Biologic theory is supported by all of the following EXCEPT

(A) the effects of certain medications on the symptoms of schizophrenia
(B) enlargement of ventricular size in significant numbers of patients with schizophrenia
(C) a strong family history in many cases of manic-depressive disorder
(D) the effect of stimulant medication on the symptoms of attention deficit disorder in children
(E) monozygotic twins discordant for schizophrenia

94. All of the following nephritides are associated with hypocomplementemia EXCEPT

(A) immunoglobulin A (IgA) nephropathy
(B) mesangioproliferative glomerulonephropathy
(C) serum sickness
(D) systemic lupus erythematosus (SLE)
(E) vasculitis

95. All of the following statements describing cell–extracellular matrix interactions are correct EXCEPT

(A) integrins are soluble nuclear proteins that directly alter gene transcription

(B) type IV collagen, which is found in basement membranes, stimulates endothelial cells to organize into tubelike structures

(C) fibronectin fragments play a pivotal role in wound healing by promoting migration of endothelial cells and fibroblasts to the damaged area

(D) laminin is a potent stimulus for inducing the replication of endothelial cells

(E) receptor glycoproteins on the surface of platelets are crucial to platelet aggregation at sites of exposed subendothelium

96. All of the following human leukocyte antigen (HLA) associations are matched correctly EXCEPT

(A) rheumatoid arthritis—HLA-DR4

(B) primary Sjögren's syndrome—HLA-DR3

(C) postgonococcal arthritis—HLA-B27

(D) 21-hydroxylase deficiency—HLA-DR4

(E) chronic active hepatitis—HLA-DR3

97. All of the following statements concerning action potentials recorded simultaneously from slow and fast myocardial fibers (illustrated below) are correct EXCEPT

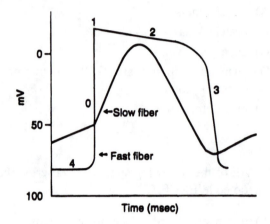

(A) the slow fiber was likely to be present in sinoatrial or atrioventricular nodes

(B) the fast fiber is typical of either atrial or ventricular myocardial cells

(C) in the fast fiber, *phase 0* is caused by opening of Na^+ channels

(D) in the fast fiber, *phase 2* coincides with an increase in conductance to Ca^{2+}

(E) application of acetylcholine (ACh) increases the slope of *phase 4* of the slow fiber

Questions 98–99

A 50-year-old woman complains of increasing fatigue over the past 2 weeks. She has a history of ovarian carcinoma and has received treatment with several courses of cyclophosphamide during the past 3 years; her last course of treatment was given 1 month previously. Physical examination shows slight hepatic enlargement. One examiner thinks the patient has some excess abdominal fluid. Laboratory examination reveals a white blood count of 2000 cells/μl, with 10% polymorphonuclear leukocytes and 90% lymphocytes. The hemoglobin concentration is 9 g/dl, and the platelet count is 50,000/μl.

98. The differential diagnosis of the cause of this patient's pancytopenia includes all of the following EXCEPT

(A) chronic lymphocytic leukemia
(B) acute myelogenous leukemia
(C) recurrent ovarian carcinoma
(D) cyclophosphamide toxicity
(E) aplastic anemia

99. Further evaluation of this patient requires all of the following studies EXCEPT

(A) radiographic studies of the abdomen
(B) cytologic examination of ascites
(C) bone marrow aspiration and biopsy
(D) immunoglobulin gene rearrangement studies
(E) liver function studies

100. Chronic type B (antral) gastritis is characterized by all of the following features EXCEPT

(A) glandular atrophy with the presence of very few short, cystically dilated glands
(B) circulating antibodies to parietal cells and intrinsic factor
(C) excess acid secretion with low intragastric pH and, frequently, duodenal ulcers
(D) low serum gastrin levels
(E) flattened or absent rugal folds

101. Asthma is characterized by an increased responsiveness of the trachea and bronchi to various stimuli and is manifested by widespread narrowing of the airway. Results of pulmonary function tests during an acute asthma attack will demonstrate all of the following EXCEPT

(A) decreased forced expiratory volume in 1 second (FEV_1)
(B) increased forced vital capacity (FVC)
(C) decreased FEV_1/FVC
(D) normal or increased total lung capacity (TLC)

102. All of the following statements about the influence of cardiovascular disease on sexuality are true EXCEPT

(A) some patients have impaired sexual functioning following a myocardial infarction

(B) myocardial infarctions that occur during intercourse are often associated with unusual and stressful circumstances

(C) the most common reason for decreased frequency of intercourse after a myocardial infarction is anginal pain associated with intercourse

(D) there is a higher incidence of return to normal sexual activity by patients who receive exercise training and education than by those who are not involved in such programs

(E) the spouse of a patient who has had a myocardial infarction needs to be involved in educational programs because his or her fears can interfere with resumption of sexual activity

103. All of the following thalamic nuclei are connected with the basal ganglia EXCEPT

(A) ventrolateral

(B) medial central

(C) pulvinar

(D) ventroanterior

104. All of the following statements concerning hormonal control of the menstrual cycle are true EXCEPT

(A) estradiol causes a proliferation and thickening in the endometrial lining

(B) progesterone induces differentiation of the endometrial lining into a secretory phase

(C) luteinizing hormone (LH) stimulates thecal cells to produce androgens that are aromatized to estrogen by the granulosa cells

(D) the LH surge immediately precedes endometrial shedding and menses

(E) follicle-stimulating hormone (FSH) couples with increasing estrogen levels to induce the synthesis of LH receptors on the granulosa cells

105. A 62-year-old man experiences crushing substernal chest pain. After 4 days of circulatory support in the intensive care unit, he dies. Histologic study of his heart would show all of the following findings EXCEPT

(A) coagulative necrosis

(B) liquefactive necrosis

(C) hypereosinophilic wavy fibers

(D) neutrophilic infiltrate

106. All of the following elements of the adult brain develop from the telencephalon EXCEPT the

(A) corpus striatum

(B) internal capsule

(C) occipital lobe

(D) hippocampus

(E) thalamus

107. Each statement below concerning the contraction of myofibrils in skeletal muscle is true EXCEPT

(A) the size of the A band decreases
(B) the size of the H band decreases
(C) the size of the I band decreases
(D) thin filaments penetrate the A band
(E) Z disks are drawn closer to the A band

108. Each of the following statements concerning intercostal nerves is true EXCEPT

(A) they are the anterior rami of the 12 thoracic spinal nerves
(B) they are connected to the sympathetic trunk by rami communicans
(C) the first intercostal nerve is joined to the brachial plexus
(D) they supply the anterior abdominal muscles
(E) they supply the parietal pleura

109. All of the following statements concerning mammalian chromosomes are true EXCEPT

(A) DNase I can be used to treat chromosomes to determine inactive regions of DNA
(B) approximately 7% of the sequences contained in the eukaryotic genome are copied into RNA
(C) heterochromatin is a term used for inactive DNA, and euchromatin is a term used for those regions of DNA that are transcriptionally active
(D) in higher eukaryotic genomes, cytosine is methylated at cytosine–guanine (CG) islands in inactive segments of DNA

110. Psychoanalysis as a form of psychotherapy includes all of the following concepts EXCEPT

(A) free association
(B) resistance
(C) countertransference
(D) interpretation
(E) meditation

111. Serious complications in a patient who has just suffered an acute myocardial infarction include all of the following EXCEPT

(A) cardiac tamponade
(B) peripheral embolism
(C) mitral valve incompetence
(D) aortic aneurysm
(E) rupture of the ventricular septum

112. Which of the following steps is NOT important in the normal synthesis of collagen?

(A) Incorporation of glycine residues into the growing polypeptide
(B) Hydroxylation of proline residues, which adds stability to the mature fiber's triple helix motif
(C) Cleavage of the globular terminal ends of soluble procollagen to make insoluble tropocollagen
(D) Secretion of the cleaved tropocollagen into the extracellular space
(E) Covalent cross-linkage of lysine residues in the nascent collagen fiber, which adds stability to both the intramolecular and intermolecular structures

113. A man is brought to the emergency room after being beaten with a baseball bat. He received one blow to the head that did not fracture the skull. At which of the following locations would a blow cause the LEAST amount of damage to the brain, assuming that all blows were delivered with equal force?

(A) The side of the head
(B) The front of the head
(C) The back of the head
(D) A glancing blow to the back of the head

Questions 114–116

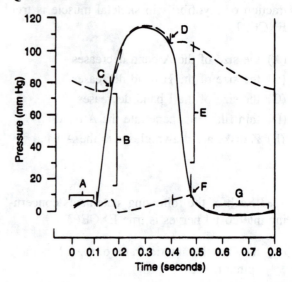

Match each of the following cardiovascular events with its correct place in the cardiac cycle.

114. Aortic valve opens

115. Left ventricle is filling

116. Isovolumic contraction of the left ventricle

117. All of the following associations regarding diseases and their signs are correct EXCEPT

(A) "rice-water" stool—cholera
(B) "rose spots" on abdomen—typhoid fever
(C) "strawberry tongue"—streptococcus
(D) tetanic contraction—botulism

118. Which one of the following families of viruses is paired with the form of nucleic acids that comprises its genome?

(A) Parvoviruses—circular, double-stranded DNA

(B) Papovaviruses—single-stranded RNA

(C) Adenoviruses—linear, double-stranded DNA

(D) Retroviruses—two linked segments of linear, double-stranded DNA

(E) Coronaviruses—linear, segmented, double-stranded RNA

(F) Herpesvirus—triplex DNA

Questions 119–121

(A) Narcissistic personality disorder

(B) Phencyclidine (PCP) ingestion

(C) Schizophrenia

(D) Borderline personality disorder

(E) Bipolar illness

For each case history described below, select the appropriate diagnosis.

119. Over the past year, Andrew, age 17, has retreated more and more often to his room. He has few friends and never calls anyone. His school performance has deteriorated during this time. His mother finds pieces of paper in his trash can with unintelligible poems written on them.

120. Margot is brought to the hospital by her husband after she has run through the family bank account by making lengthy long-distance telephone calls and by purchasing expensive jewelry and clothing.

121. George is indignant when his graduate school thesis committee refuses to approve his project. ''They're just jealous of me because they know I'll be the most brilliant anthropologist in history,'' he remarks. This is the attitude he has had all of his life.

122. Agammaglobulinemias are diseases resulting from the absence of antibodies due to mutations of B lymphocytes. People who lack antibodies have an increased risk for

(A) recurrent viral infections

(B) recurrent infections by extracellular bacteria

(C) recurrent viral infections and infections caused by extracellular bacteria

(D) recurrent infections by fungi and viruses

(E) nothing, because the immune system has redundant mechanisms that make up for the lack of antibodies

123. Immunologic memory is the name given to the body's ability to better fight pathogens that it has been exposed to previously. Antibodies play a large role in mounting an immune response to a new antigen (primary antibody response) as well as a previously encountered antigen (secondary antibody response). All of the following differences between the primary antibody response and the secondary antibody response are correct EXCEPT

(A) antibody affinity for the antigen is greater in the secondary antibody response than in the primary response

(B) immunoglobulin M (IgM) is the predominant class of antibody made during the initial antigen encounter

(C) IgG is the predominant class of antibody made during the secondary antigen encounter

(D) antibodies are produced more quickly during the secondary antibody response than during the primary response

(E) the amount of antibody made in the primary response is greater than the amount made in the secondary response

Questions 124–127

(A) Incidence
(B) Prevalence
(C) Specificity
(D) Sensitivity
(E) Validity/accuracy
(F) Reliability/precision

Match each biostatistical concept with the definition that best describes it.

124. Ability of a test to correctly identify a true positive in a patient with a disease

125. Ability of a test to consistently reproduce measurements of the same entity

126. Number of cases of the disease at any moment in time (per 100,000 population)

127. Ability of a test to correctly produce a negative result in a patient without disease

128. Which one of the following segments of the nephron is NOT paired with the appropriate type of epithelium?

(A) The parietal portion of Bowman's capsule—simple squamous epithelium
(B) Proximal tubules—simple cuboidal epithelium
(C) The thin ascending limb of the loop of Henle—simple cuboidal epithelium
(D) The cortical thick ascending limb of the loop of Henle—simple cuboidal epithelium
(E) The papillary ducts—pseudostratified columnar epithelium

129. A 28-year-old man is brought into the emergency department after having been lost in the desert for 2 days. The patient complains of a headache and pain from multiple wounds. On examination, the patient has a fever and is severely dehydrated. Which one of the following statements is most likely correct?

(A) The patient should be given a nonsteroidal anti-inflammatory drug to relieve his headache and fever
(B) The patient's levels of angiotensin II are low
(C) The patient's antidiuretic hormone levels are below normal
(D) The patient's kidneys are producing higher levels of prostaglandins than normal
(E) The patient has reduced serum sodium levels and bradycardia

130. Which one of the following descriptions is typically associated with a nephrotic syndrome?

(A) Red blood cell casts, a low level of proteinuria, and granular casts
(B) Heavy proteinuria, oval fat bodies, and fatty casts
(C) Hematuria, granular casts, and broad waxy casts
(D) A proliferative glomerulonephritis on renal biopsy
(E) Hematuria, oval fat bodies, and a proliferative glomerulonephritis on renal biopsy

131. A renal biopsy has been performed on an elderly woman with chronic renal failure and edema. Ultrasound demonstrated that the patient's kidneys were enlarged. On light microscopy, the glomeruli are of normal cellularity but have a waxy material that expands the mesangium and basement membrane. By performing a Congo red stain, areas of apple-green birefringence under polarized light are seen. Which one of the following is most likely true?

(A) On an immunofluorescence stain for immunoglobulin A (IgA), a linear pattern of fluorescence would be seen

(B) On an immunofluorescence stain for IgE, a linear pattern of fluorescence would be seen

(C) The Congo red stain is binding to the cross–β-pleated configuration of amyloid fibrils

(D) The patient should be informed that she has amyloidosis, and that it will likely respond to immunostimulatory agents

(E) The patient should be informed that she has sarcoidosis, and that it will likely respond to treatment with steroids

(F) Electron microscopy would not be helpful in confirming a diagnosis

132. Which one of the following statements about the replication cycle of viruses is correct?

(A) During the eclipse period, infectious virus particles accumulate within the cell, but none are released

(B) During the latent period, the infecting viral particles are completely inactive and waiting for an opportunity to produce new viral particles

(C) The elevated period is the time when infectious viral particles accumulate intracellularly, but none have been released from the cell

(D) Cell lysis is always the final step of a viral infection

(E) During the eclipse period, no infectious viral particles have been made

133. A 24-year-old man who returned from India a few weeks ago has a mild fever and is noticeably jaundiced. The patient has not been feeling well for approximately 10 days. The patient's symptoms are vomiting, anorexia, fatigue, a sore throat, and joint pain. Laboratory results are significant for elevated aspartate aminotransferase (AST), alanine aminotransferase (ALT), and bilirubin. Test results show positive for anti-hepatitis A virus immunoglobulin G. All of the following statements are correct EXCEPT

(A) the most common mode of transmission of the causative organism is the fecal–oral route

(B) the prognosis for this patient is poor because his condition frequently progresses to a chronic disease

(C) prophylactic measures are available for this disease

(D) this patient does not require treatment and should recover completely over the next couple of weeks

(E) anti-hepatitis A virus immunoglobulin G is never found in people who do not have a history of severe hepatitis

134. A 44-year-old African-American woman presents to her physician in Tempe, Arizona, with the following symptoms: chest pain, fever, cough, and malaise. A few weeks ago this fourth-grade teacher took her class on a rock-hunting trip. A few of the students have also recently become ill. A chest radiograph showed hilar adenopathy, and a biopsy contained spherules. Which one of the following is the most likely diagnosis?

(A) Candidiasis
(B) Aspergillosis
(C) Coccidioidomycosis
(D) Histoplasmosis
(E) Blastomycosis

135. A 22-year-old man complains of a urethral discharge and urethral itching. The patient claims to have had only one sexual partner in the past 3 years, but he has experienced similar symptoms on two other occasions during this period. The discharge is noted to be whitish in color, but the result of the Gram stain is negative; however, leukocytes are present. The patient is told that he has nongonococcal urethritis and is given a prescription for tetracycline. All of the following statements are correct EXCEPT

(A) the organism that is most likely causing his symptoms is *Chlamydia trachomatis*

(B) the sexual partner should also be examined and treated; his partner may be an asymptomatic carrier, causing the patient to become reinfected

(C) the selected antibiotic is appropriate for this case

(D) the organism that is most likely causing this disease is an extracellular pathogen

(E) the organism that is most likely causing this disease can cause serious complications, including death, in women

136. Which one of the following statements about leprosy is true?

(A) It is caused by *Mycobacterium leprae,* an extremely fast- growing organism that is easily cultured

(B) It is one of the most contagious diseases known

(C) Affected patients usually die because there is no effective treatment

(D) The disease-causing organism is able to survive being phagocytosed by a macrophage

(E) The disease exists in two distinct forms, lepromatous and tuberculoid, and there is no crossover of these typical patterns within one individual

Questions 137–140

(A) Cerebrovascular accident in the motor cortex

(B) Guillain-Barré syndrome

(C) Amyotrophic lateral sclerosis (ALS; Lou Gehrig disease)

(D) Neurosyphilis

(E) Duchenne muscular dystrophy

(F) Friedreich's ataxia

(G) Myasthenia gravis

Match the following patient presentations with the most likely clinical diagnosis.

137. A 39-year-old man presents to his physician because of progressive muscle weakness of 1 week's duration. His medical history is unremarkable, although he reports having had an influenza-like episode approximately 2 weeks ago. He has been sexually active since age 16. During the physical examination, the physician notes a marked decrease in reflexes and a loss of light touch and vibration sensation in the distal extremities.

138. A 6-year-old boy is brought to the physician's office by his mother. His mother is concerned that he can no longer keep up with his friends, and she notes that he is using his hands to pull himself up from the floor. Medical history reveals that an uncle on her side of the family died in his late teens. During the physical examination, the physician notes that the boy's calf muscles appear enlarged and that his heel tendon is unusually taut. His muscle strength is extremely impaired.

139. A 55-year-old man with no previous medical problems visits a physician because his arms have become progressively weaker over the past 2 months. He is divorced and has been sexually active with more than one partner. The weakness and fatigue began first in one arm and developed later in the other. During the physical examination, the physician notes hyperreflexia, as well as generalized muscle weakness, in all four extremities. The man has no sensory dysfunction, and his gait is normal, considering his weakness.

140. A 34-year-old woman presents with muscular weakness of 3 months' duration and says that she "tires easily" when she's trying to work. After she rests for a while, some of her strength returns. She reports having some trouble with her vision, particularly diplopia; her speech appears to be dysarthric. During the physical examination, the physician notes bilateral facial weakness and a somewhat asymmetric distribution of proximal limb weakness. The woman's tendon reflexes are normal.

Questions 141–148

(A) Septic arthritis
(B) Osteoarthritis (degenerative joint disease)
(C) Rheumatoid arthritis
(D) Lyme disease
(E) Systemic sclerosis
(F) Reiter's syndrome
(G) Gout

Match each of the following historical, physical, or laboratory findings with the appropriate form of arthritis.

141. The roentgenogram and the computed tomography scan (p. 39) of a femoral joint taken from a 40-year-old mail carrier

142. The synovial biopsy of the wrist showed invasive pannus tissue eroding the cartilage.

143. This condition is associated with human leukocyte antigen B27 (HLA-B27).

144. Obesity predisposes a person to this disease; occurrences are often preceded by gluttonous alcohol consumption and heavy eating.

145. Cloudy synovial fluid with a leukocyte count of 110,000/mm^3 (95% polymorphonuclears) was drained from the hip of an elderly woman who experienced acute warmth and tenderness in the joint.

146. Cloudy, hypercellular synovial fluid shows negatively birefringent crystals.

147. Arthritic symptoms in the knee following an episode of *Chlamydia trachomatis* urethritis

148. Polyarthritis in a 9-year-old girl following a maculopapular erythematous rash

Questions 149–152

(A) Cataracts
(B) Astigmatism
(C) Presbyopia
(D) Myopia
(E) Hyperopia

Match each visual defect described with the condition that causes it.

149. A progressive decrease in the power of accommodation

150. A progressive loss of lens transparency

151. Focusing point of light rays is in front of the retina

152. Focusing point of light rays is behind the retina

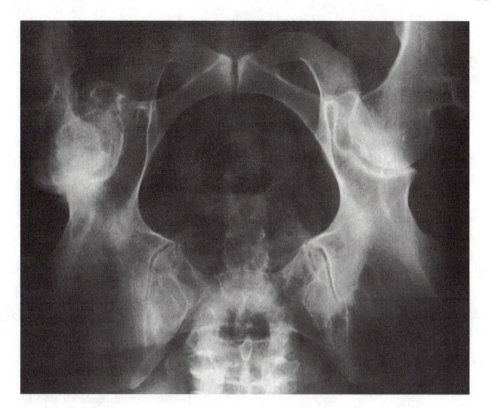

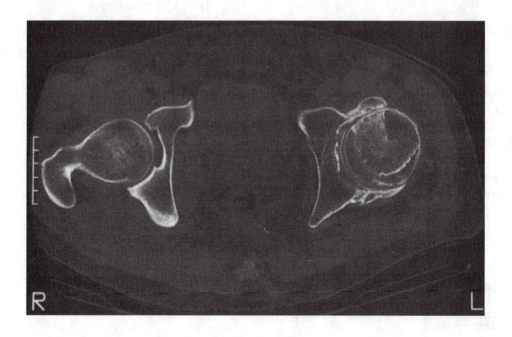

Questions 153–157

(A) Continuous
(B) Fenestrated
(C) Discontinuous
(D) Lymphatic

Match each characteristic listed below with the most appropriate type of capillary.

153. Abundant in skeletal muscle

154. Predominant in areas producing blood filtrates such as urine

155. Line bone marrow sinusoids

156. Present in the choroid plexus

157. Form the blood–brain barrier

Questions 158–161

(A) Maximal effect
(B) K_D
(C) $-1/K_D$
(D) 1/Maximal effect
(E) None of the above

A drug experiment was conducted, and the results have been plotted in two different ways. Match each number in the figures with the most appropriate term.

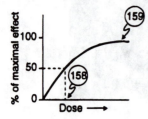
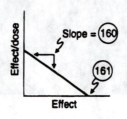

Questions 162–167

(A) Gene mapping
(B) Linkage
(C) Linkage disequilibrium
(D) Genetic polymorphism
(E) Synteny

For each of the descriptions listed below, select the most appropriate term.

162. Usually identified by a lod score of $+3$ or greater at a recombination distance of $< 50\%$

163. Restriction fragment length polymorphisms (RFLPs) are a commonly used example

164. Can be performed by somatic cell genetic and cytogenetic methods

165. The occurrence of two or more alleles at a locus in frequencies greater than can be maintained by mutation

166. The tendency in a population for specific alleles at two loci to occur together more often than is expected by chance

167. The occurrence of two loci on the same chromosome regardless of how far apart they may be

Questions 168–170

(A) 3–12 months
(B) 1–3 years
(C) 4–5 years
(D) 6–9 years

Match each of the following developmental milestone(s) with the appropriate age range in a child who is progressing normally

168. Can use two- and three-word phrases

169. Reaches for objects not in the immediate range of grasp

170. Can group objects on the basis of common features; understands that mass or volume is conserved, despite a change in shape or form (i.e., fixed volume of water is the same regardless of whether it is in a tall or short glass)

Questions 171–175

(A) Anaphase
(B) Early prophase
(C) Late prophase
(D) Telophase
(E) Metaphase

Match each of the following stages of mitosis with the appropriate term.

171. Dissolution of the nuclear envelope

172. Separation of the centromeres

173. First appearance of chromosomes

174. Alignment of chromosomes in the equatorial plane

175. Occurrence of cytokinesis

Questions 176–180

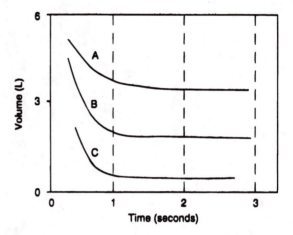

Match each of the following clinical presentations with the appropriate spirographic tracing of forced expiration.

176. A 65-year-old man who has smoked two packs of cigarettes per day for 50 years comes to the office short of breath. His breath sounds are decreased bilaterally.

177. A 58-year-old man presents with a cough that has persisted for 3 months. A chest x-ray shows irregular opacities in the lower and middle lung fields. The man believes he was exposed to asbestos for approximately 5 years when he was in his early forties.

178. A 9-year-old girl with a history of asthma presents to the emergency room with an acute exacerbation, after her albuterol inhaler ran out the day before.

179. A healthy, 30-year-old woman visits the office for a life insurance physical. She has never smoked, and her breath sounds are normal.

180. A 30-year-old man has been hospitalized for Guillain-Barré syndrome and is now short of breath.

ANSWER KEY

1-A	32-A	63-B	94-A	125-F
2-B	33-E	64-B	95-A	126-B
3-D	34-C	65-A	96-D	127-C
4-D	35-D	66-C	97-E	128-C
5-A	36-C	67-D	98-A	129-D
6-C	37-D	68-B	99-D	130-B
7-C	38-A	69-B	100-B	131-C
8-A	39-C	70-C	101-B	132-E
9-E	40-E	71-A	102-C	133-B
10-C	41-B	72-A	103-C	134-C
11-A	42-B	73-E	104-D	135-D
12-C	43-A	74-D	105-B	136-D
13-C	44-C	75-C	106-E	137-B
14-C	45-C	76-D	107-A	138-E
15-D	46-B	77-E	108-A	139-C
16-A	47-C	78-B	109-A	140-G
17-B	48-D	79-A	110-E	141-B
18-E	49-B	80-C	111-D	142-C
19-A	50-A	81-D	112-D	143-F
20-B	51-C	82-A	113-A	144-G
21-A	52-C	83-E	114-C	145-A
22-C	53-C	84-B	115-G	146-G
23-A	54-B	85-C	116-B	147-F
24-B	55-E	86-D	117-D	148-D
25-D	56-B	87-A	118-C	149-C
26-D	57-C	88-E	119-C	150-A
27-B	58-B	89-B	120-E	151-D
28-B	59-C	90-E	121-A	152-E
29-D	60-B	91-C	122-B	153-A
30-B	61-B	92-E	123-E	154-B
31-C	62-E	93-E	124-D	155-C

156-B	161-A	166-C	171-C	176-A
157-A	162-B	167-E	172-A	177-C
158-B	163-D	168-B	173-B	178-A
159-E	164-A	169-A	174-E	179-B
160-C	165-D	170-D	175-D	180-C

ANSWERS AND EXPLANATIONS

1–5. The answers are: 1-A, 2-B, 3-D, 4-D, 5-A. (*Pharmacology; synaptic neurotransmission*)

Acetylcholine (ACh) is among the first of the neurotransmitters to have its synthesis, localization, signal transduction, and pharmacology described. Presynaptic neurons frequently have receptors for the transmitter that they release, and these autoreceptors are often important for regulating the subsequent amount of transmitter release. Cholinergic neurons are found in the cerebral cortex and the anterior horn of the spinal cord. All preganglionic neurons in the autonomic nervous system release ACh, and postganglionic neurons of the parasympathetic branch are also cholinergic. A small subset of postganglionic neurons in the cholinergic sympathetic branch release ACh onto eccrine sweat glands and blood vessels. Alzheimer's dementia is correctly characterized by a relatively focal loss of cholinergic neurons in the basal nucleus of Meynert. Tetanus toxin is rapidly transported in a retrograde fashion from peripheral nerve terminals to the anterior horn cell bodies where it is released; inhibitory interneurons take up the toxin in the spinal cord, and the tetanus protein blocks the inhibitory transmission of these neurons.

Release of inositol triphosphate and diacylglycerol is not a direct result of nicotinic receptor activation. Nicotinic receptors are found in the cerebral cortex and in the neuromuscular junction as well as postsynaptically in the autonomic ganglia. They are complex proteins with an ACh-binding site coupled to a cation-permeable channel. When activated, the receptors conduct sodium and potassium ions. Drugs like succinylcholine produce paralysis during intubation by blocking the nicotinic receptors at neuromuscular junctions. Muscarinic receptors are universally coupled to either excitatory or inhibitory G proteins. They are important in mediating the effects of parasympathetic activation; thus, their blockade with drugs such as atropine results in decreased salivation (as well as other effects). Both receptor types are activated endogenously by ACh.

Nicotinic receptor activation during physiologic conditions principally causes sodium (not potassium) influx, with a resultant depolarization and increase in excitability. Sufficient depolarization leads to the activation of voltage-sensitive calcium channels and an influx of calcium. Muscarinic activation can be inhibitory or excitatory; however, this is not dependent on its function as an ion channel (because these receptors are not ion channels). G proteins can be excitatory or inhibitory, and muscarinic receptors can be coupled to either type of G protein. The particular G protein that is activated determines the effect of muscarinic activation. Different G proteins lead to depolarization or hyperpolarization, and, thus, muscarinic activity can and does change the neuron's resting potential. Muscarinic receptors were initially identified by the muscarine toxin; however, they activate (not inhibit) the receptor and, thus, mimic ACh. The symptoms described (i.e., bradycardia, salivation, flushing of the skin, bronchoconstriction) are the symptoms of mushroom poisoning (parasympathetic activation). The toxin activates the receptors for a longer period because it is not as easily degraded as ACh.

The influx of calcium is a prerequisite for the release of any neurotransmitter from any axonic terminal. ACh release is blocked by the toxin from *Clostridium botulinum*. Whereas high-affinity uptake of choline is important for the synthesis of new ACh, termination of the cholinergic transmission is mainly the function of fast-acting acetylcholinesterase (AChE). Cholinesterase inhibition is an important therapy in patients with myasthenia gravis. Myasthenic patients have an autoimmune disorder directed against their nicotinic receptors, not their nerve terminals. Inhibitors of monoamine oxidase (MAO) are important therapeutics for depression because of their effects on the dopaminergic and adrenergic systems.

All proteins—and, therefore, most enzymes, including ChAT—are synthesized in cell bodies (not axons) of neurons, because ribosomes are confined to the neuronal soma. In the cholinergic neuron, choline acetyltransferase (ChAT) creates a covalent link between choline and acetyl coenzyme A (acetyl CoA) before transport of newly synthesized ACh into storage vesicles. ChAT must be present in all cholinergic nerve terminals. Cholinergic nerve terminals are widely distributed throughout the nervous system in all animals. As mentioned previously, cholinergic neurons selectively degenerate in patients with Alzheimer's dementia, and a subsequent decrease in the ChAT levels of these patients is easily detected.

6. The answer is C. *(Microbiology; anaerobic flora)*
Pseudomonads are gram–negative, aerobic motile rods. Propionibacterium organisms are anaerobes found in the skin. Bacteroides are anaerobes found in the mouth, colon, and vagina. Fusobacterium organisms are anaerobes that live in the mouth. Clostridia are anaerobes found in the colon.

7. The answer is C. *(Microbiology; Clostridium difficile)*
The patient developed psuedomembranous colitis caused by *Clostridium difficile,* an anaerobic, gram-positive, spore-forming rod. The patient has been receiving clindamycin to treat the abscess. The clindamycin suppressed the normal colonic flora, permitting multiplication of the *C. difficile*. The patient should stop taking the clindamycin, and should be prescribed vancomycin or metronidazole. Aminoglycosides are not appropriate, because they are not effective against anaerobes. If untreated, *C. difficile* pseudomembranous colitis can be fatal. *C. difficile* produces at least two toxins (A and B). These toxins are monoglucosyltransferases specific for mammalian Rho protein, which is involved in cytoskeletal assembly (disassembly and signal transduction).

8. The answer is A. *(Microbiology; Corynebacterium diphtheriae)*
Corynebacterium diphtheriae is recognized by its unusual "Chinese letter" shape. Disposing the infecting organisms and administering the proper antitoxin are treatments for diphtheria. The gene that encodes the diphtheria toxin is located on the β–corynephage, which lysogenizes into the *C. diphtheriae* chromosome. The only known host for *C. diphtheriae* is the human body. The diphtheria toxin is produced only in low-iron environments, like the human body, and is transmittted by aerosolization. Prevention of diphtheria is possible with the diphtheria-pertussis-tetanus (DPT) vaccine.

9. The answer is E. *(Cardiology; myocardial infarction)*
The patient's history, particularly chest pain for 20 minutes or longer, is consistent with a myocardial infarction. Both creatine kinase (CK-MB) and lactate dehydrogenase (LDH_1) levels are typically elevated after a myocardial infarction; however, the timing of these changes is not the same for both markers. CK-MB levels increase several hours after an infarction, peak approximately 24 hours after the infarction, and may return to normal by 48 hours. Thus, CK-MB levels may be normal in a patient presenting a few days after having symptoms. Myoglobin is one of the first cardiac markers to increase after a myocardial infarction, but blood levels return to normal within 24 hours. LDH_1 levels do not peak until 48–72 hours after onset, but they remain elevated for 7–10 days. ST-segment elevation is also commonly seen after a myocardial infarction. Although changes in leads I, V_5, and V_6 are characteristic of involvement of the left circumflex coronary, changes in leads II, III, and aVF usually are associated with inferior infarcts with right coronary involvement.

10. The answer is C. *(Cardiology; cardiomyopathies)*
Idiopathic hypertrophic cardiomyopathy occurs as either an autosomal dominant or sporadic disease, most often in young men. It commonly causes syncopal attacks, and it is recognized pathologically by the presence of a disproportionately enlarged interventricular septum, which differs from the concentric left ventricular hypertrophy of hypertensive heart disease. Sarcoidosis, amyloidosis, and hemochromatosis are not associated with hypertrophy, but rather are restrictive cardiomyopathies that can be differentiated from each other on the basis of myocardial biopsies. Acute respiratory distress syndrome (ARDS) is a condition characterized by acute hypoxemic respiratory failure due to pulmonary edema caused by increased permeability of the alveolar capillary barrier. As the name implies, this is an acute, not a chronic, syndrome.

11. The answer is A. *(Cardiology; cardiac valvular diseases)*
Diagnosis of mitral valve prolapse can be made on the basis of the presence of a mid-systolic click with confirmation by echocardiography. This abnormality occurs in approximately 7% of the population, and even more frequently in those with connective tissue diseases. Its clinical importance is questionable, as it is often asymptomatic. Mitral regurgitation and infective endocarditis are rare complications.

12. The answer is C. *(Cardiology; rheumatic heart disease)*
Rheumatic heart disease is a complication of a group A β-hemolytic streptococcal pharyngitis characterized by carditis, polyarthritis, chorea, erythema marginatum, and subcutaneous nodules as major diagnostic criteria. It is a pancarditis, affecting all three layers of the heart. The mitral valve is most commonly affected, followed by the aortic valve. On microscopic examination, Aschoff bodies, which are areas of fibrinoid necrosis with histiocytes and Anitschkow cells, are pathognomonic.

13. The answer is C. *(Pharmacology; log–dose response relationships)*
Curves A, C, and D all reach approximately the same maximal response and, thus, are similar in efficacy. However, curve A is more potent than C, which, in turn, is more potent than D. Potency is based on the relative positions of the curves along the X axis. A competitive inhibitor would shift the curve to the right. For instance, curves A and C might be responses to an agonist in the absence (curve A) and presence (curve C) of a competitive inhibitor. Noncompetitive inhibitors decrease the efficacy (like a partial agonist might do). Thus, curves A and B might be the response to an agent in the absence (curve A) and the presence (curve B) of a noncompetitive inhibitor.

14. The answer is C. *(Biochemistry; Ehlers-Danlos syndrome)*
Ehlers-Danlos syndrome represents a spectrum of disordered collagen biosynthesis. The clinical features of Ehlers-Danlos syndrome depend on the exact underlying abnormality but can include hyperextensible skin, hypermobile joints, large vessel fragility, and vulnerability to retinal detachment. The defect in type VI Ehlers-Danlos syndrome involves the collagens that predominate in the skin, bone, tendons, and vessels (i.e., types I and III). The syndrome results from decreased lysyl hydroxylase activity. Since hydroxylysine residues are critical to proper crosslinking, the structural stability of collagen in patients with Ehlers-Danlos syndrome is compromised. There are no common Ehlers-Danlos syndromes that principally involve the cartilage and vitreous humor, which are structures that contain type II collagen. The characteristics describing laminin, proteoglycans, and fibronectin are all correct; however, none of these macromolecules are implicated in any of the Ehlers-Danlos syndromes.

15. The answer is D. *(Pathology; serous intermediate ovarian tumor)*
The papillary tumor pictured is a serous intermediate (borderline) tumor of the ovary, which is commonly seen in young women. The tumor behaves in an indolent fashion, with repeated recurrences but rare metastases outside of the abdominal cavity, resulting in a high incidence of intestinal obstruction and long survival. The tumor is characterized by edematous papillae lined by stratified cuboidal to columnar cells, which have atypical cytology. Unlike serous adenocarcinomas, serous intermediate tumors do not invade ovarian stroma.

16. The answer is A. *(Pathology; myocardial infarction)*
Immediately after a person suffers a myocardial infarction, changes are often evident on an electrocardiogram. Alterations in electrical events in the ventricles, including prolonged depolarization, are common and are manifested by abnormalities in the T wave. Although changes in circulating enzyme levels are helpful for diagnostic and prognostic purposes, they usually occur 6 hours or more after the attack and are more helpful 24 to 72 hours after the myocardial infarction.

17. The answer is B. *(Infectious diseases; hepatitis A)*
Hepatitis A has a short incubation period of between 15 and 40 days. The infection is transmitted by the fecal–oral route and takes hold very quickly. The virus replicates in the gastrointestinal tract and is shed in the feces during both the incubation and acute phases of the disease.

18. The answer is E. *(Physiology; gas exchange and partial pressure of oxygen)*
The change in cabin air pressure will cause a modest reduction in arterial Po_2. The partial pressure of a gas is proportional to the fractional concentration of the gas and total gas pressure. Predictably, Po_2 would decrease from the normal range of 97 to 100 mm Hg to approximately 67 mm Hg following decreases in alveolar Po_2. This decrease is partially due to water vapor pressure, which remains constant at 47 mm Hg, and Pco_2, which may decrease slightly due to stimulation from ventilation. This modest decline in Po_2 would not be associated with a decrease in oxygen saturation of arterial hemoglobin. A compensatory response would shift the oxyhemoglobin dissociation curve to the right because of the production of 2,3- diphosphoglycerate (2,3-DPG); however, this response usually takes more time than the average plane flight.

19. The answer is A. *(Immunology; type IV hypersensitivity)*
Type IV, or delayed, hypersensitivity reactions involve reactive lymphocytes recognizing an antigen and directing the immune response by the release of cytokines. Antibodies are not involved in this type of immune response. Neutrophils and mast cells are part of the nonspecific immune response, so they would not be major mediators of the specific response to the tuberculin test. Cytotoxic CD8 + T cells recognize antigen presented only by major histocompatability complex (MHC) I, which would not present proteins that the cell obtained from its environment but only proteins made within the cell. Therefore, these cells would not be part of the type IV response.

20. The answer is B. *(Immunology; immune suppression)*
Interleukin-2 (IL-2), also known as T-cell growth factor, is produced by T cells and leads to T-cell activation by recognition of a combination of peptide and major histocompatability complex (MHC) in the presence of costimulator molecules. IL-2 stimulates (not suppresses) the activated T cells to proliferate, as well as to differentiate to effector T cells. IL-2 has no effect on somatic cells of the body or on macrophages. Although other T-cell cytokines can influence the type of antibody made by plasma cells (e.g., IL-4 directs IgE synthesis, IL-5 directs IgA synthesis), IL-2 does not have this role.

21. The answer is A. *(Immunology; lymphoid tissues)*
The central lymphoid tissues are the bone marrow and the thymus. Both T cells and B cells develop in the bone marrow. B cells also mature in the marrow, whereas T cells migrate to the thymus for maturation. Gut-associated lymphoid tissue, bronchial-associated lymphoid tissue, and other mucosal-associated lymphoid tissues are peripheral lymphoid tissues. The gut-associated lymphoid tissue collects any antigens entering the body through the gastrointestinal tract, and the proper immune response may begin. The spleen is the site of filtration of antigens in the blood, and the site of red blood cell destruction. Most plasma cells migrate to the bone marrow, making it the site for the majority of antibody production. Germinal centers are sites for B-cell proliferation after they encounter antigen in the context of the proper cytokines.

22. The answer is C. *(Immunology; functions of antibodies)*
Antibodies have two active ends, Fab and Fc. The Fab (for antigen binding) portion binds specifically to one antigen. If the antibody is attached to the immature B cells that synthesized it, then binding of the antigen to the Fab portion can lead to activation of the B cell. Free antibodies in the blood can bind to bacteria or their toxins. Then, macrophages or other cells can ingest the antibody–antigen complexes using Fc receptors for recognition. The Fc (for constant) portion is responsible for the effector functions of antibodies. It binds to Fc receptors on neutrophils or macrophages to trigger phagocytosis of the antibody–antigen complex. Bound antibodies that cross-link their Fc portions can trigger the classical complement pathway. Antibody-dependent, cell-mediated cytotoxicity occurs when antibodies attach to specific antigens on tumor cells (or other cells recognized as foreign) and designate those cells to be killed by either natural killer (NK) cells or macrophages. The NK cells and macrophages have Fc receptors that allow them to identify the cells that are to be killed.

23–25. The answers are: 23-A, 24-B, 25-D. *(Pathology; hemochromatosis and clinical findings in cirrhosis)*
Identification of hemochromatosis in its early stages facilitates effective treatment of this otherwise relentlessly progressive disease. Although he is being treated, this patient has already progressed to late stages of the disease, and he is now displaying the classic signs of cirrhosis. The bleeding is most likely the result of ruptured esophageal varices. Portal hypertension chronically diverts blood through the esophagus veins, and those vessels dilate to support the increased flow. Portal hypertension causes the development of several collateral circulations; these other vessels offer less resistance to flow, and they enlarge over time to accommodate the increased volume. The rectal and esophageal veins dilate to become varices, which may allow significant blood loss if they tear. The caput medusae vascular pattern over the abdomen represents the enlargement of another collateral circulation. Portal hypertension also causes blood flow to back up in the spleen, which results in splenomegaly. Hemoglobin synthesis is limited by iron availability. A hemochromatosis patient has excess iron and will probably not be hemoglobin deficient. Protein C is an anticoagulant whose exact mechanism of action remains unknown. Deficiency of protein C has been demonstrated in some cases of disseminated intravascular coagulation. Although neither eroded gastric ulcer nor bronchogenic carcinoma is excluded by hemochromatosis, hemochromatosis does not predispose to either of those conditions. The patient's bleeding is more likely the result of portal hypertension.

Hepatic encephalopathy is an important complication in cirrhosis of the liver. It causes no irreversible pathology, and clinical symptoms recede as soon as metabolic corrections are made. The clinical findings can range from mild disturbances in consciousness to frank coma. The flapping tremor of asterixis (i.e., rapid extension–flexion movements of the head and arms) is most distinctive. Parkinson's disease is primarily confined to the motor system. Alterations in consciousness are rarely attributable to Parkinson's pathology. Shy-Drager syndrome is a degenerative disease characterized by autonomic neuropathy and Parkinsonian-like motor abnormalities; the man would not be showing signs of sympathetic activation. The neuronal degeneration in vitamin B_{12} deficiency is characterized by demyelination in the spinal cord and leads to peripheral sensorimotor deficits without changes in consciousness. Patients usually characterize subarachnoid hemorrhage as the ''worst headache of my life.''

Hemochromatosis is an autosomal recessive disorder that is five times more common in men, and it is related to the human leukocyte antigen A3 in 70% of cases. Renal excretion of iron is inherently limited to approximately 1 mg/day. Thus, in developed countries, the regulation of iron homeostasis requires absolute control of absorption. Unfortunately, the normal mechanisms of regulation are not well understood. The iron buildup seen as a physiologic response to anemia is almost entirely confined to phagocytic cells of the reticuloendothelial system. Yet, in hemochromatosis patients, parenchymal cells of the liver, pancreas, and heart accumulate large amounts of iron, whereas phagocytes remain normal. Thus, although there is clearly a regulatory problem at the absorptive stage, the reticuloendothelial system is also functioning improperly. Patients with various erythropoietic difficulties, and a resultant physiologically normal iron accumulation, almost never experience the extensive pathology seen in patients with primary hemochromatosis. Involvement of the pancreas commonly leads to diabetes mellitus, and skin pigmentation is a routine finding.

26. The answer is D. *(Microbiology; structure of viruses)*
Viruses have either RNA or DNA, not both. Bacteria in the genus *Chlamydia* contain both types of nucleic acid. Both *Chlamydia* and viruses are obligate intracellular parasites, which depend on the host cell for energy. Because some viruses require arthropod vectors, but other viruses (and *Chlamydia*) do not need arthropod vectors, this is not a dependable differentiating characteristic.

27. The answer is B. *(Biostatistics; probability of hepatitis B)*
Given that $P(D+) = .20$, $P(D-) = .80$, $P(T+|D+) = .90$, and $P(T-|D-) = .95$, the probability that a patient with a negative test result does not have hepatitis B, $P(D-|T-)$, is

$$P(D-|T-) = \frac{P(T-|D-)P(D-)}{P(T-|D-)P(D-) + P(T-|D+)\,P(D+)}$$
$$= \frac{(.95)(.80)}{(.95)(.80) + (1 - .90)(.20)}$$

28–29. The answers are: 28-B, 29-D. *(Physiology; acid–base disturbances)*
The blood findings indicate that this patient has a respiratory alkalosis, an acid–base disturbance characterized by increased arterial pH (or decreased $[H^+]$), decreased Pa_{CO_2} (hypocapnia), and decreased plasma $[HCO_3^-]$. It should be noted that both $[H^+]$ and $[HCO_3^-]$ are decreased in this patient, which is consistent with the axiom that $[H^+]$ and $[HCO_3^-]$ change in the same direction in respiratory acid–base imbalances. The decline in $[HCO_3^-]$ indicates that renal compensation has begun.

In alkalotic states, the $[HCO_3^-]/S \times P_{CO_2}$ ratio exceeds the normal 20:1, because of either an increase in $[HCO_3^-]$ (metabolic alkalosis) or a decrease in P_{CO_2} (respiratory alkalosis). S is a solubility constant. The normal ratio of 20:1 is derived as

$$\frac{[HCO_3^-]}{S \times P_{CO_2}} = \frac{24 \text{ mmol/L}}{0.03 \times 40 \text{ mm Hg}} = \frac{24 \text{ mmol/L}}{1.2 \text{ mmol/L}} = \frac{20}{1}$$

In this alkalotic patient, the $[HCO_3^-]/S \times P_{CO_2}$ ratio is 30:1. This ratio can be determined by substituting the patient's blood data into the preceding equation, as

$$\frac{[HCO_3^-]}{S \times P_{CO_2}} = \frac{22.5 \text{ mmol/L}}{0.03 \times 25 \text{ mm Hg}} = \frac{22.5 \text{ mmol/L}}{0.75 \text{ mmol/L}} = \frac{30}{1}$$

30. The answer is B. *(Cardiology; valvular heart disease)*
Aortic stenosis commonly presents with symptoms of angina, syncope, and dyspnea on exertion. On physical examination, a delayed upstroke of the carotid pulse may be noted, as well as a late-peaking systolic ejection murmur and soft A_2 on auscultation. Over time, left ventricular hypertrophy may develop, leading to an S_4 gallop and electrocardiogram (ECG) abnormalities. Aortic stenosis may be differentiated from mitral stenosis and aortic regurgitation by the systolic murmur rather than the diastolic murmurs caused by these two lesions. Similarly, the murmur heard in mitral regurgitation is holosystolic rather than ejection type, and it does not vary with changes in the cardiac cycle length. However, mitral regurgitation intensity does vary with the administration of amyl nitrite, a vasodilator that causes decreased intensity of the murmur.

31. The answer is C. *(Cardiology; cardiac conduction abnormalities)*
High-grade atrioventricular (AV) block is characterized by blockage of several P waves ("skipped beats") but a normal PR interval and a normal QRS complex when a P wave is conducted to the ventricles. Second-degree AV block, Mobitz type II, is characterized by single skipped beats without a prolonged PR interval and, frequently, a wide QRS complex.

32–36. The answers are: 32-A, 33-E, 34-C, 35-D, 36-C. *(Neuroanatomy, pathology, hematology; stroke, lateral neglect syndrome, anticoagulation)*

The absence of motor defects rules out much of the frontal lobe, and the presence of partial visual field defects (as well as the striking cognitive disturbance) indicates temporal or parietal lesions. The patient is displaying signs of lateral neglect syndrome, in which lesions to the nondominant parietal lobe cause severe disturbances in a person's ability to respond to any stimuli contralaterally. Thus, sensory stimuli administered to the left side are attributed to the homologous region on the right side of the body; persons or objects in the left visual field are ignored. However, there is clearly no primary sensory loss—the deficit is purely perceptual (i.e., secondary and tertiary processing are dysfunctional). The visual deficit described is commonly referred to as "pie-on-the-floor" because the two homologous lower quadrants are lost. This pattern of visual loss coupled with the features of lateral neglect strongly suggest a parietal lesion, because half of the optic radiations from the thalamus proceed upward through the parietal lobe before reaching the calcarine cortex.

The correct localization of optic tract lesions can be instrumental in isolating tumors, infarctions, and other sources of neurologic disorders. Lesions of the optic nerve (*A*) result in unilateral blindness and are generally not difficult to identify. Severance of the chiasm at *B* results in the unique finding of bitemporal hemianopsia. There is complete loss of the nasal visual fields because the temporal retinal fibers cross over to the other hemisphere at this point. Section of the fibers at *C* results in a unilateral visual loss of the contralateral visual field (again, retinal areas always "look at" the contralateral field). The fibers at *D* and *E* are the optic radiations that relay information from the thalamus to the calcarine cortex. Cutting the fibers at *D* causes a "pie-in-the-sky" lesion opposite to the one described because the two homologous upper quadrants are lost. Information from the lower half of the retinal ganglion cells projects through the temporal lobe—the lower retina "looks at" the upper visual field. The correct lesion interrupts the parietal optic radiation, which conducts information from the superior retinal ganglia and causes pie-on-the-floor deficits. Thus, the characteristic visual deficit coupled with the lateral neglect syndrome give adequate reason to suspect a parietal lobe lesion.

Perhaps the most important reason for identifying the cause of a cerebrovascular accident (CVA) is to prevent the next one from happening. Berry aneurysms in the circle of Willis cause a different set of symptoms (most commonly, subarachnoid hemorrhage and what patients describe as "the worst headache of my life"). Berry aneurysms would have been detected by angiography. In some cases, deep venous thrombosis might indicate a coagulopathy, which could also cause local thrombosis in the cortex. However, in this 75-year-old woman, it is more likely that deep venous thrombosis is the result of decreased physical activity. Thrombi breaking off of a deep venous thrombosis would most directly give rise to a pulmonary (not cerebral) embolus and infarction. Congestive heart failure can cause low-flow ischemia and infarction, especially in patients with severe atherosclerotic disease. However, low-flow ischemia generally targets the areas of the brain that are most susceptible to hypoxia—the large pyramidal cells of the motor cortex (i.e., Betz cells) and the large hippocampal neurons. This woman has neither focal motor deficits nor memory dysfunction. Arteriovenous malformations would have been found on routine angiography, and they usually cause frank hemorrhage or hemorrhagic infarction, which were not seen on a computed tomography (CT) scan. Atrial fibrillation with mural thrombosis is the likely cause of this woman's thromboembolic event. Thrombi breaking off of a large clot in the left atrium have easy and direct access to the vessels of the cerebral cortex. Areas without collateral circulation are quickly infarcted after embolic occlusion of the small vessel serving that region of tissue. Multi-infarct dementia is often related to a large clot in the left atrium, the common carotid, or one of the major branches of the carotids. The clot serves as a ready source of tiny emboli, which continually break off and cause focal lesions in the tissue served by the small vessel that they occlude. The region of tissue is often small enough that the deficit is not immediately noted; instead, a large number of individual deficits produce substantial functional loss over time. This woman needs to be evaluated as a candidate for anticoagulant and antiarrhythmic therapy.

The liver synthesizes most of the substances in the clotting cascade as zymogen (inactive) proteins, which are either cofactors or enzymes. Many of the enzymes are members of a class known as serine proteases, because a serine residue forms the active site and cleaves the ester or amide linkage on the substrate. Tissue factor, which is derived from endothelial cells, is released after tissue damage to activate the extrinsic pathway. High molecular weight kininogen, prekallikrein, and Hageman factor interact to activate the intrinsic cascade. The final common pathway is activation of the serine protease thrombin by factor V; thrombin cleaves platelet-bound fibrinogen to create the fibrin monomer. Vitamin K is essential in the liver synthesis of γ-carboxyglutamate. The large negative charge afforded by the extra carboxylic acid is critical in the calcium-binding properties of several clotting factors. Antithrombin III is an important regulatory protein, but, as its name implies, it antagonizes the clotting cascade by irreversibly binding to activated thrombin. Antithrombin III is similar to the protein α_1-antitrypsin, which inhibits elastase in the lung.

Heparin, a large, negatively charged polysaccharide, acts by increasing the speed of binding of antithrombin III to thrombin (i.e., increasing the effectiveness of antithrombin III). Because it directly affects the clotting cascade, heparin's onset of action is relatively acute. Tissue plasminogen activator and urokinase both cleave plasminogen to plasmin, the active form. Plasmin cleaves the cross-linked fibrin clot in the connector rod regions, converting the clot into a multitude of fibrin monomers. Thus, tissue plasminogen activator and urokinase act in an extremely direct fashion to dissolve established clots (which may be growing); therefore, they are the mainstay in the treatment of acute myocardial infarction. Aspirin irreversibly inhibits cyclooxygenase in all the cells of the body. For platelets, this irreversible enzyme inhibition means irreversible platelet inhibition because platelets have no protein synthesis machinery. Because platelet activation depends on enzymatic release of arachidonic acid metabolites, such as thromboxane, inhibition of the enzyme permanently inactivates the platelet. Streptokinase acts by aiding the enzymatic cleavage of inactive plasminogen to active plasmin. Its action is similar to urokinase and tissue plasminogen activator; however, it is much less specific, markedly antigenic, and no longer the drug of choice. Dicumarol (warfarin) competitively inhibits vitamin K from binding to the liver enzymes that are responsible for carboxylation. Vitamin K antagonists like dicumarol have a slow onset of action, are easily overcome by vitamin K injections, and are important therapeutics in patients with a need for chronic anticoagulation.

37–38. The answers are: 37-D, 38-A. *(Biostatistics; genetic disorders)*
The patient had a brother with poliodystrophy; therefore, the patient's mother and father must be carriers of the disorder. The patient herself may be heterozygous or homozygous for the dominant allele of the poliodystrophy gene. The probability that a child born to two known carriers will be healthy is 3/4; the probability that such a child is also a carrier is 1/2. Thus,

$$P(\text{patient carrier}|\text{patient healthy}) = \frac{P(\text{patient carrier and patient healthy})}{P(\text{patient healthy})}$$
$$= (1/2) \div (3/4)$$
$$= 2/3$$

In the absence of information on his family history of poliodystrophy, the probability that the patient's husband is a carrier is assumed to equal that of the general population (i.e., 1/20). The probability that both the patient and her husband are carriers is, therefore,

$$P(\text{patient carrier and husband carrier}) = P(\text{patient carrier}) P(\text{husband carrier})$$
$$= (2/3) (1/20)$$
$$= 1/30$$

39–42. The answers are: 39-C, 40-E, 41-B, 42-B. *(Microbiology; bacterial meningitis)*
The findings of fever, headache, nuchal rigidity, and lethargy with an acute onset and the lack of dramatic neurologic manifestations suggest acute bacterial meningitis. Viral meningitis causes much of the same symptomatology, but the onset typically is more insidious and the patient usually is less acutely ill. Patients with viral encephalitis display the same general symptomatology as those with viral meningitis, but encephalitis is differentiated by dramatic neurologic manifestations and a much poorer prognosis. Fungal meningitis is more chronic and frequently is seen with other systemic signs of mycotic disease. Brain abscess usually is seen with other foci of infection, and the patient typically has deficits that reflect the location of the lesion.

Streptococcus pneumoniae is the most common cause of bacterial meningitis among the elderly. *Haemophilus influenzae* type b is the most common cause of bacterial meningitis overall. Its incidence is highest in children 6 to 12 months old and decreases with age; the incidence of meningitis caused by *H. influenzae* is low in adults. Meningococcal meningitis occurs primarily among young adults, and *Neisseria meningitidis* serogroups A, B, C, and Y cause most cases. *Staphylococcus aureus* occasionally causes meningitis but is a common cause of brain abscess. *Actinomyces israelii* is a rare cause of meningitis associated with trauma to the jaw and gingiva or gastrointestinal tract.

The cell count in the cerebrospinal fluid (CSF) is elevated during acute bacterial meningitis to 1,000–10,000 cells/mm^3; neutrophils are the predominant cell type. Normal cell counts are 0–5 cells/mm^3 CSF. Mononuclear cells are predominant in the CSF late in viral meningitis and in patients with late manifestations of neurosyphilis; lymphocytes are prominent in early manifestations of neurosyphilis. A few erythrocytes may contaminate the CSF during the lumbar puncture; many erythrocytes can indicate brain hemorrhage. Segmented neutrophils are predominant in the CSF during viral meningitis, but the count rarely exceeds 1,000 cells/mm^3.

CSF chemistry is an important tool in determining the general diagnosis of meningitis. During bacterial meningitis, CSF protein characteristically is increased in relation to the cell count; glucose levels are low with a concentration of approximately 40% of simultaneous serum glucose levels. Elevated protein and a very low glucose level usually are found in fungal meningitis. In viral meningitis, protein levels are moderately elevated and glucose concentrations are normal or slightly decreased.

43–44. The answers are: 43-A, 44-C. *(Pharmacology; pharmacokinetics)*
The volume of distribution (V_d) is the ratio of the amount injected to the extrapolated concentration (C_0) at time zero. Because equal amounts of X, Y, and Z were injected, V_d is inversely related to C_0. Therefore, X and Z have an identical V_d, and $V_d Y > V_d X$ or $V_d Z$. Clearance is proportional to the ratio of V_d to half-time ($t_{1/2}$). Because $V_d Y > V_d X$, clearance of Y > clearance of X. Because $t_{1/2} Z > t_{1/2} X$ (which is identical to $t_{1/2} Y$), clearance of Z < clearance of X.

The time to reach steady state is purely a function of $t_{1/2}$. Because $t_{1/2} Z > t_{1/2} X$ or $t_{1/2} Y$, it will take Z longer to reach a steady state than either X or Y. However, X and Y will reach a steady state at precisely the same time. The steady-state concentration (C_{SS}) is a function of the ratio of infused rate to clearance. The infused rates are constant; therefore, C_{SS} is inversely related to clearance. Because clearance of Y > clearance of X or clearance of Z, steady-state concentrations will be [Z] > [X] > [Y].

45. The answer is C. *(Microbiology; infectious hepatitis)*
Hepatitis B surface antigen (HBsAg) is the earliest serologic marker of the hepatitis B virus (HBV) infection. It indicates active infection (acute or chronic) and usually appears before the onset of symptoms. By the end of 6 months, HBsAg has declined to undetectable levels in most patients. Hepatitis C (HCV; also called non-A, non-B, or transfusion-associated hepatitis) progresses to chronic hepatitis in as many as 60% of infected individuals; as many as 2%–3% of the general population may be HCV carriers. Hepatitis D infection requires coexisting hepatitis B infection because it needs the HBV encapsulation (i.e., surface antigen). Hepatitis B causes subclinical disease in two thirds of infected individuals; fulminant hepatitis occurs in fewer than 1% of affected individuals, and progression to hepatocellular carcinoma occurs in fewer than 5%.

Hepatitis A is not common in the United States but is very common in developing countries because it is spread by the fecal–oral route. The carrier state does not exist for hepatitis A infections.

46. The answer is B. *(Histology; mitochondrial intracellular localization)*
Mitochondria typically exist in cell areas that use substantial amounts of adenosine triphosphate (ATP). They are abundant in the apices of ciliated cells because the beating action of cilia consumes ATP. Mitochondria are distributed evenly throughout the cytoplasm of smooth muscle cells, steroid-secreting cells, skeletal muscle cells, and liver parenchymal cells rather than existing in apical concentrations.

47. The answer is C. *(Behavioral science; medical ethics)*
The man's highly emotional state indicates that he might not be competent. Providing counseling and educating him about his options make a reasoned decision possible. Until he appears competent, his demand for testing is overridden by the physician's duty to prevent a suicide (beneficence). Lying to him about test results would disrespect his autonomy, as would refusing to test him without attempting to facilitate a state of mind in which he could make a reasoned decision. Testing for other diseases would be irrelevant as well as impractical.

48. The answer is D. *(Cardiology; coronary artery disease)*
The risk factors for coronary artery disease include hypertension, hyperlipidemia, smoking, and diabetes mellitus. Angina is a symptom of the disease. Assessment of a patient for coronary artery disease is aided by an exercise test because the clinically detectable manifestations of this disease often are not present at rest. Such an assessment is important before either performing surgery or releasing someone with a high risk of sudden death. Dipyramidole is a vasodilator that acts by inhibiting adenosine metabolism. It causes increased coronary blood flow and can be used to assess coronary artery blockage. Thus, more invasive techniques may be put on hold.

49. The answer is B. *(Pharmacology; pharmacokinetics, pH partitioning)*
A weak acid such as phenobarbital tends to be in its ionized form at a higher pH. Therefore, alkalinizing the urine with $NaHCO_3$ has the desired effect of hastening renal elimination. In addition, urine flow increases in an alkaline situation, further increasing the amount of phenobarbital that is eliminated. Alkalinization of plasma also tends to move un-ionized phenobarbital out of the central nervous system (CNS) and into the plasma by creating a transient gradient in which movement can occur. Phenobarbital and other barbiturates tend to induce P_{450} enzymes, which should aid the elimination of these drugs. However, the induction of P_{450} enzymes is somewhat slower than desired in an emergency situation.

50. The answer is A. *(Physiology; pulmonary mechanics)*
Pleural pressure is not equally distributed from the base to the apex. For a variety of reasons, the pleural pressure is more negative at the apex and, therefore, the transpulmonary pressure (i.e., alveolar–pleural pressure) is greater at the apex. The pressure–volume relationship shown is dependent on the lung's elastic properties, which are constant from base to apex. If it is correctly interpreted, the graph answers the question. The alveoli at different places in the lungs experience different pressures and thus have different volumes. At lung volumes close to functional residual capacity (FRC), which is the resting lung volume, the pressure–volume relationship is steep. Thus, the alveoli at the base, which have slightly smaller pressures, have much smaller volumes. At volumes close to VC, the transluminal pressure has reached the flat portion of the curve, so that the small pressure differences from base to apex no longer matter; alveoli are uniformly inflated. The transluminal pressure is actually negative (therefore closing the alveoli) at the base when the lungs are near residual volume. Not until the lungs have begun filling elsewhere do these alveoli open up again. Alveoli

in the apex are more full at FRC than are alveoli at the base; therefore, they receive less ventilation than the alveoli at the base. In other words, alveoli that are already full do not have much room for more ventilation.

51. The answer is C. *(Physiology; neuromuscular transmission)*
Motoneurons innervate many skeletal muscle fibers. In large muscles, thousands of fibers may be innervated by one neuron. However, each fiber receives only one axon terminal. Depolarization of the nerve terminal releases acetylcholine (ACh) into the synaptic cleft, where it binds directly to Na^+ channels, causing an end-plate potential. The end-plate itself is not electrically excitable, but passive spreading of end-plate potential to a nearby membrane leads to propagation of the action potential and contraction of all muscle fibers innervated by the motoneuron. When ACh is the neurotransmitter, termination of transmission is accomplished by hydrolysis via acetylcholinesterase.

52. The answer is C. *(Physiology; pulmonary mechanics)*
According to the equal pressure point theory, expiratory effort increases flow until airways are actually closed off by the pressure of the effort. Inspiratory efforts that lead to vital capacity inflate the lungs to a large end-inspiratory pressure. Therefore, there is sufficient positive alveolar pressure to maintain patency through all airways, even with a large expiratory effort. Thus, from vital capacity, increased expiratory efforts (i.e., increased positive pleural pressures) are rewarded with increased flow. However, at 50% of VC, increased expiratory efforts only increase the resistance of the airways because the pleural pressure exceeds the alveolar pressure and closes the airways. Because airway resistance decreases with increasing size of the airway, resistance is lowest at vital capacity, where the airways are at their largest calibre. At residual volume, the elastic properties of the chest wall are directed outward. (Try holding your lungs at residual volume for a moment to see how much elastic recoil exists.)

53. The answer is C. *(Microbiology; anatomy; herpes simplex virus infection of the nervous system)*
"Cold sores" are caused by the herpes simplex virus (HSV), which usually infects the lips, philtrum, and the areas around the nares of affected individuals. After the primary infection, HSV establishes a latent state in the ganglia of cranial nerve (CN) V where the second (CN V_2) and third (CN V_3) branches of this nerve innervate the areas described above. CN VII is not infected by this virus.

54. The answer is B. *(Endocrinology; hormonal regulation of pregnancy)*
Human chorionic gonadotropin (hCG) can be detected within 10 days of conception, providing a rapid and specific test for pregnancy. Human chorionic somatomammotropin (hCS) directs maternal metabolism to maintain a continuous nutrient flow to the fetus and is first detected 4 weeks after conception. Luteinizing hormone (LH), follicle-stimulating hormone (FSH), and hCG [as well as thyroid-stimulating hormone (TSH)] share α subunits; their β subunits have approximately 70% homology. The first function of hCG is to maintain the corpus luteum steroid production. Without hCG, the corpus luteum dies from lack of LH, and menses begin. After the first 8–12 weeks of gestation, placental production of steroids is sufficient, and the corpus luteum is no longer needed. The hCG level declines somewhat to a plateau, where it remains for the remainder of pregnancy. The hCG actually suppresses pituitary LH secretion, which is already low by the time of conception (i.e., 1–3 days after ovulation).

55. The answer is E. *(Genetics; DNA replication)*
DNA replication begins at specific sites. In *Escherichia coli*, DNA replication starts at a unique origin and proceeds sequentially in opposite directions. Because of the size of the eukaryotic genome, multiple replication origins are important for timely DNA replication. DNA polymerase cannot start chains de novo; all known DNA polymerases add mononucleotides to the 3' hydroxyl end of an RNA primer, or, as in the case of adenovirus replication, DNA synthesis begins from a serine residue on a protein primer. DNA replication occurs during the S phase of the cell cycle.

56. The answer is B. *(Physiology; pulmonary mechanics)*
Compliance is defined as a change in volume over change in pressure. The steeper the curves of the static volume–pressure relationships shown in the figure, the more compliant the lungs. A compliant, or flabby, lung is typical of emphysema, in which recoil pressures are lower at any given lung volume and the functional residual capacity tends to be higher. In contrast, a fibrotic, stiff lung (subject C) has decreased compliance and increased elastic recoil and tends to have a lower functional residual capacity. This increased elastic recoil pulls the chest wall in until the outward recoil of the chest wall equals (but is opposite) the inward recoil of the lung, therefore lowering functional residual capacity.

57. The answer is C. *(Pathology; microbiology; diagnosis of syphilis)*
A Venereal Disease Research Laboratory (VDRL) test and dark-field examination would be the most appropriate combination of tests for determining the cause of the penile lesion. A painless penile lesion that is crateriform, moist, and indurated is suggestive of primary syphilis. The organism responsible, *Treponema pallidum*, cannot be cultured or detected by Gram stain. It can, however, be visualized by dark-field observation of scrapings from the lesion. Some, but not all, patients with primary syphilis have serologic evidence of infection, readily detected by the VDRL test. The fluorescent treponemal antibody absorption (FTA-ABS) test is only used to confirm diagnosis and is not appropriate here.

58. The answer is B. *(Genetics; radiolabeled nucleic acid uptake)*
One of the best methods for measuring cellular proliferation is measuring the uptake of radiolabeled nucleic acid. Dividing cells require nucleotides for DNA synthesis, and the uptake of labeled thymidine and its incorporation in DNA are excellent indicators of cell proliferation. Uracil, which is only used in RNA synthesis, except for some reconstituted through a salvage pathway, would not be indicative of cell division, only of messenger RNA (mRNA) synthesis. Likewise, uptake and incorporation of radiolabeled methionine would involve protein synthesis, not cell division. Trypan blue exclusion is used for quantitating viability and would not be useful in this experiment.

59–60. The answers are: 59-C, 60-B. *(Cardiology; physiology; congestive heart failure, cardiac mechanics)*
The major signs of congestive heart failure are fatigue and dyspnea. Vascular congestion confirmed by physical examination (i.e., neck veins, rales) and third heart sounds due to abnormally high diastolic flow to a normal ventricle or normal flow into a dilated ventricle are also consistent with congestive heart failure. The enlarged cardiac silhouette with pulmonary vascular markings is strongly suggestive of left-sided heart failure. Neither the heart rate nor blood pressure is elevated significantly enough to consider this a malignant arrhythmia or emergency hypertensive crisis.

In the control subject (X), end-diastolic pressure is low, and ejection is well-maintained during systole. In the failing heart, end-diastolic pressure and volume are greatly elevated, and ejection is poorly maintained (stroke volume is reduced). Digitalis (Y) exerts a positive inotropic effect by inhibiting Na^+-K^+ ATPase and indirectly elevating intracellular Ca^+. The effect is to decrease diastolic pressures and volumes and increase stroke volume.

61. The answer is B. *(Neuroanatomy; structures of the brain)*
The limbic system is concerned with unconscious biologic drives and emotions and, therefore, is considered the most primitive part of the brain. It contains the limbic lobe, hippocampus, anterior thalamic nucleus, hypothalamus, and the amygdala.

62. The answer is E. *(Biochemistry; RNA structure and function)*
In eukaryotes, messenger RNA (mRNA) is formed in the nucleus and must be exported into the cytosol for

translation. The initial product of transcription includes all of the introns and flanking regions, which must be removed by splicing before correct translation can occur. The splicing reaction involves hydrolysis of phosphodiester bonds and formation of new phosphodiester bonds within the mRNA molecule. Other processing reactions include additions at both the 5′ and 3′ ends. A guanosine triphosphate (GTP) molecule is added in reverse orientation to form a cap at the 5′ end, and the cap is further modified by the addition of methyl groups. A polyadenylate tail is added at the 3′ end.

63–64. The answers are: 63-B, 64-B. *(Microbiology, pharmacology; Lyme disease)*
Lyme disease is a recently described tick-borne disease in which the infectious agent is a spirochete, *Borrelia burgdorferi*. Erythema chronicum migrans and positive antibody to the spirochete are presumed to be diagnostic for this condition, which may be manifested by flu-like symptoms that may ultimately progress toward arthritic, cardiac, and central nervous system (CNS) symptoms. The causative spirochete is sensitive to several antibiotics, including penicillin, tetracycline, and erythromycin.

65. The answer is A. *(Biochemistry; structure and function of amino acids in proteins)*
The physical and chemical properties of the peptide reflect the properties of the constituent amino acids. At pH 7.4, the positive and negative charges of the α-amino and α-carboxyl terminal groups cancel one another. The side chains of the two aspartate and one glutamate residues are negatively charged; the side chain of arginine is positively charged. Cysteine and methionine both contain sulfur atoms. Any of the amino acids that contain a hydrogen atom attached to a sulfur, nitrogen, or oxygen atom, or containing an atom with an unshared pair of electrons, could form hydrogen bonds. The amino acids valine, phenylalanine, methionine, and cysteine contribute hydrophobic character to the peptide. The specificity of chymotrypsin is for peptide bonds in which the carboxyl group is donated by an aromatic amino acid.

66. The answer is C. *(Pharmacology; treatment of arrhythmias)*
Lidocaine is often the drug of choice for the treatment of ventricular arrhythmia. It suppresses Na^+ currents in the infarct area that have abnormal resting membrane potentials and elevated K^+ levels. If lidocaine fails, the most frequently chosen agent is another Na^+-channel blocker, procainamide. The Ca^{2+}-channel blockers (diltiazem, verapamil) and β-blockers (propranolol) have a greater effect on supraventricular disturbances in which slow Ca^{2+} channels are involved more significantly than Na^+ channels.

67. The answer is D. *(Pathology; renal cell carcinoma)*
The renal mass pictured is classic clear cell carcinoma of the kidney. The cells have round to oval nuclei and inconspicuous nucleoli. The cytoplasm is abundant; it is clear because of the large amounts of glycogen and lipid within these cells (the glycogen accounts for the yellow color). Renal cell carcinomas may be hemorrhagic, and they tend to invade the renal veins and inferior vena cava, from which they may metastasize to the bones and lungs.

68. The answer is B. *(Biochemistry; urea cycle)*
Urea is the principal compound by which ammonia is excreted from the body. The nitrogens in urea come from ammonia and aspartate. Ammonia reacts with carbon dioxide and adenosine triphosphate (ATP) to form carbamoyl phosphate in a reaction catalyzed by carbamoyl phosphate synthetase (ammonia). This enzyme requires N-acetylglutamate as a positive allosteric effector. Without this reaction, urea would not be formed, and ammonia levels would be high. The next step in the urea cycle is the reaction of carbamoyl phosphate with ornithine to form citrulline. In the absence of carbamoyl phosphate, ornithine levels are high, citrulline is undetectable, and neither argininosuccinate nor arginine is formed.

69. The answer is B. *(Neurology; assessment)*
Cerebellar disease manifests as dystonia to palpation but does not alter grip strength. Pain elicited by touching

the chin to the chest is known as Brudzinski's sign and usually indicates inflammation of the meninges. Cerebellar disease is indicated by decreased resistance of the limbs to passive movement. Deep tendon reflexes continue for longer than usual; in the patellar tendon this is known as the "pendular knee jerk" due to the motion of the limb when the reflex is elicited. Patients with cerebellar disease also show voluntary ataxia, dysdiadochokinesia, nystagmus, and dysarthria of the larynx. Cerebellar lesions usually affect the ipsilateral body.

70–71. The answers are: 70-C, 71-A. *(Physiology; electrical activity of the heart)*
The traces shown in *A*, *B*, and *C* are of cells from the left ventricle, sinoatrial (SA) node, and left atrium, respectively. The refractory period, during which the cell cannot fire another action potential, occurs during the first one half to two thirds of *phase 3* in each of the traces. Contraction of the left ventricle occurs during the calcium plateau (*phase 2*) of myocytes in the left ventricle.

   Phase 0 of cells in the ventricles and atria is marked by the opening of voltage-gated, tetrodotoxin-sensitive sodium channels. These "fast" sodium channels are responsible for the rapid upstroke of action potentials in the contractile cells; however, these channels do not seem to play a role in the action potentials of cells in the SA or atrioventricular (AV) nodes where Ca^{2+} channels conduct phase 0 of depolarization. The fast sodium channels inactivate almost as rapidly as they activate, so that the increase in sodium conductance, which leads to depolarization, is soon terminated. No sodium currents are activated until the next action potential. The resting potential of contractile myocytes is maintained by a large potassium conductance. An increase in the potassium conductance does not result in rapid depolarization but rather mild hyperpolarization caused by a small potassium efflux. However, during the action potential, repolarization (*phase 3* of both traces *A* and *B*) is characterized by an increase in the potassium conductance, leading to an outward potassium current (efflux). Because the cell is depolarized at this time, the increase in potassium current quickly moves the cell toward the resting potential. Calcium- activated potassium currents seem to be particularly important in the ventricular repolarization (*phase 3*); these currents may be the site at which the calcium increases result in an increased heart rate (staircase effect). SA node automaticity (the unique pacemaker potential) occurs in *phase 4* (slow depolarization).

72. The answer is A. *(Cardiology; fourth heart sound)*
Under certain pathologic conditions, the fourth heart sound (S_4) is a low-frequency presystolic sound that is produced in the ventricle during filling. It occurs on atrial contraction with the flow of blood into a stiffened, noncompliant ventricle. An S_4 is almost never heard during atrial fibrillation. An S_4 is commonly associated with ischemic heart disease, severe hypertension, aortic stenosis, and hypertrophic cardiomyopathies. However, the incidence of S_4 sounds increases with age, and S_4 sounds are often benign findings in a healthy, athletic person. Therefore, whether audible S_4 sounds are in themselves abnormal remains unclear.

73. The answer is E. *(Physiology; cardiac physiology)*
The upstroke of the ventricular action potential is primarily due to a fast inward Na^+ current. Blockage of the rapid upstroke by tetrodotoxin (TTX) and other studies have demonstrated this point. The plateau phase of the action potential is maintained by a combination of K^+, Ca^{2+}, and Na^+ currents, whereas repolarization is mainly due to increased K^+ conductance.

74. The answer is D. *(Cardiology; regulation of blood flow)*
The muscles have a much higher oxygen demand during exercise than they do at rest. Although active muscles are able to extract a higher proportion of the delivered oxygen, increased perfusion is also required to satisfy the enormous demand for oxygen. Metabolic by products such as H^+, CO_2, adenosine, phosphate, and prostaglandins act as signals within the exercising muscles to cause vasodilation. These metabolic signals can even overcome the vasoconstrictive signal of increased sympathetic outflow; however, the sympathetic outflow does result in vasoconstriction of the vascular beds that are not directly involved with the exercise

(e.g. the vessels in the arms of someone on a stationary bicycle). Another signal mechanism is the release of nitric oxide from endothelial cells when blood flow is increased due to the metabolic signals. Nitric oxide is an inhibitor of smooth muscle contraction; therefore, it acts to further decrease the resistance and increase perfusion in the vessels leading to the active skeletal muscles.

75–79. The answers are: 75-C, 76-D, 77-E, 78-B, 79-A. *(Pathology; cholecystitis and cholelithiasis)*
Fat, forty, and female are the features of a patient with a classic case of symptomatic gallstone disease. The pain is correctly described as biliary colic; that is, severe pain lasting for up to 20 minutes and then subsiding, only to return several more times in the hours following. Such a characterization is highly specific to cholelithiasis. Nausea and vomiting frequently accompany biliary colic, and mild elevation of serum bilirubin occurs in 25% of these patients. However, none of these are specific signs for biliary calculi. Ultrasonic radiography is diagnostic in more than 90% of cases and, if available, it is the evaluation of choice. Abdominal rigidity and rebound tenderness are the signs of "acute abdomen," a surgical emergency that is frequently the result of visceral perforation. Hemoccult-positive stool is a nonspecific indicator of a more emergent problem that requires additional workup. Excessive postprandial flatulence needs to be evaluated with other more specific signs of abdominal disease. Steatorrhea and lactose intolerance are two fairly common conditions associated with a tremendous amount of abdominal gas.

The fever and elevated white blood cell count are explained by an acute infection in the patient's gallbladder. Enterococci, *Escherichia coli*, *Klebsiella*, and *Clostridium* are commonly occurring enteric pathogens. *Neisseria* species are not commonly found in the gut, but rather cause urinary tract infections and meningitis.

In autopsies performed in the United States, more than 20% of women and 8% of men over the age of 40 are found to have had asymptomatic gallstones. There has been substantial debate over the appropriate management of asymptomatic gallstones found incidentally when imaging the abdomen for other problems. Currently, surgical intervention is not indicated for asymptomatic disease.

Cholesterol and mixed stones account for more than 80% of biliary calculi, with the remaining 20% being pigment stones. The risk factors for the more common cholesterol stones fall into two groups: factors that increase cholesterol output and factors that decrease bile salt secretion. Clofibrate therapy, obesity, pregnancy, and diabetes mellitus all tend to increase cholesterol output. Oral contraceptive use and ileal disease or resection result in fewer bile salt secretions (the ileum is the principal site of bile salt recycling, which is a major source of secreted bile salts). Alcoholic cirrhosis and chronic hemolysis are examples of disease processes that result in elevations of unconjugated serum bilirubin. Insoluble bilirubin can be converted to calcium bilirubinate, which is the major component of pigment stones.

Cholesterol stones are formed when an imbalance between bile acid secretion and cholesterol output occurs. Increases in cholesterol output or decreases in the cholesterol-solubilizing bile acids result in an increased likelihood of stone formation. HMG CoA reductase performs the rate-limiting step in cholesterol synthesis and, therefore, it is the target of a family of cholesterol-reducing drugs (e.g., lovastatin). Hence, decreases in the activity of HMG CoA coupled with increased bile acid secretion markedly decrease the stone-forming potential. Gallbladder hypomotility associated with severe trauma, total parenteral nutrition, and oral contraceptives is an important factor in the genesis of bile calculi. Infection of the biliary tree with certain pathogens can result in cleavage of the conjugation moieties, turning soluble, conjugated bilirubin into insoluble, unconjugated forms.

80–84. The answers are: 80-C, 81-D, 82-A, 83-E, 84-B. *(Pathology, pharmacology; Graves' disease and hyperthyroidism)*
Severe illness or physical trauma can cause changes in thyroid hormone regulation that are referred to as sick euthyroid syndrome (SES). Euthyroid indicates that the patient has sufficient but not excess thyroid hormone function. Clinically, the patient appears normal; however, the different thyroid laboratory tests return values that indicate hypo- or hyperthyroidism, depending on the variant of SES. Hashimoto's thyroiditis

is characterized in the chronic phase by thyroid insufficiency. Symptoms common in hypothyroidism include lethargy, constipation, cold intolerance, menorrhagia, and weight gain. Dry skin and patchy hair loss emerge as the disease progresses. Graves' disease, thyroid adenomas, and the extremely rare overproduction of thyrotropin-releasing hormone (TRH) by the hypothalamus all result in the hyperthyroid symptoms described. However, the ocular pathology described (i.e., exophthalmos, extraocular ophthalmoplegia) is characteristic of the autoimmune disorder known as Graves' disease. The inflammatory reaction against the muscles and connective tissue in the orbit causes edema, muscular weakness, and fibrosis leading to the symptoms described.

The complete triad of Graves' disease also includes pretibial myxedema, an inflammatory thickening of the dermis most often found over the dorsum of the legs and feet. The skin is raised and thickened; it may be itchy and often has a peau d'orange appearance. Pericardial effusion and patchy loss of hair are both consistent with hypothyroidism. Diffuse hyperpigmentation is often found with adrenal insufficiency (e.g., Addison's disease) or pituitary adrenocorticotropic hormone (ACTH)-producing adenomas. Jaundice is not a finding commonly related to Graves' disease.

The TRH challenge is particularly useful in demonstrating thyrotoxicosis. The pituitary thyroid-stimulating hormone (TSH) response to TRH is significantly blunted by high serum T_3 levels. Serum TSH is a less useful indicator but should be low or undetectable in this woman. Thyrotoxicosis coupled with the ocular signs described gives strong evidence for Graves' disease, in which autoantibodies against the TSH receptor provide unregulated stimulation of the thyroid gland. The triiodothyronine resin uptake (T_3RU) test is useful in describing the relation between total and free T_3. In this in vitro test, excess radiolabeled T_3 is introduced into the patient's serum, and a particulate resin is used to collect any unbound T_3 (labeled or unlabeled). The resin uptake is inversely proportional to the number of available binding sites on the patient's thyroid-binding globulin (TBG). If the patient's own T_3 occupies most of the available sites (as it has in this case), much of the labeled T_3 remains for the resin to "soak up." If, on the other hand, there is an excess of available TBG-binding sites (i.e., in patients with low serum T_3), the labeled T_3 first binds the sites, and less labeled T_3 is left for the resin (decreased T_3 resin uptake).

Multinodular goiter, autonomous adenomas, and single carcinoma all have distinctive scintiscan results that are inconsistent with the description given (i.e., uniform radioiodine uptake). Multinodular goiter and autonomous adenomas show areas of particular brightness or dullness on a scintiscan; the carcinoma is often nonfunctional and dark. Lymphocytic infiltration with atrophic follicles usually shows up on a scintiscan as uniformly dull, but the radiographic description alone does not rule out this condition. However, follicular atrophy is characteristic of Hashimoto's disease (i.e., thyroid insufficiency), not Graves' disease. Lymphocytic infiltration is common to Hashimoto's disease and Graves' disease, although it is much more striking in Hashimoto's disease.

Propylthiouracil (PTU) and methimazole share a common mechanism of action in inhibiting the synthesis of thyroxine, but methimazole is more potent. However, PTU offers the advantage of reducing the peripheral conversion of T_4 to T_3; it is, therefore, equipped to give faster relief from the symptoms of thyrotoxicosis because T_3 has substantially more biologic activity. Radioactive iodine is a useful alternative to surgery in the patient who might have perioperative complications (e.g., the elderly, those with severe thyrotoxicosis). No carcinogenic effects have been documented, but radioactive iodine may be contraindicated in women who want to become pregnant in the future. Because the mechanical components of the ocular pathology in Graves' disease are inflammatory in nature, they are relieved with large doses (120 mg/day) of prednisone. Propranolol provides the fastest symptomatic relief of the nervousness, tachycardia, lid lag, and other sympathetic manifestations.

85–89. The answers are: 85-C, 86-D, 87-A, 88-E, 89-B. *(Endocrinology, pathology; paraneoplastic syndromes)*

Paraneoplastic syndromes represent an important source of morbidity in the spectrum of cancer pathophysiology. The varied signs and symptoms that fall into this category cannot be directly related to the physical tumor but are instead a result of the tumor's presence in the body. Although the mechanisms involved are not completely understood, in some cases the tumor produces a substance and, in other cases, the signs and symptoms are probably related to the body's immunologic reaction against the tumor.

This patient presents with the classic symptoms of Cushing's syndrome, which is indicated by an excess of corticosteroids. In this case, the lack of libido is the result of cortisol suppression of the pituitary's secretion of gonadotropin-releasing hormone (GnRH). The muscle wasting and abdominal stria are caused by deranged protein metabolism, which results in degradation of the connective tissue. The characteristic patterns of weight gain (e.g., buffalo hump, moon facies) are due to ill-defined effects of excess steroids on lipid metabolism. The signs and symptoms of a paraneoplastic syndrome can often present at the same time as (or earlier than) the symptoms associated with the tumor (e.g., hoarseness, cough). The two sets of signs together are a strong indicator of a bronchogenic tumor.

The best confirming tests are a chest x-ray and dexamethasone suppression test. The suppression test helps to differentiate between endocrine dysregulation and completely autonomous steroid production (i.e., no regulation). Although urinary glucocorticoids can indicate that steroids are being produced in excess, physical examination is needed to confirm a diagnosis. The water restriction is useful for diagnosing syndrome of inappropriate ADH (SIADH), which is characterized by hyponatremia and water retention. The other tests are useful for diagnosing primary thyroid and glucose abnormalities, which are not likely given this clinical scenario.

When Cushing's syndrome coexists with a bronchogenic tumor, it is almost always a result of tumor ACTH production. Tumors almost never produce steroids—the synthesis pathway is too complex for a dysfunctional cell. Autonomous secretion of parathyroid hormone causes a syndrome known as hypercalcemia of malignancy, which is associated with hypercalcemia and lytic lesions of the bone. There is no indication of thyroid dysfunction. Although glucose metabolism is almost certainly altered, the glucose derangement is a result of the excess steroids; insulin alone could not be responsible for the other metabolic abnormalities.

Ectopic, unregulated ACTH production causes bilateral hypertrophy of the adrenal cortices. Focal enlargement in any organ indicates neoplasia. Carcinoid tumors are nonbronchogenic lung tumors that cause a paraneoplastic syndrome associated with serotonin and histamine release. Pituitary hypertrophy is the result of excess hypothalamic secretion of corticotropin-releasing hormone (CRH), and it may indicate the presence of an ACTH adenoma. Such an excess gives rise to Cushing's syndrome, but tumor production of CRH is uncommon.

Lung cancer occurring in families with members who smoke is not definitive epidemiologic evidence for either a genetic or an environmental hypothesis of lung carcinoma. In trying to establish a correlation between a variable (cigarette smoking) and a disease (lung cancer), one needs to look for a confounding relationship (i.e., a positive family history for both).

With the exception of hyperaldosteronism, the other signs and symptoms listed are all common in various bronchogenic carcinomas. Squamous cell carcinomas are most frequently associated with hypercalcemia; small cell carcinomas tend to cause Cushing's syndrome or SIADH. The dermatomyositis is less common and is thought to be related to an immunologic reaction against the tumor. Hypertrophic osteodystrophy with clubbing involves unknown mechanisms but is a common manifestation of lung cancer.

90. The answer is E. *(Histology; protein structure, receptors)*
Known receptors for physiologic growth factors and effectors display a small group of structures that are shared among different proteins and are found on either the external or internal domain of the protein. These structures are recognizable at a primary amino acid sequence level. This allows receptors to be classified into groups that resemble ion channels; groups that resemble kinases, especially tyrosine, serine, and threonine kinases; and cyclases. Several plasma membrane receptors require interactions with guanosine triphosphate (GTP)–binding proteins (G proteins) to function in signal transduction. Metallothioneins are good acceptors for zinc and heavy metal, but have not been reported to be receptors or elements in signal transduction systems.

91. The answer is C. *(Biochemistry; nucleotides)*
Three nucleotides are required to specify the insertion of an amino acid into a polypeptide chain. These groups of three nucleotides comprise a codon that is represented in the 5′ to 3′ direction. Because there are four different bases in RNA, the maximum number of codons is sixty-four. Sixty-one of these codons specify the twenty amino acids; some amino acids have more than one. The triplet AUG serves as a start signal, and three triplets that do not code for any amino acid serve as stop signals. The genetic code is virtually universal; all organisms use the same codons to translate their genomes into proteins. A transcription unit can be influenced by promoter and enhancer elements as well as methylation of nucleotides.

92. The answer is E. *(Neurology; excitatory amino acids)*
Decreased GABA-ergic activity is associated with increased seizure activity, and antiepileptic drugs are GABA-ergic. Baclofen, used for multiple sclerosis, reduces muscle spasms. Benzodiazepines have agonist activity at a macromolecular receptor complex that includes a γ-aminobutyric acid (GABA) receptor, and the activity of this receptor appears to be overactive in hepatic encephalopathy.

93. The answer is E. *(Behavioral science; biologic theory)*
Biologic theory proposes some alteration of brain function as underlying mental disorder. If schizophrenia is considered a genetic disorder, monozygotic twins would be concordant for the disorder.

94. The answer is A. *(Nephrology, pathology; hypocomplementemia-associated renal disease)*
Complement levels are normal in immunoglobulin A (IgA) nephropathy and diffuse proliferative glomerulo-nephritis (poststreptococcal glomerulonephritis). Nephritides associated with hypocomplementemia include cryoglobulinemia, membranoproliferative glomerulonephropathy, and a variety of visceral infections, includ-ing infections of peritoneal and central nervous system (CNS) shunts (''shunt'' nephritis).

95. The answer is A. *(Biochemistry; extracellular matrix)*
Cell–cell interactions and cell–matrix interactions are essential for normal development and wound healing. The integrins are part of the supergene family, which also includes leukocyte adhesion molecules and receptors on the platelet membrane surface. These transmembrane glycoproteins have extracellular domains that bind matrix molecules (e.g., fibronectin) and intracellular domains that interact with cytoskeletal elements to activate signals in the cytosol and nucleus. The integrins do stimulate gene transcription indirectly as a result of their mobilization of cytosolic signal-transducing pathways. Platelet aggregation requires a fibrinogen bridge between two transmembrane receptors. Adhesion to the damaged surface requires that a different receptor interacts with von Willebrand factor and the subendothelium. Laminin is thought to be important in the developing nervous system, and several extracellular matrix molecules are crucial to the formation of proper relationships between cells (e.g., endothelial cells making tubes).

96. The answer is D. *(Immunology; HLA-associated disorders)*
The major histocompatibility complex, which is also known as the human leukocyte antigen (HLA) complex, has been associated with a variety of diseases. Probably the best known association is between HLA-B27 and ankylosing spondylitis. All of the HLA associations in the question are matched correctly except for 21-hydroxylase deficiency, which is associated with HLA-BW47, not HLA-DR4.

97. The answer is E. *(Physiology; myocardial cells)*
Application of acetylcholine (ACh) or vagal stimulation decreases the slope of phase 4 of a slow fiber (or pacemaker cell) that is likely to be found in the sinoatrial or atrioventricular nodal tissue. This is owing to increased permeability to K^+ and causes a decrease in heart rate in situ. Fast fibers like those found in non-nodal atrial or ventricular tissue have a rapid depolarization (phase 0) caused by the opening of fast Na^+ channels, followed by a plateau (phase 2) secondary to the opening of slow Ca^{2+} channels.

98–99. The answers are: 98-A, 99-D. *(Pathology; acute leukemia)*
The presence of pancytopenia is not associated with chronic lymphocytic leukemia. Patients with acute myelogenous leukemia, recurrent ovarian carcinoma, and aplastic anemia can have pancytopenia. Cyclophosphamide, which is used to treat some patients with ovarian carcinoma, does cause bone marrow depression, and recovery can be delayed.

An immunoglobulin gene rearrangement analysis would not be useful for this patient unless she had shown evidence of a lymphoproliferative disorder. Radiographic and cytologic studies could confirm the presence of ascites and possible recurrent ovarian carcinoma. Bone marrow aspiration is essential to establish the diagnosis. With hepatic enlargement, it is necessary to evaluate the patient for evidence of liver damage. Some agents that damage the liver can also damage the bone marrow.

100. The answer is B. *(Pathology; chronic type B gastritis)*
Chronic type B gastritis is four times more common than type A (fundal) gastritis, the form of chronic gastritis in which there are circulating antibodies to the parietal cells and intrinsic factor. Type B gastritis may result from chronic alcohol or aspirin use, bile reflux, ulcer disease, or postgastrectomy states. Type A is found in elderly individuals and individuals with pernicious anemia. Levels of gastrin tend to be low, and there may be antibodies to gastrin-producing cells in type B gastritis, in contrast to type A gastritis. In type B gastritis, the stomach wall loses its rugal folds and becomes flattened, glazed, and red.

101. The answer is B. *(Physiology, pulmonology; asthma, pulmonary mechanics)*
The forced vital capacity (FVC) is unchanged or decreased during an acute asthma attack. An important spirometric manifestation of asthma is a decrease in forced expiratory volume in 1 second (FEV_1) by itself or normalized to FVC. Total lung capacity (TLC) will be normal, or elevated possibly, because of loss of elastic recoil.

102. The answer is C. *(Behavioral science; cardiovascular disease and sexuality)*
The most common reasons for a decreased frequency of sexual intercourse after a myocardial infarction are psychological. Patients who have had a myocardial infarction can have decreased self-esteem and concerns about impotence. The stress associated with an unusual circumstance (e.g., an atypical sexual activity, inebriation, a new sexual partner) is often responsible for myocardial infarction during intercourse. Exercise and educational programs have been effective in helping cardiac patients resume a normal life, but the involvement of the partner in these programs is important.

103. The answer is C. *(Neuroanatomy; thalamic connections)*
The pulvinar nucleus receives input from the superior colliculus and pretectal areas and projects to visual cortex areas 18 and 19. It does not connect with the basal ganglia or the vagus.

104. The answer is D. *(Endocrinology; endocrinology of menstruation)*
A detailed understanding of the hormonal control of menstruation is especially important to evaluate vaginal bleeding and the choice of oral contraceptives. The surge of luteinizing hormone (LH) immediately precedes ovulation; LH, estradiol, and progesterone levels are all declining at the beginning of menses, whereas follicle-stimulating hormone (FSH) is rising to recruit the follicle for the subsequent cycle. Early in the cycle, FSH renders cells sensitive to LH, which later causes ovulation. The follicles that were not sufficiently sensitive to FSH to mature do not develop sensitivity to LH for ovulation.

105. The answer is B. *(Histology; liquefactive necrosis)*
Coagulative necrosis follows hypoxic death in most body tissues except those of the central nervous system (CNS). For example, the necrotic process that ensues following a myocardial infarction is coagulative necrosis,

due to occlusion of the coronary vessels. Liquefactive necrosis occurs only in the CNS, as a result of vascular occlusion. It is more commonly caused by pyogenic bacterial infection or septic emboli.

106. The answer is E. *(Neuroanatomy; telencephalon)*
Elements that develop from the telencephalon, which includes the internal capsule and the area lateral to it, include the forebrain; parietal, temporal, and occipital lobes; the hippocampus; and the corpus striatum. The thalamus is considered part of the diencephalon.

107. The answer is A. *(Physiology; skeletal muscle contraction)*
The length of the A band remains constant during the contraction of myofibrils in skeletal muscle. The sarcomere of the myofibril is composed of thick and thin filaments. According to the sliding filament hypothesis, thick and thin filaments slide past one another during contraction, increasing the amount of overlap between them; they do not change length. The H band contains only thick filaments; the A band contains thin and thick filaments. The I band contains only thin filaments, which are anchored in the middle of the I band by components of the Z disk. During contraction, thin filaments slide into the A band, reducing the size of both the H band and I band and drawing the Z disks closer to the A band.

108. The answer is A. *(Neuroanatomy; intercostal nerves)*
Intercostal nerves are the anterior rami of the first 11 thoracic spinal nerves; the twelfth thoracic nerve gives rise to the subcostal nerve.

109. The answer is A. *(Genetics; transcriptional activation of chromosomes)*
Mammalian DNA utilizes only about 7% of the genome to transcribe RNA. Inactive DNA is referred to as heterochromatin, and it is tightly wound in an organized fashion in conjunction with nucleosomes. Inactive DNA is also methylated at cytosine–guanine (CG) islands, but the exact relation between inactivation and methylation is not clear. Active segments of DNA are referred to as euchromatin. Euchromatin is not wound as tightly and is less protein bound than heterochromatin. Because it is less organized, euchromatin also happens to be more sensitive to enzymatic digestion by DNase I, which can be used to determine active regions of DNA.

110. The answer is E. *(Behavioral science; psychoanalysis)*
Free association is the major method of communication in psychoanalysis. Interpretation is a method of intervention, and resistance and countertransference are processes that develop during the treatment. Meditation is not involved in the psychoanalytic process.

111. The answer is D. *(Pathology; acute myocardial infarction)*
Aortic aneurysm is usually related to peripheral atherosclerotic disease; therefore, it is related to coronary atherosclerotic disease. Cystic medial necrosis can cause a dissecting form of aortic damage without much aortic dilation. Syphilis can cause aneurysmal dilation, especially in the ascending aorta. However, there is no common relationship between acute myocardial infarction and any of these aortic diseases. Cardiac tamponade, mitral valve incompetence, and rupture of the ventricular septum represent serious complications following damage to the myocardial wall or the papillary muscles. Peripheral embolism can occur as a result of mural thrombosis after infarctions involving the cardiac endothelium. Not mentioned are cardiac arrhythmias, which account for 75% of complications in acute myocardial infarction.

112. The answer is D. *(Biochemistry; collagen formation)*
Collagen, which is widely distributed in all animals, is important because it has been studied extensively as a model of the relationship between protein structure and function. Glycine is critical to collagen's structure

because of glycine's small size: The triple helix motif could not contain a large side chain on the inside, so the Gly-X-Y repeat puts a small glycine in the center of each turn. The degree of hydroxylation on proline residues is directly correlated with the thermodynamic stability of the collagen fiber. Because the strength of the triple helix is largely dependent on hydrogen bonding and other weak cooperative interactions, it is important to have a large number of these weak interactions to achieve high overall stability. Cleavage of the globular ends is important in making the insoluble tropocollagen molecule. However, this step must occur after secretion. Otherwise, secretion of the insoluble molecule would be much more difficult. Thus, it is the uncleaved procollagen molecule that is secreted. Cross-linkage of lysyl and hydroxylysyl residues occurs both within and between the collagen monomers. As discussed previously, ineffective cross-linkage can lead to disease.

113. The answer is A. *(Neurology; cranial injury)*
The amount of injury to the brain is proportional to the amount of distance the brain moves within the skull before being forcibly halted by fixed structures within the skull. Blows to the front or back of the head cause more displacement of the brain and, hence, more trauma than blows directed to the side of the head. A blow that glances off the head causes considerable rotation of the brain within the skull and, thus, is potentially more dangerous than blows to the sides, front, or back of the head.

114–116. The answers are: 114-C, 115-G, 116-B. *(Physiology; cardiac cycle)*
The cardiac cycle illustrated shows the simultaneous measurement of three entities. At the *top* is aortic pressure, left ventricular pressure is the *solid bold line*, and left atrial pressure is the *dashed line* at the bottom. At the end of the phase marked *A* (atrial systole), the mitral valve closes, giving rise to the S_1 sound. Mitral valve closure marks the beginning of isovolumic left ventricular contraction (*B*). When ventricular pressure is equal to aortic pressure, the aortic valve is forced open (*C*), and the rapid ejection phase begins. Ejection then begins to slow and later ends abruptly with aortic valve closure (*D*); the S_2 sound is generated at this time. *E* marks the phase of isovolumic relaxation in the left ventricle, until pressure is low enough that the mitral valve opens (*F*). The left ventricle can then begin refilling (*G*).

117. The answer is D. *(Microbiology; bacterial infections)*
Botulism is associated with flaccid, not tetanic, paralysis because it blocks acetylcholine (ACh) release at the neuromuscular junction. *Clostridium tetani* is associated with tetanic contraction, as tetanus toxin acts in the central nervous system to block the release of inhibitory neurotransmitters. Cholera is caused by *Vibrio cholera,* a gram-negative, comma-shaped rod that produces a toxin that increases cyclic adenosine monophosphate (cAMP) in the intestine, leading to ''rice-water'' diarrhea and dehydration. *Salmonella typhi,* a gram-negative facultative rod, is the causative agent of typhoid fever. ''Rose spots'' are associated with this disease. A ''strawberry tongue'' is a common symptom of group A streptococcal infection. This manifestation is caused by an erythrogenic toxin that also causes a red rash that starts at the chest and spreads.

118. The answer is C. *(Microbiology; viral genomes)*
The adenoviruses have a linear, double-stranded DNA genome with a molecular weight of approximately $20–30 \times 10^6$. Coronaviruses and papovaviruses are DNA, not RNA, viruses. Parvoviruses have a linear, single-stranded genome and are the smallest of the DNA viruses. Retroviruses are RNA viruses with unlinked segments of single-stranded RNA. Herpes have a linear, double-stranded DNA genome.

119–121. The answers are: 119-C, 120-E, 121-A. *(Behavioral science; personality disorders)*
Andrew's deterioration in performance, his social withdrawal, and his apparent difficulties in cognition have lasted longer than 6 months. These symptoms, as well as his age, suggest a diagnosis of schizophrenia.

Spending sprees and grandiosity that extend to energetic dysfunctional actions are characteristic of manic episodes. Although acute states such as these can be present in patients with narcissistic personality disorder, they usually are of brief duration.

The type of reaction to major disappointments that is exhibited by George is typical of individuals with narcissistic personality disorders. These individuals are given to a sense of self-importance and entitlement. Fantasies concerning success and infinite capabilities also are characteristic.

122. The answer is B. *(Immunology; agammaglobulinemia)*
Antibodies are a main defense against extracellular bacteria. Antibodies bind the bacteria and enable phagocytic cells (e.g., macrophages and neutrophils) to "get a grip" on the pathogen. This process is especially important for phagocytosis of bacteria that have antiphagocytic capsules. Intracellular pathogens (e.g., viruses) are eliminated primarily by the cell-mediated immune system, which contains natural killer cells and cytotoxic T lymphocytes. The immune system has many redundancies, but the lack of antibodies is not fully compensated for in patients with agammaglobulinemia. Thus, they are susceptible to infections by *Haemophilus influenzae*, *Streptococcus pneumoniae*, *Streptococcus pyogenes*, and *Staphylococcus aureus*. Treatment includes prophylactic antibiotics and gamma globulin.

123. The answer is E. *(Immunology; primary versus secondary immune responses)*
Approximately 5 days after the immune system encounters an antigen, the B lymphocytes begin producing antibody. This lag time is required for the antigen to be recognized by the naive immune cells and for sufficient numbers of B cells to be activated to begin antibody synthesis. The primary response consists of primarily immunoglobulin M (IgM) antibodies. During the initial antibody response, antibody affinity maturation occurs, so that memory B cells, which can make antibodies with a stronger affinity for the antigen, are formed. Additional encounters of the antigen, these memory B cells begin to synthesize IgG antibodies in only 1–2 days because they had been activated previously. During this secondary antibody response, a much larger quantity of antibodies is produced.

124–127. The answers are: 124-D, 125-F, 126-B, 127-C. *(Biostatistics; clinical reasoning)*
Understanding definitions is crucial to reading and critically evaluating the literature. Sensitivity and specificity are terms frequently used to describe clinical tests. A test with high sensitivity finds the abnormality if it is there; however, many tests with a high sensitivity have a low specificity (i.e., they are often positive in the absence of disease). A test with high specificity is very useful as a confirmation (because it is rarely positive in the absence of disease), but it may not be useful as a screening tool (where false positives are usually better than false negatives).

Validity reflects a test's ability to accurately assess a given element. For example, if urine glucose is below normal, a valid test reveals low urinary glucose. Sometimes a test's validity must first be established by active research. This is often true of tests that seek to assess psychiatric disease or cognitive development. Reliability refers to the test's ability to reproduce values that it already measured. A reliable test delivers relatively constant values when measuring the same entity. Again, tests of more nebulous entities must be examined for reliability before their results can be meaningfully interpreted.

Incidence and prevalence are essential concepts for the clinician to understand. Incidence is the number of new cases of a disease diagnosed in a given year (per 100,000 population). Prevalence is the number of diagnosed cases at any given moment in time (per 100,000 population). The prevalence of chronic diseases (e.g., rheumatoid arthritis) is generally higher than the incidence. Similarly, the incidence of diseases that can be rapidly lethal (e.g., disseminated intravascular coagulation) is usually higher than the prevalence.

128. The answer is C. *(Histology; renal histology)*
The parietal layer of Bowman's capsule is simple squamous epithelium, whereas the visceral layer is made up of specialized podocytes. The proximal tubule contains simple cuboidal epithelium with an apical brush border. The thin portions of the loop of Henle are lined with simple squamous epithelium, whereas the thick sections contain simple cuboidal epithelium. The distal convoluted tubule is also simple cuboidal. The collect-

ing tubule begins as simple cuboidal epithelium, but it changes to columnar and then pseudostratified columnar epithelium as it travels to the papillary ducts.

129. The answer is D. *(Physiology; renal response to volume depletion)*
Dehydration, as well as volume-depleted states due to other causes, induces the release of renin, which leads to an increase in angiotensin II. Antidiuretic hormone release is also stimulated by both the volume depletion and the angiotensin II. In an effort to maintain blood pressure, the angiotensin II functions as a vasoconstrictor, whereas the antidiuretic hormone acts in several ways to formulate concentrated urine and to minimize water loss. The vasoconstricting effects of angiotensin II in the afferent arterioles of the kidney cause a decrease in renal plasma flow. Increased prostaglandin synthesis counterbalances the decrease in renal plasma flow by causing afferent arteriole dilation. Thus, giving a volume-depleted patient a nonsteroidal anti-inflammatory drug, which works by blocking prostaglandin synthesis, could cause the patient to go into renal failure. The angiotensin II would cause the afferent arteriole to constrict, and renal plasma flow would decrease dramatically. Severe dehydration results in an increase in serum sodium and tachycardia.

130. The answer is B. *(Nephrology; glomerulonephritis)*
A nephrotic syndrome is normally associated with 3–4+ proteinuria, fatty casts, oval fat bodies, free fat droplets, and a nonproliferative glomerulonephritis. Typically hematuria and red blood cell casts are indicative of a nephritic syndrome and a proliferative glomerulonephritis. Chronic glomerulophritis is characterized by proteinuria, variable hematuria, broad waxy casts, and granular casts.

131. The answer is C. *(Pathology; amyloidosis)*
Amyloidosis is a life-threatening disease for which there currently is no effective treatment. It is characterized by large, pale kidneys on autopsy; apple-green birefringence with a Congo red stain under polarized light; autofluorescence with a thioflavin stain; immunoperoxidase staining for amyloid P and sometimes amyloid A; short nonbranching rods on electron microscopy; and mesangial and glomerular basement membrane expansion, as well as deposits in the arteries. Congo red binds to amyloid fibrils. IgA or IgE deposition is not commonly seen. This disease typically affects multiple organs including the liver, heart, and blood vessels. There is no evidence that immunostimulation affects amyloidosis; however, recent clinical trials suggest combinations of prednisone, colchicine, and melphalan can prolong the lives of these patients. Sarcoidosis is characterized by mononuclear cell granulomatous inflammation, which rarely affects the kidneys. The lungs are frequently affected, and sarcoidosis is usually responsive to glucocorticoids.

132. The answer is E. *(Microbiology; viral replication)*
The viral replication cycle begins with the eclipse phase, during which the viral genome is present within the cell, but no infectious viral particles have been made. The second phase is the intracellular accumulation period, during which nucleocapsids are being made, but are not released from the cell. There will only be infectious viral particles if the virus does not need to make its envelope from the plasma membrane of the cell. The latent period includes the eclipse phase and the intracellular accumulation period and ends when the first virus particle is released from the cell. When the latent period ends, the elevated period begins and continues as long as the extracellular virus particles continue to increase. Lysis of the infected cell may be the final step of an infection, but persistent infection and latent infection are two other options.

133. The answer is B. *(Microbiology; hepatitis A)*
Hepatitis A virus (HAV) is an acute infection that is most common in children and young adults. It is frequently transmitted by fecal–oral contamination. Although it is associated with a wide variety of symptoms, no treatment is required. The disease usually resolves completely within a few weeks. A vaccine is available for hepatitis A, and immunoglobulin (Ig) injections may also be used for propylaxis in some cases. Anti-

HAV IgG is present in a large number of individuals who have not had a symptomatic episode of hepatitis A; however, the prevalence has been declining since the 1970s, leaving more adults susceptible.

134. The answer is C. *(Microbiology; fungal infections)*
Coccidioidomycosis is endemic to the American southwest and other arid climates. It is caused by the fungus *Coccidioides immitis,* which is found in soil. Often, several people may become infected when soil is disturbed and the dust carries the fungus. Symptoms include those common to other pulmonary diseases, as well as possible hypersensitivity reactions and dissemination to the central nervous system, skin, and joints. Frequently the disease is progressive in African Americans, Native Americans, and Filipinos. Infiltrates, hilar adenopathy, and pleural effusion may be been seen on radiograph, and spherules may be seen on biopsy. Candidiasis and aspergillosis are rare in immunocompetent people. Histoplasmosis is endemic to regions with moist soil, such as the Midwest. Blastomyces is also rare in the Southwest; it is more common in the Southeast, Midwest, and in men rather than in women.

135. The answer is D. *(Microbiology; Chlamydia)*
Chlamydia trachomatis is the most common cause of nongonoccocal urethritis. This organism exists in two forms: reticulate bodies, which are the metabolically active intracellular form, and elementary bodies, which are the extracellular, infectious form. The organism is spread by sexual contact, and it may exist asymptomatically in women. Untreated carriers may continue to reinfect their partners. The organism is also capable of causing serious harm to women, including salpingitis and pelvic inflammatory disease, which can lead to infertility, ectopic pregnancy, and death. Tetracycline and other antibiotics (e.g., erythromycin, doxycycline) that can penetrate into eukaryotic cells are appropriate treatments, because this organism is metabolically active only inside cells.

136. The answer is D. *(Microbiology; leprosy)*
Leprosy is a disease caused by *Mycobacterium leprae,* a slow-growing, strict aerobe that is an obligate intracellular pathogen and is difficult to culture. It can survive being phagocytosed by a macrophage. In fact, macrophages may be the vehicles that enable spread of the disease through the body. Leprosy exists in two forms: lepromatous, which is characterized by ineffective cell-mediated immunity, and tuberculoid, which is characterized by an effective cell-mediated immunity. However, there is a great deal of overlap between these two forms, even within one individual. Transmission of the disease requires prolonged exposure to infected individuals, even those who are not receiving treatment. Effective treatments for leprosy are dapsone, rifampin, and clofazimine. In untreated patients, death is more commonly due to secondary infections than the leprosy itself.

137–140. The answers are: 137-B, 138-E, 139-C, 140-G. *(Neurology; differential diagnosis of neuromuscular disease)*
The differential diagnosis of muscular weakness is an essential skill for both a neurologist and a general practitioner. In ascertaining a diagnosis, it is important to distinguish between purely motor difficulties and sensorimotor difficulties, and to localize the problem (i.e., upper versus lower motor neuron disease, neuromuscular junction, muscular atrophy). Cerebrovascular accidents in the motor cortex almost always give rise to two distinct phases: flaccid paralysis of the affected areas, followed by distinct upper motor neuron signs (e.g., hyperreflexia, hypertonia, minimal muscular atrophy). Generally, the affected areas are well demarcated and most cerebrovascular accidents do not cause bilateral symptoms. Furthermore, only the 55-year-old man would be in the age range in which cerebrovascular accidents would be high in the differential.

Guillain-Barré syndrome is an autoimmune disorder frequently triggered by a preceding viral infection or surgery. Herpes-type viruses are thought to be involved in an unusually large percentage of cases. The principal feature of the disease is peripheral demyelination, and the clinical presentation is generally gradual at first, leading later to fulminant symptoms that require hospitalization (many patients need ventilatory support). Early clinical findings are related to the demyelination, including hyporeflexia, hypotonic paralysis (especially in the distal extremities), and loss of light touch and vibration sensation. Although the motor symptoms mimic upper motor neuron disease, the findings are actually related to the decreased muscle spindle fiber (i.e., inhibitory) input to the anterior horn cells. Recovery is usually complete within 1 month.

Duchenne muscular dystrophy is a primary myopathy whose clinical course is severe, resulting in death from respiratory failure by the middle to late teens. Age of onset is usually 3 to 7 years. The mother observed all of the common symptoms of Duchenne muscular dystrophy. Earlier difficulties are noticed in children who are more active (e.g., difficulty running, frequent tripping, difficulty climbing). The pseudohypertrophy seen principally in the calf is nearly pathognomonic at the age of 6, and biopsy reveals significant fibrosis with almost no normal muscle fibers. Most children are confined to a wheelchair by age 12.

Amyotrophic lateral sclerosis is slightly more common in men than in women and rarely has its onset before age 50. It is a relentlessly degenerating disease that attacks both upper and lower motor neurons. One of the cardinal features of amyotrophic lateral sclerosis, as is seen in this man, is that it occurs in the complete absence of any sensory loss. The cause of this disease is unknown, and there is currently no treatment. The clinical onset includes weakness and fatigue that generally begin in one extremity and progress to include the entire body. Hyperreflexia is usually apparent early and is a sign of upper motor neuron disease. Babinski sign is often present (i.e., upgoing). As the underlying disease progresses, the lower motor neuron degenerates so that areflexia and flaccid paralysis predominate in the later stages. Muscle wasting eventually leads to the amyotrophy that gives the disease its name.

Myasthenia gravis is much more common in women than in men and is an autoimmune disorder with antibodies directed against nicotinic cholinergic receptors of the neuromuscular junction. Treatment is available and somewhat effective, so that early diagnosis of this disease is critical. The features described, particularly weakness that subsides after rest, are cardinal symptoms of the disease. The characteristic distribution of fatigue that affects facial musculature earlier is a hallmark of the myasthenia pathology. Because this is not an upper motor neuron disease, reflexes are maintained. Also, note that there are no sensory deficits.

Neurosyphilis, or tabes dorsalis, is the tertiary (late) stage of the sexually transmitted syphilis organism. It appears in patients 20 to 30 years following infection and was, at one time, part of every differential diagnosis of muscular weakness. Sensory manifestations are almost universally reported, so that only the 39-year-old man had signs even remotely related to neurosyphilis. Severe gait disturbances (caused by loss of proprioception) and recurrent fleeting pains radiating down the legs are common presentations. Hyporeflexia, impaired light touch and vibration sensation, and bladder disturbance occur in many patients. The Argyll Robertson pupils, which accommodate but do not react to light, are also a frequent sign.

Friedreich's ataxia (i.e., spinocerebellar degeneration) is characterized by degeneration of the spinocerebellar tracts, with accompanying loss of the peripheral neurons that synapsed with the now dead spinocerebellar neurons. In its true form, Friedreich's ataxia is generally inherited as a recessive trait (although it is sometimes dominant), and the clinical picture first appears in the legs. Clumsiness in the hands follows later, and general weakness marks the final stages. Survival beyond early adulthood is rare, and death is frequently the result of an associated cardiomyopathy.

141–148. The answers are: 141-B, 142-C, 143-F, 144-G, 145-A, 146-G, 147-F, 148-D. *(Rheumatology, radiographic anatomy; differential diagnosis of arthritis)*
Osteoarthritis is a degenerative disease that most commonly affects the large weight-bearing joints. Osteoarthritis is related to use; therefore, mail carriers are more susceptible than office administrators. The x-ray shows classic radiographic findings in osteoarthritis including asymmetrical involvement of joints (i.e., only the left), segmental narrowing of the medial and superior joint space, subchondral sclerosis of the bone, and osteophyte formation. The osteophyte formation is striking and can be best seen on the computed tomography scan: The normal femoral head has been completely dislodged from the joint space by the large femoral

osteophyte, and the acetabulum is covered with its own distinct osteophyte. This is an advanced case, and these radiographs were taken immediately prior to total joint replacement. Generally speaking, inflammatory changes are not a feature of osteoarthritis.

Rheumatoid arthritis is an autoimmune disease in which cellular inflammation and antibody complex formation destroy normal synovial tissue and articular cartilage. The disease has a propensity toward small joints of the wrists, hands, ankles, and feet. The lymphokines and hydrolytic enzymes found in the synovial fluid of a patient with rheumatoid arthritis combine with activated inflammatory cells to destroy articular cartilage. Chronic rheumatoid arthritis is characterized by the formation of pannus, which is a form of granulation tissue with inflammatory cells, proliferating fibroblasts, and small blood vessels. This destructive tissue ultimately replaces articular cartilage with a fibrous scar, which frequently results in joint ankylosis. Two other histopathologic features of rheumatoid arthritis are large lacunae in the cartilage (the result of invasive pannus) and inflammatory cells in the marrow, which can destroy bone. Rheumatoid arthritis is associated with the DR4 haplotype of the human leukocyte antigen (i.e., HLA-DR4).

Reiter's syndrome is a seronegative arthritis following an episode of infectious urethritis, cervicitis, or dysentery. When initially described, the complete triad also included noninfectious conjunctivitis. The inflammation associated with the ocular and joint symptoms is reactive and probably related to an autoimmune phenomenon triggered by the urethritis. Other documented symptoms include hyperkeratotic lesions of the skin and painless shallow ulcers of the penis, urethral meatus, and mouth. Human leukocyte antigen B27 (HLA-B27) occurs in approximately 80%–90% of all patients with Reiter's syndrome. The knee and ankle joints are commonly involved, and sacroiliitis occurs in about 25% of patients. Most episodes of Reiter's arthritis last less than 6 months and are rarely debilitating.

Gout is a poorly understood disease that results from urate crystal formation in joints (i.e., arthritis), renal tubules (i.e., gouty nephropathy, urate renal calculi), and soft tissues (i.e., tophi). Although hyperuricemia is usually necessary for the manifestations of gout, it is not sufficient; hyperuricemia can exist without the clinical findings of gout. Two common characteristics are described in the questions. The first association pairing gout with diet and alcohol intake is well documented. Obesity and hyperlipidemia are much more common in patients with gout, and excess intake of ethanol during the course of a heavy meal may be adequate to incite a painful attack. The second question describing synovial fluid from the wrist is diagnostic for gout. Being negatively birefringent, urate crystals produce a bright yellow color under polarized light. The cellular infiltrate seems to be a response to the crystals, and leukocyte counts between 2000 and 75,000/mm^3 are routine.

Septic arthritis is most common in elderly people and individuals who are immunocompromised. It is most frequently caused by *Staphylococcus aureus*, although *S. epidermidis* and group A streptococci are also encountered. People with connective tissue diseases and those with chronic arthritis are more inclined to develop coincidental septic arthritis. Disseminated gonococcal infection is the most common bacterial arthritis in urban populations and complicates as many as 0.5% of all gonococcal infections. However, disseminated gonococcal infection is usually distinguished from other forms of septic arthritis because of its route of transmission. In general, infectious arthritis is characterized by the acute onset of a warm, swollen joint, most commonly the knee (involvement of more than one joint is indicative of disseminated gonococcal infection). A synovial leukocyte count greater than 50,000 with 80% (or more) polymorphonuclears (PMNs) is strongly suggestive of septic arthritis. Although other inflammatory arthritides can elevate synovial cell counts to that level, the high percentage of polymorphonuclears is relatively specific to infections. A Gram's stain or culture is necessary for definitive diagnosis. Treatment of infectious arthritis requires immediate and complete drainage of the synovial fluid. Intravenous antibiotics administered without delay can help reduce the potentially irreversible joint damage associated with such a large inflammatory response. Even with prompt therapy, complete functional recovery following *S. aureus* arthritis is less than 60%, and infectious arthritis remains a significant cause of joint deformity.

Lyme disease is an infectious process caused by the tick-borne spirochete *Borrelia burgdorferi*. The first stage of the illness occurs within 1 month of exposure and is characterized by erythema migrans at the site of the tick bite. Flu-like symptoms can accompany the rash, and the rash frequently spreads to other sites. In about 10% of patients, neurologic or cardiac involvement occurs within weeks to months. As many as 67% of patients develop frank arthritis following the initial rash. Intermittent attacks of arthritis in the large joints, particularly the knee, are typical. Synovial fluid examination reveals an average leukocyte count of 25,000 (predominantly PMNs), which is similar to the chronic inflammatory arthritides. The clinical symptoms of Lyme disease have a slower onset than do the symptoms of acute infectious arthritis. Lyme disease can cause irreversible damage if the disease is not discovered until its later stages (weeks to months after the initial rash). However, most patients respond to oral tetracycline in the early stages, and complete recovery is not uncommon.

Systemic sclerosis is another disorder that has an unknown cause. Convincing evidence has implicated the overproduction of collagen as a factor, but the trigger for this disease continues to elude investigators. Two variants, CREST (i.e., *c*alcinosis cutis, *R*aynaud's phenomenon, *e*sophageal dysfunction, *s*clerodactyly, *t*elangiectasia) syndrome and diffuse cutaneous scleroderma, have been described, and usually Raynaud's phenomena or polyarthritis of the small joints is the presenting complaint. Laboratory and clinical findings are usually much different than those provided in the questions. Synovial fluid often contains less than 10,000 leukocytes/mm^3. In most cases, the radiographic findings show atrophy of disuse and osteopenia. Finally, fibrin deposition and chronic inflammatory cell infiltration are the only significant changes in synovium biopsy. Later, fibrosis of the connective tissue can occur, but rarely does one see the erosion that is characteristic of rheumatoid arthritis in a patient with systemic sclerosis.

149–152. The answers are: 149-C, 150-A, 151-D, 152-E. *(Neurophysiology; visual science)*
Presbyopia (impairment of vision due to old age) is caused by a decrease in the elasticity of the lens. As a result, the eyes are unable to accommodate for near vision. Another condition associated with aging is cataracts, in which the lens becomes progressively less transparent. Myopia is caused by an overall refractive power that is too great for the axial length of the eyeball. It causes distant objects to be focused in front of the retina and can be corrected by a diverging lens. In hyperopia, the overall refractive power is too low for the axial length of the eyeball, therefore the eyes must continuously accommodate to see distant objects clearly.

153–157. The answers are: 153-A, 154-B, 155-C, 156-B, 157-A. *(Anatomy; types of capillaries)*
Continuous capillaries are present in skeletal muscle, the lungs, and the brain. They form a continuous endothelial barrier that restricts diffusion of materials from the blood into the tissues.

Fenestrated capillaries are present in renal glomeruli. The fenestrations are holes through the walls of capillary endothelial cells.

Discontinuous capillaries are present in the liver, bone marrow, and spleen. Gaps large enough to allow passage of cells exist between the endothelial cells of discontinuous capillaries. In the bone marrow, for example, mature erythrocytes move from the hematopoietic compartment into the blood through intercellular gaps in the discontinuous capillaries.

Cerebrospinal fluid (CSF), a blood filtrate containing some of the proteins found in whole blood, is produced in the choroid plexus. Fenestrated capillaries in the choroid plexus allow a select subset of blood proteins to enter CSF.

Continuous capillaries in the brain form the blood–brain barrier by restricting the flow of some substances in blood into the brain parenchyma.

158–161. The answers are: 158-B, 159-E, 160-C, 161-A. *(Biochemistry; quantitative dose–response curves)*
The figure on the *left* represents an ideal dose–response curve for a drug and shows the typical hyperbolic effect. The dose that gives the half-maximal effect (K_D) can be estimated from the figure, but the maximal effect cannot easily be determined because of the hyperbolic nature of the data. The figure on the *right* is

a mathematical transformation of these data to a linear form that is more useful—a Scatchard plot that allows the maximal effect to be determined from the intercept at the X axis. The concentration of K_D is the reciprocal of the slope.

162–167. The answers are: 162-B, 163-D, 164-A, 165-D, 166-C, 167-E. *(Genetics)*
Lod scores are the usual statistical method of measuring linkage. Loci that are separated by recombination less than 50% of the time are said to be linked. This recombination fraction corresponds to a genetic distance of 50 cM.

Common examples of genetic polymorphisms include restriction fragment length polymorphisms (RFLPs), variable number of tandem repeats (VNTRs), chromosome heteromorphisms, inherited enzyme variants, and antigenic variants of proteins.

Several methods are available for the assignment of genetic loci to specific chromosomes (i.e., for gene mapping). Family studies to demonstrate linkage are widely used, but somatic cell genetic methods are often easier to perform when there is no knowledge of the location of the gene. Cytogenetic methods of gene mapping are particularly useful for regional localization within a chromosome.

Genetic polymorphism is defined as the occurrence of two or more alleles at a locus in a frequency greater than can be maintained by mutation alone. In practice, polymorphism is often said to exist when the most common allele at a locus accounts for less than 99% of all alleles. Many genes exhibit polymorphism of their coding regions, but polymorphic DNA variation in noncoding regions is even more common.

Linkage describes the close physical proximity of two or more loci on a chromosome, but the specific alleles present at each locus are irrelevant to the identification of linkage. If a certain allele at one locus tends to be found more often than expected by chance with a certain allele at another locus linked to the first, linkage disequilibrium is said to be present. Linkage disequilibrium is specific for a given population, and the same alleles may or may not be similarly associated in a different population.

Synteny occurs when two or more loci are on the same chromosome. Syntenic loci may or may not be linked, but linked loci are always syntenic. Syntenic loci may be far enough apart on a chromosome for crossing over to occur between them. By definition, linked loci are so close that recombination usually does not occur between them.

168–170. The answers are: 168-B, 169-A, 170-D. *(Behavioral science; childhood development)*
Effective monitoring of childhood developmental milestones is critical for the early detection and management of developmental delay. A number of helpful charts are available to allow the primary care physician to make an assessment of normal cognitive development. Infants reach for objects outside of their immediate grasp as early as 3 months but should certainly have achieved this task by 8 months. Similarly, some precocious toddlers use intelligible phrases by 2 years of age, but the sole use of single words in a child of 3 years is clearly abnormal. Piaget described the concrete operations phase, during which children learn to categorize and mentally manipulate tangible objects. Before this stage, they are easily fooled by the short glass–tall glass trick. For some children, achievement of this milestone marks their final cognitive development, as some adults never become proficient at abstract thinking.

171–175. The answers are: 171-C, 172-A, 173-B, 174-E, 175-D. *(Histology; cell division)*
The beginning of prophase is marked by the appearance of chromosomes within the nucleus. Throughout prophase, the chromosomes condense further; dissolution of the nuclear envelope marks the end of this phase. During metaphase, the kinetochore becomes attached to tubulin, the major component of the mitotic spindle. Metaphase is marked by the alignment of chromosomes along the equatorial (metaphase) plane. The next stage of cell division is anaphase, and it is marked by the separation of the centromeres. By the addition of tubulin to the mitotic spindle, the chromosomes are drawn toward opposite poles of the cell. Anaphase ends when the chromosomes are clustered at opposite poles of the cell. During the final stage, telophase, the

chromosomes uncoil, the nuclear envelope reforms, and the cell divides. As the cell divides, the cytoplasm also divides by a process known as cytokinesis; these processes continue until two daughter cells are produced. During telophase, cell division is thought to occur by the constriction of a ring of actin filaments.

176–180. The answers are: 176-A, 177-C, 178-A, 179-B, 180-C. *(Pulmonology; pulmonary function tests in disease)*
Forced expiration spirometry provides valuable information for the classification of pulmonary disease. Specific variables assessed include forced vital lung capacity, forced expiratory volume in the first second (FEV_1), forced expiratory volume between 25% and 75% of total lung capacity (FEV_{25-75}; also called maximum midexpiratory flow rate), and residual capacity. The traces shown represent classic spirometric results for people with (*A*) obstructive disease, (*B*) normal function, and (*C*) restrictive disease.

The hallmarks of obstructive disease are increased forced vital capacity, decreased FEV_1 and substantially increased residual volume. The most striking feature is usually the increased residual volume, for which obstructive disease is named. The increase in residual volume is responsible for the characteristic "barrel-chested" appearance of someone with chronic obstructive pulmonary disease. The hallmarks of restrictive disease are reduced forced vital capacity, normal to increased FEV_1, and decreased residual volume.

To correctly answer the question, the classic clinical features of two different manifestations of each broad disease type must be recognized. More than 20% of life-long, heavy smokers progress to emphysema or chronic bronchitis (chronic obstructive pulmonary disease). Decreased breath sounds are a result of the substantial increase in residual volume coupled with a decrease in tidal volume and vital capacity.

A child with an active asthma exacerbation produces a spirometric tracing that also has the features of obstructive disease. Although only directed at the symptoms, the bronchodilation afforded by a β_2-selective adrenergic agonist (e.g., albuterol) results in a more normal spirometric tracing. Effective treatment of the disease process requires the use of inhaled or systemic corticosteroids.

Progressive pulmonary fibrosis can follow chronic exposure to a variety of environmental and industrial hazards, including asbestos. The clinical picture of dyspnea on exertion, unproductive cough, and diffuse radiographic opacities, which are first apparent in the lower lung fields, is characteristic of the interstitial fibrosis process that occurs following chronic exposure to any one of the known irritants.

Although particulars about the spirometric tracing may vary, disorders associated with diaphragmatic weakness produce the picture of restrictive disease. Guillain-Barré, muscular dystrophy, myasthenia gravis, and impingement of the phrenic nerve all can result in diaphragmatic weakness and a spirometric picture of restrictive lung disease in an individual with normal lungs.

Test II

QUESTIONS

DIRECTIONS: *Single best answer questions* consist of numbered items or incomplete statements followed by answers or by completions of the statement. Select the ONE lettered answer or completion that is BEST in each case.

Matching questions consist of a list of four to twenty-six lettered options (some of which may be in figures) followed several numbered items. For each numbered item, select the ONE lettered option that is most closely associated with it. Each lettered option may be selected once, more than once, or not at all.

1. In patients with Barrett's esophagus, factors responsible for the morphologic changes in the distal portion of the esophagus from normal squamous cell epithelium to columnar epithelium include all of the following EXCEPT

(A) incompetence of the lower esophageal sphincter
(B) the ingrowth of immature pluripotent stem cells
(C) increased exposure to acid and pepsin
(D) the absence of inflammatory processes
(E) increased exposure to bile acids and lysolecithin

2. Of the following effects, drug binding to plasma proteins generally

(A) limits glomerular filtration
(B) is highly drug-specific
(C) is an interaction between drug and immunoglobulins
(D) is irreversible
(E) limits renal tubular secretion

Questions 3–4

A 36-year-old woman is brought to the emergency room because a friend found her unresponsive on the floor at home. Her friend relates a recent history of depression. An empty prescription bottle for thirty 100-mg amitriptyline tablets was found nearby. The woman's amitriptyline level is 2300 ng/ml, and her serum ethanol level is 250 mg/100 ml.

3. The physician's first step would be to

(A) prepare involuntary commitment documents
(B) order an immediate electroencephalogram
(C) insert a nasogastric tube
(D) administer physostigmine
(E) place the patient on a respirator

The patient is placed on a cardiac monitor, the results of which are shown below.

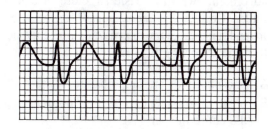

4. This electrocardiogram reveals which of the following patterns?

(A) Widened QRS complexes consistent with quinidine-like effects of tricyclics
(B) Bradycardia consistent with the cholinergic effects of tricyclics
(C) Premature ventricular contractions consistent with the toxic effects of ethanol
(D) S-T segment elevation consistent with the ischemic effects of ethanol
(E) Shortened P-R interval consistent with the toxic effects of tricyclics

5. All of the following are clinical and laboratory features of T-cell acute lymphoblastic leukemia EXCEPT

(A) patients are often in their teens or young adulthood
(B) patient population has a male predominance
(C) the leukemic population in the thymus forms a mediastinal mass
(D) patients usually have a high white blood cell count
(E) leukemic cells are positive for terminal deoxynucleotidyl transferase (TdT)
(F) leukemic cells are positive for Sudan black stain

6. The plasma membrane is composed of lipids and proteins with the basic structure of a lipid bilayer. Correct statements regarding the structure and function of the plasma membrane include all of the following EXCEPT

(A) phospholipids are amphipathic
(B) proteins may penetrate either portion of or the entire bilayer
(C) phospholipids promote free diffusion of ions and small water-soluble molecules
(D) proteins are amphipathic
(E) some large proteins are free to diffuse laterally in the plane of the membrane

7. A polymerase chain reaction can increase the sensitivity of certain genetic tests. Necessary components of a polymerase chain reaction include all of the following EXCEPT

(A) the DNA to be amplified is denatured in the presence of an equimolar ratio of primers
(B) a heat-resistant DNA polymerase is used for strand synthesis
(C) multiple heating and cooling cycles are required for amplification of the DNA
(D) the sequence of the segment of DNA to which the primers will bind must be known

8. Of the following statements about messenger RNA (mRNA) transcription, the most accurate is that it

(A) proceeds by synthesis of the RNA in the 3' to 5' direction
(B) involves the removal of internal regions of DNA from the genome
(C) only occurs in the cytoplasm of the human cell
(D) may be regulated by hormones
(E) involves the post-transcriptional addition of adenylate nucleotides to the 5' end of the molecule

9. An individual with a gastric carcinoma is likely to present with any of the following skin lesions EXCEPT

(A) seborrheic keratosis
(B) acanthosis nigricans
(C) erythema nodosum
(D) amyloidosis
(E) Paget's disease

10. Which sequence below is the correct order of epidermal maturation?

(A) Stratum basale, stratum spinosum, stratum lucidum, stratum granulosum, stratum corneum
(B) Stratum basale, stratum spinosum, stratum granulosum, stratum lucidum, stratum corneum
(C) Stratum basale, stratum granulosum, stratum spinosum, stratum lucidum, stratum corneum
(D) Stratum basale, stratum lucidum, stratum spinosum, stratum granulosum, stratum corneum
(E) Stratum basale, stratum lucidum, stratum granulosum, stratum spinosum, stratum corneum

11. A 25-year-old sexually active woman is evaluated for her fourth acute urinary tract infection during the past 12 months. Her infections are characterized by frequency, urgency, dysuria, and *Escherichia coli* bacteriuria. Her recurrent infections are most likely due to

(A) overgrowth of highly resistant *E. coli* in her fecal reservoir

(B) passage of an infected renal calculus

(C) resistance of the bacteria to the drugs selected for treatment

(D) presence of a foreign body within the genitourinary tract

(E) colonization of the vaginal introitus with fecal Enterobacteriaceae

12. A 2-year-old child is hospitalized with splenomegaly, anemia, hypersplenism, hepatomegaly, and progressive nervous system dysfunction. Enzyme studies show an absence of glucocerebrosidase with an accumulation of β-glucosylceramide in macrophages and hepatocytes. The lipid storage disease most likely to be diagnosed in this child is

(A) Niemann-Pick disease

(B) Gaucher's disease, type II

(C) Krabbe's disease

(D) Tay-Sachs disease

Questions 13–15

The micrograph below is of the male reproductive system.

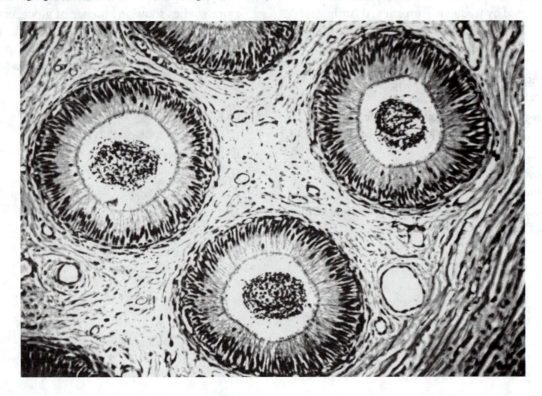

13. Which of the following organs is pictured in the micrograph?

(A) Testis
(B) Epididymis
(C) Vas deferens
(D) Seminal vesicle
(E) Bulbourethral gland

14. The epithelium of the organ pictured in the micrograph can best be described as

(A) simple cuboidal
(B) simple columnar
(C) stratified columnar
(D) pseudostratified columnar with stereocilia
(E) stratified squamous

15. Which adjective below best describes the function of the epithelium in the micrograph?

(A) Gametogenic
(B) Proliferative
(C) Secretory and absorptive
(D) Inactive
(E) Apoptotic

16. What condition is marked by formation of a malignant pustule?

(A) Enteritis necroticans
(B) Lockjaw
(C) Cutaneous anthrax
(D) Pseudomembranous colitis
(E) Woolsorter's disease

17. A 52-year-old man presented with painless swelling of his right testis. An orchiectomy was performed. A sample of the tissue is pictured in the photomicrograph below. The correct diagnosis is

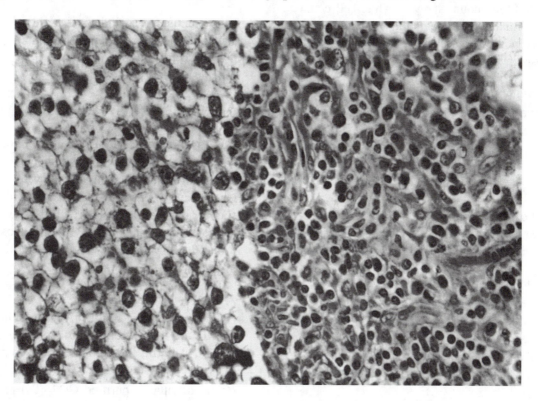

(A) seminoma

(B) mumps orchitis

(C) immature teratoma

(D) choriocarcinoma

18. A patient must be evaluated because of thrombocytopenia. The patient is a 55-year-old, previously well man, who was admitted to the hospital yesterday because of pneumonia. Antibiotic therapy was started; and, although his temperature continues to spike, it is lower than it was on admission. On admission, his hemoglobin was reported to be 13 g/dl, his white blood cell count was 9000/μl, and his platelet count was 70,000/μl. The next laboratory study that should be done is

(A) bone marrow examination

(B) bleeding time

(C) examination of the peripheral smear

(D) platelet aggregation studies

(E) antiplatelet antibody detection tests

19. An infant is brought to the emergency room with severe oral thrush and hypocalcemia. A complete blood count shows a white cell count within normal limits. The mother admits to being an intravenous drug user. What is the most likely diagnosis in this case?

(A) Chronic mucocutaneous candidiasis
(B) Severe combined immunodeficiency disease
(C) DiGeorge syndrome
(D) Chronic granulomatous disease

20. All of the following are clinical and laboratory features of acute myeloblastic leukemia (AML) EXCEPT

(A) patients present with pancytopenia
(B) patient often develop hypernatremia and hyperkalemia
(C) presence of Auer rods in the cytoplasm of leukemic cells
(D) leukemic cells are positive for myeloperoxidase
(E) leukemic cells are positive for terminal deoxynucleotidyl transferase (TdT)
(F) leukemic cells are positive for Sudan black stain

21. All of the following are true statements about chronic lymphoblastic leukemia (CLL) EXCEPT

(A) the disease is usually seen in patients older than 50 years of age
(B) it is the most common form of chronic leukemia in the United States
(C) it represents a clonal expansion of neoplastic B lymphocytes
(D) the disease is more frequent in females than males
(E) the cells commonly have trisomy 12 chromosomal abnormality
(F) most patients develop hypogammaglobulinemia

22. After osmotic equilibrium, infusion of several liters of a hypertonic saline solution will

(A) decrease intracellular osmolality
(B) not affect intracellular volume
(C) increase extracellular fluid volume
(D) decrease the plasma osmolarity

23. The Food and Drug Administration (FDA) has announced that it will test the vaccines against human immunodeficiency virus (HIV) with the least potential for causing the disease and the best chance of inducing protective immunity. Which of the vaccination reagents listed is most likely to be tested?

(A) An attenuated virus that does not cause disease in monkeys
(B) A recombinant HIV DNA in a vaccinia virus to induce host cells to produce only the HIV p24 protein, and then antibodies to p24 protein
(C) A denatured, purified CD4 (T4) protein to cause the host to mount an immune response to the HIV-infected CD4+ cells
(D) A human monoclonal antibody that reacts with the intact CD4 (T4) receptor

24. All of the following statements concerning immunogenicity are true EXCEPT

(A) compounds with a molecular weight greater than 6000 daltons are generally immunogenic
(B) haptens become immunogenic only when coupled to high molecular weight carriers
(C) a homopolymer of lysine with a molecular weight of 30,000 daltons would not be immunogenic
(D) a polymer of lysine, methionine, and glutamate with a molecular weight of 10,000 daltons would not be immunogenic

25. The most important allosteric activator of glycolysis in the liver is which one of the following compounds?

(A) Fructose 2,6-bisphosphate
(B) Acetyl coenzyme A (acetyl CoA)
(C) Adenosine triphosphate (ATP)
(D) Citrate
(E) Glucose 6-phosphate

26. Ingestion of 150 mEq Na^+/day is usually balanced by excretion of a similar amount in urine. Because the glomerular filtrate normally contains 26,000 mEq Na^+/day, several important Na^+- reabsorbing mechanisms have evolved, including all of the following EXCEPT

(A) active transport of Na^+ from inside proximal epithelial cells to interstitial spaces
(B) passive cotransport of Na^+ with glucose or amino acids in the proximal tubular epithelium
(C) active transport in the thick segment of the loop of Henle
(D) hormone-independent passive reabsorption in the distal tubular epithelium

27. The thyroid tumor pictured here was removed from a 60-year-old woman whose medical history likely includes

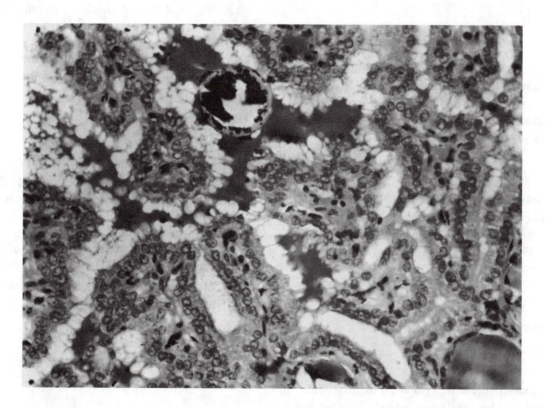

(A) hyperthyroidism
(B) hypothyroidism
(C) irradiation to the head and neck
(D) a pituitary adenoma

28. When comparing pertussis and diphtheria, true statements include which one of the following?

(A) Both pertussis and diphtheria are caused by bacteria that must adhere to respiratory tract cells

(B) Diphtheria symptoms are caused by an exotoxin, but no symptoms of pertussis result from an exotoxin

(C) The bacteria responsible for diphtheria and pertussis both produce endotoxin

(D) Pertussis is caused by an intracellular pathogen, but diphtheria is caused by an extracellular pathogen

(E) The neurologic problems observed with the current DTP (diphtheria-tetanus-pertussis) vaccine are caused by the diphtheria component of this vaccine

Questions 29–31

A 68-year-old widower complains of headaches, forgetfulness, decreased appetite, weight loss, insomnia, constipation, and anhedonia. An electrocardiogram shows first-degree heart block; he also has prostatic hypertrophy.

29. Considering side effect profiles, the best choice of medication would be

(A) imipramine
(B) phenelzine
(C) lithium carbonate
(D) clonazepam
(E) chlorpromazine

The patient's psychiatric symptoms improve with treatment, but his headaches persist. They occur daily and are bifrontotemporal, nonthrobbing, and bring him to tears when the pain is severe, but they do not disrupt his sleep. Physical examination reveals tenderness near the eye ridges.

30. The most appropriate test would be

(A) computed tomography scan of the head
(B) biopsy of the temporal artery
(C) electroencephalogram
(D) examination of the cerebrospinal fluid

31. Medication for migraine headache includes all of the following agents EXCEPT

(A) lithium carbonate
(B) ergotamine
(C) methysergide
(D) amitriptyline
(E) propranolol

32. Which of the following statements concerning the maturation of T cells is true?

(A) It occurs earliest in the thymic medulla
(B) It is independent of thymic epithelial cells
(C) It is independent of antigen
(D) None of the above

33. Each condition below is a diagnostically significant abnormality in Zellweger syndrome EXCEPT

(A) absent or grossly reduced numbers of peroxisomes
(B) catalase in the cytosol of hepatocytes
(C) overproduction of platelet activating factor (PAF)
(D) elevated plasma C26:0/C22:0 ratio
(E) accumulation of phytanic acid in central nervous system (CNS) tissues

34. A 24-year-old man presented to his family practitioner with a purulent penile discharge. Gonorrhea was diagnosed based on the finding of intracellular gram-negative cocci in his discharge. He was given amoxicillin and probenecid. The infection improved, but 1 week later the patient still complained of a persistent urethral discharge and pain on urination. On a visit to a local clinic for sexually transmitted diseases, a diagnosis of postgonococcal urethritis was made. What is the most likely cause of his latest syndrome?

(A) A common side effect of probenecid administered during the initial treatment
(B) A lingering gonococcal infection caused by a penicillin-resistant strain of *Neisseria gonorrhoeae*
(C) An improper therapy regimen, which did not treat a coinciding chlamydial infection
(D) A side effect of the correct therapy regimen, which suppressed the patient's normal flora and allowed the establishment of a secondary infection

35. A 38-year-old man with AIDS develops meningitis. Microscopic examination of his spinal fluid shows yeast cells. India ink staining of these yeasts shows a visible clear halo surrounding each cell. Which one of the following pathogens is responsible for the man's meningitis?

(A) A virus
(B) *Cryptococcus neoformans*
(C) *Haemophilus influenzae*
(D) *Neisseria meningitidis*
(E) *Candida albicans*

36. All of the following are properties of acetylsalicylic acid (aspirin) EXCEPT

(A) inhibits lipoxygenase activity
(B) analgesic activity
(C) antipyretic effects
(D) anti-inflammatory activity

37. Captopril is useful in the treatment of systemic hypertension because it

(A) blocks the effect of angiotensin II at its receptor in the central nervous system (CNS)
(B) directly relaxes vascular smooth muscle
(C) inhibits the movement of extracellular calcium into myocardial cells
(D) decreases the activity of angiotensin-converting enzyme (ACE)
(E) inhibits the production of renin

38. All of the following statements concerning insulin-dependent diabetes mellitus (type I; IDDM) are correct EXCEPT

(A) sulfonylureas may be a useful adjuvant to insulin therapy
(B) use of recombinant ''human'' insulin has eliminated problems of immunologic toxic effects
(C) insulin levels are routinely monitored
(D) ingestion of carbohydrates may be required to offset undesired hypoglycemia
(E) insulin therapy usually reverses the course of the disease

39. All of the following statements about allosteric enzymes are true EXCEPT

(A) positive cooperativity sensitizes the enzyme to small changes in substrate concentration
(B) they frequently catalyze the slowest step in a metabolic pathway
(C) the allosteric site can be located on a different subunit from the catalytic site
(D) the binding of a ligand to the allosteric site induces a conformational change in the active site
(E) they have substrate saturation curves that frequently show first-order kinetics

40. A patient presents with a torn medial collateral ligament of the left knee. Which of the following signs may be elicited on physical examination?

(A) Posterior displacement of the tibia
(B) Abnormal lateral rotation during extension
(C) Abnormal passive abduction of the extended leg
(D) Inability to lock the knee on full extension

41. The female reproductive viscera are best characterized by which of the following statements?

(A) The mesosalpinx contains the tubal branches of the uterine vessels
(B) The ovarian veins drain directly into the inferior vena cava
(C) Lymph from the cervix drains into the inguinal nodes
(D) Visceral afferent nerves from the body of the uterus course along the pelvic splanchnic nerves

42. The uterine cervical tissue shown in the photomicrograph below shows features of which one of the following infections?

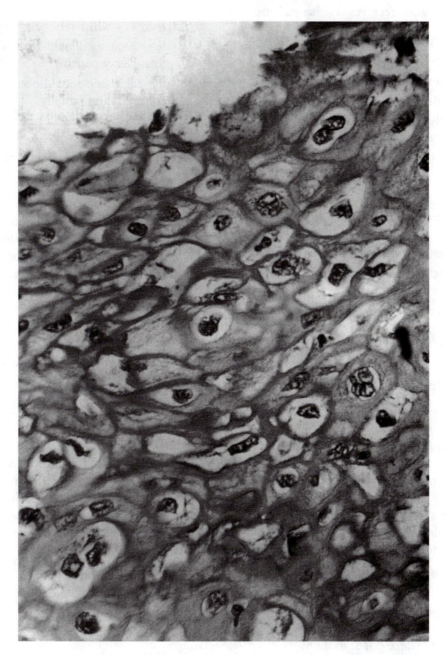

(A) Papillomavirus
(B) Herpes genitalis
(C) Gonorrheal cervicitis
(D) Carcinoma in situ

43. Tetracycline, a broad-spectrum antibiotic used in treating rickettsial, mycoplasmal, and chlamydial infections, receives widespread use because it

(A) is particularly useful in children
(B) causes minimal gastrointestinal side effects
(C) is bactericidal
(D) is selectively toxic to prokaryotes
(E) inhibits DNA-dependent RNA polymerase

44. Hepatic gluconeogenesis from alanine requires the participation of

(A) glucose 6-phosphatase and pyruvate kinase
(B) phosphofructokinase and pyruvate carboxylase
(C) pyruvate carboxylase and phosphoenolpyruvate carboxykinase
(D) fructose 1,6-diphosphatase and pyruvate kinase
(E) transaminase and phosphofructokinase

Questions 45–47

A resident has been assigned to the operating room for a 2-month rotation. The staff surgeon under whom he will work is a stickler for theory, and on the first day of the new rotation, he asked the resident the following questions.

45. With regard to anesthetics, MAC refers to

(A) maximum allowable concentration
(B) minimum alveolar concentration
(C) maximum alveolar concentration
(D) minimum arterial concentration
(E) maximum arterial concentration

46. If an anesthetic has a high blood:gas partition coefficient, it means that

(A) recovery will likely be prolonged
(B) lean patients should receive a lower dose than heavy patients
(C) the anesthetic should be delivered at a low concentration initially
(D) the anesthetic should be mixed with an inert gas or oxygen
(E) none of the above should occur

47. Nitrous oxide cannot be used alone to produce surgical anesthesia but is often used in conjunction with a more powerful agent, such as halothane, because nitrous oxide is

(A) explosive
(B) slow in onset of action due to a low blood:gas partition coefficient
(C) not very potent (i.e., has relatively low lipid solubility)
(D) rapidly metabolized

48. A 52-year-old middle school teacher has chronic peptic ulcer disease that has been treated for several years with ranitidine (Zantac) and metoclopramide (Reglan). On examination, the physician notes that the patient has involuntary, irregular chewing movements and repetitive tongue protrusion. The most likely cause of these movements is

(A) dystonic reaction
(B) Wilson's disease
(C) Huntington's disease
(D) cerebellar degeneration
(E) tardive dyskinesia

49. All of the following are true statements about hairy cell leukemia EXCEPT

(A) it represents an expansion of neoplastic T lymphocytes
(B) patients usually present with symptoms caused by splenomegaly
(C) neoplastic lymphocytes often produce monoclonal immunoglobulin
(D) cells are positive for tartrate-resistant acid phosphatase (TRAP)
(E) the disease is more frequent in males than females
(F) the disease is usually seen in patients older than 40 years of age

50. All of the following are true statements about chronic myelogenous leukemia (CML) EXCEPT

(A) there is an increased production of granulocytes
(B) it is characterized by marked splenomegaly
(C) Auer rods are present in the myeloblasts
(D) a prominent laboratory finding is leukocytosis
(E) there is a marked decrease of serum vitamin B_{12} levels
(F) the disease occurs equally in both sexes

51. Glycine is a diprotic amino acid containing two ionizing groups available for titration. If the pK$_a$ values for these groups are pK$_1$ = 2.4 and pK$_2$ = 9.60, what is the isoelectric point (pI) for glycine?

(A) 1.5
(B) 6.0
(C) 7.0
(D) 9.0
(E) 12.9

52. A decrease in blood glucose levels produces all of the following effects EXCEPT

(A) an increase in liver glycogen breakdown
(B) secretion of glucagon
(C) a decrease in insulin release
(D) inhibition of glucose breakdown
(E) inactivation of glycogen phosphorylase

53. Which one of the following statements about competitive enzyme inhibitors is NOT true?

(A) They bind to the enzyme irreversibly
(B) A reaction usually does not occur once the inhibitor is bound
(C) They bind to the active site of the enzyme
(D) They often resemble the substrate of that enzyme
(E) They compete with substrate for the active site of the enzyme

54. A mildly obese 20-year-old man presents to the emergency room at 5:00 A.M. He had ingested several six-packs of beer the evening before and had awakened at home with a sharp pain in his wrist at the radial–carpal articulation. The wrist is swollen and tender. The patient is slightly disoriented and ataxic but does not remember falling. X-rays of the wrist are negative. A slight fever is present. For long-term therapy, the patient should be treated with

(A) acyclovir
(B) allopurinol
(C) amantadine
(D) acetazolamide
(E) ampicillin

55. Which of the following statements concerning primitive aortic arches and their derivatives is true?

(A) The left fourth aortic arch forms the arch of the aorta
(B) The right sixth aortic arch forms the right subclavian artery
(C) The left fifth aortic arch forms the ductus arteriosus
(D) The first aortic arch forms the common carotid artery

56. If forbidden clones are not deleted during T-cell development, a person may develop

(A) hypogammaglobulinemia
(B) a type I hypersensitivity reaction to exogenous antigens
(C) an autoimmune disease
(D) tolerance to autoantigens

57. A 60-year-old woman is brought to the hospital because of fever and confusion. One week earlier, she received chemotherapy for lymphoma. In the emergency room, she is noted to have rapid breathing; cool, clammy skin; and a blood pressure of 70/40. Complete blood count shows a white blood cell count of $200/\mu l$. Gram stain of urine and sputum is negative. Which of the following empiric therapies would be most appropriate for this patient?

(A) Gentamicin
(B) Amikacin
(C) Chloramphenicol–gentamicin
(D) Piperacillin–gentamicin

Questions 58–60

A physician who has recommended urography for her competent, 68-year-old male patient is trying to decide whether or not to disclose the remote risk (1 in 10,000) of a fatal reaction.

58. If the physician favors nondisclosure, reasoning that it would not be in the patient's best interest to worry him with such remote risks, the physician is guided by

(A) beneficence but not nonmaleficence
(B) nonmaleficence but not beneficence
(C) both beneficence and nonmaleficence
(D) justice
(E) gratitude

59. If the physician believes that her decision should be determined by what other physicians would do in similar circumstances, she is guided by

(A) both beneficence and nonmaleficence
(B) strong paternalism
(C) weak paternalism
(D) respect for autonomy
(E) the professional practice standard

60. If the physician bases her decision on her assessment of whether or not the patient would want to learn about such remote risks, the physician is guided by

(A) respect for autonomy
(B) beneficence
(C) nonmaleficence
(D) both beneficence and nonmaleficence
(E) the professional practice standard

61. A scientist in the year 2350 is advising the NASA genetic engineering department concerning its attempts to engineer humans who can better survive the harsh climate of a planet that has high levels of ultraviolet (UV) light. The NASA engineers want to incorporate a group of genes that will allow epidermal cells to produce a light-absorbing pigment. Of the following genetic manipulations, which would be most advantageous in cells in a UV-rich environment?

(A) Removing intron DNA from the engineered genes
(B) Introducing the engineered genes in an overlapping fashion into the human genome
(C) Altering a theoretical human equivalent of the bacterial RecA protein in the cells to decrease RecA activity
(D) Producing genes with a low thymidine content

62. The photomicrograph below shows an adrenal mass that was resected from a 2-year-old child. This lesion most likely is

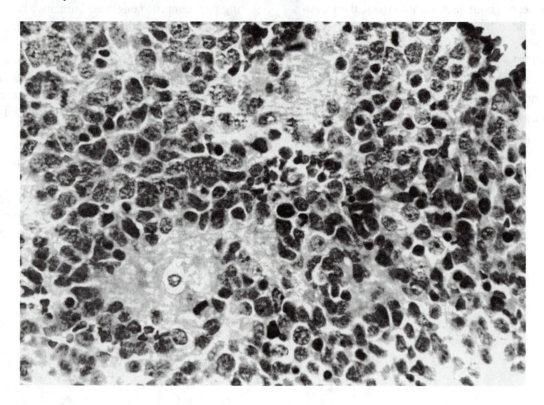

(A) Wilms' tumor

(B) a neuroblastoma

(C) a ganglioneuroma

(D) a pheochromocytoma

63. A 15-year-old girl presents for evaluation of short stature. She has not yet begun to menstruate. Examination reveals an intellectually normal child with short stature, webbing of the neck, a broad chest, and cubitus valgus. Which of the following tests will provide the best evaluation of this patient?

(A) Amino acid analysis of urine

(B) Organic acid analysis of urine

(C) Serum long-chain fatty acids

(D) Chromosome analysis

(E) Tissue glycogen content

64. Based on the Michaelis-Menten equation, V_0, the initial velocity, equals V_{max} when

(A) $[S] >> K_m$

(B) $K_m = [S]$

(C) $K_m >> [S]$

(D) $[S] = 0$

65. Of the following amino acids, which one is released from skeletal muscle in amounts that exceed its relative abundance in muscle protein?

(A) Aspartate
(B) Alanine
(C) Glutamate
(D) Leucine
(E) Tyrosine

66. Rapid diagnosis and determination of the causal species are essential because of the immediately life-threatening nature of which one of the following parasitic infections?

(A) Malaria
(B) Chronic Chagas disease
(C) Amebic dysentery
(D) Mucocutaneous leishmaniasis
(E) Giardiasis

Questions 67–68

A patient who weighs 50 kg is given a 20-mg/kg dose of a new drug. The plasma concentrations determined over time are illustrated in the graph below.

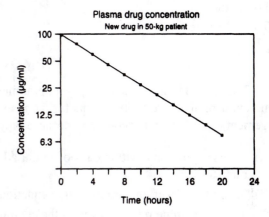

67. The drug's volume of distribution (V_d) is approximately

(A) 200 ml
(B) 1 L
(C) 2 L
(D) 10 L
(E) insufficient information to answer

68. The half-life of elimination of this drug is approximately

(A) 1 hour
(B) 2 hours
(C) 4 hours
(D) 10 hours
(E) insufficient information to answer

69. *N*-glycosylation of proteins occurs on which of the following amino acids?

(A) Asparagine
(B) Aspartate
(C) Lysine
(D) Serine
(E) Threonine

70. Tricyclic antidepressants (e.g., imipramine and amitriptyline) are useful agents for the management of endogenous depression because they

(A) reverse symptoms within days of initial administration
(B) have little effect on cardiovascular function
(C) affect dopamine receptors within the central nervous system (CNS)
(D) affect neuronal amine uptake mechanisms
(E) deplete brain serotonin levels

Questions 71–72

Cystic fibrosis is an autosomal recessive disease with an incidence of 1 per 1600 in the Caucasian population.

71. What is the frequency of the cystic fibrosis gene?

(A) 1/4
(B) 1/20
(C) 1/40
(D) 1/200
(E) 1/400

72. Of the following values, what proportion of the normal siblings of individuals with cystic fibrosis would most likely be carriers?

(A) 1/4
(B) 1/2
(C) 2/3
(D) All
(E) None

73. A 50-year-old woman with diabetes has an almost complete loss of renal function within 3 hours of a seemingly successful kidney transplant. All of the following statements concerning this type of rejection are true EXCEPT

(A) the patient had preformed antibodies to the graft
(B) the patient's rejection histologically resembles the classic Arthus reaction
(C) T cells are not directly involved
(D) administration of an immunosuppressive agent will restore kidney function

74. A 23-year-old woman with borderline personality disorder is hospitalized on a surgery ward to recover from fractures sustained in a motor vehicle accident. The patient states that her resident physician is wonderful and caring, but her primary nurse is cold and cruel. The psychologic mechanism being displayed is best termed

(A) denial
(B) projection
(C) manipulation
(D) displacement
(E) splitting

75. Baroreceptors are highly branched nerve endings that generate receptor potentials that are proportional to the rate of change in arterial blood pressure; they can also adapt to changes in arterial blood pressure over a prolonged period of time (hours to days). Which of the following statements concerning the specific properties of baroreceptors is most accurate?

(A) Baroreceptors are important for long-term regulation of blood pressure

(B) Clamping both carotid arteries after cutting both vagus nerves results in a decrease in arterial blood pressure

(C) Massaging the carotid sinus area leads to bradycardia and a decrease in arterial blood pressure

(D) A decrease in blood pressure activates baroreceptors, which, in turn, directly activate the vasomotor center

76. Lidocaine is the prototype of an amide local anesthetic and as such is

(A) free of potential central nervous system (CNS) side effects

(B) free of potential cardiac adverse effects

(C) rapidly metabolized by plasma cholinesterases

(D) a Na^+-channel blocker, especially in small, myelinated nerve fibers

(E) inappropriate for use in spinal anesthesia

77. Actin is a microfilament that is involved with all of the following activities EXCEPT

(A) endocytosis

(B) exocytosis

(C) cell locomotion

(D) mitotic spindle formation

(E) acrosome reaction

78. Mitochondria are important to the cells of eukaryotes for generating the adenosine triphosphate (ATP) necessary to carry out all energy-requiring processes. All of the following statements concerning mitochondria are true EXCEPT

(A) they contain a DNA molecule in a ring conformation

(B) mitochondrial proteins come solely from the cell nucleus

(C) the codons used by mitochondrial transfer RNA (tRNA) are not identical to those used in other mammalian genes

(D) mitochondrial proteins are encoded by gene sequences that overlap one another

79. A very painful, spreading, cutaneous edematous erythema is clinically descriptive of

(A) erysipeloid

(B) diphtheria

(C) Pontiac fever

(D) listeriosis

(E) nocardiosis

80. All of the following statements concerning gene duplication are true EXCEPT

(A) gene duplication involves unequal crossover between homologous repetitive DNA sequences during mitosis

(B) pseudogenes are nonfunctional duplications

(C) β-tubulins and β-like globins are perfect examples of duplicated gene families

(D) gene duplications are necessary to meet the cell's requirements for some RNA transcripts

81. Tay-Sachs disease occurs almost exclusively among Ashkenazi Jews, with an incidence of 1/3600. The frequency of carriers of the Tay-Sachs gene, which can be calculated by using the Hardy-Weinberg law ($p^2 + 2pq + q^2 = 1$), is which of the following?

(A) 1/4
(B) 1/30
(C) 1/60
(D) 1/600
(E) None of the above

82. Which of the endogenous substances listed is derived from the cyclooxygenase pathway of arachidonic acid metabolism?

(A) Platelet activating factor (PAF)
(B) Leukotriene D_4
(C) Eosinophil chemotactic factor (ECF)
(D) Thromboxane (TXA_2)

Questions 83–84

A 25-year-old medical student is buried by an avalanche of snow while skiing. Upon rescue, it is necessary to revive him from cardiopulmonary arrest. Although resuscitated, he remains in a coma for several hours before regaining consciousness.

83. It is known that the patient has suffered global hypoxia. The function most likely to have been lost under this condition is the ability to

(A) move facial muscles
(B) walk
(C) move arms
(D) move eyes

84. Which test of higher cortical functions would the patient most likely fail because of the hypoxic event?

(A) Remembering the name of the hospital or his physicians
(B) Reading a sentence
(C) Recognizing his cousins
(D) Adding two numbers together

85. A 65-year-old woman with degenerative joint disease secondary to rheumatoid arthritis has been admitted to the hospital for insertion of a prosthesis in her right hip (total hip arthroplasty). The physician is aware that *Staphylococcus aureus* and *Staphylococcus epidermidis* are likely to cause postoperative infection after total hip replacement. In addition, the hospital has reported a significant increase in beta-lactamase–resistant *S. aureus* isolates. Which of the following drugs is LEAST likely to be effective as prophylactic therapy in this patient?

(A) Cefazolin
(B) Methicillin
(C) Vancomycin
(D) Ampicillin
(E) Imipenem

86. A pregnant woman who is primigravida with blood type O-negative comes to the obstetrician's office for a routine visit. The patient states that her husband is AB-positive, and she is concerned about the incompatibility of the Rh factors. Her isohemagglutinin titers are normal. What would the most appropriate treatment be?

(A) Administer human anti-D globulin (Rho-GAM) to the mother after the birth of the child

(B) Administer RhoGAM to the child immediately after birth

(C) Administer RhoGAM to the child if the blood is Rh-positive

(D) Do nothing at this time

87. In the figure below, the oxyhemoglobin dissociation curve is shown for a normal patient and for an anemic patient. A true statement concerning these patients is which one of the following?

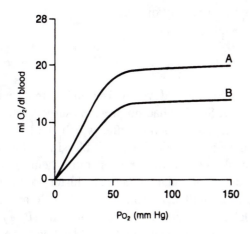

(A) Patient A is anemic

(B) Arterial Po_2 is likely to be similar for both subjects

(C) Venous Po_2 of the anemic subject will be greater than that of the normal subject at rest or during exercise

(D) If cardiac output is identical, oxygen delivery will be identical in subjects A and B

88. A 45-year-old woman has eaten some home-canned vegetables. Two days later she has blurred vision and difficulty swallowing. This is followed by respiratory distress and flaccid paralysis. The symptoms of her illness result from an intoxication caused by a bacterial toxin whose action involves which one of the following effects?

(A) Adenosine diphosphate (ADP)-ribosylation of elongation factor 2

(B) Blockage of release of inhibitory neurotransmitters

(C) Blockage of release of acetylcholine (ACh)

(D) Stimulation of adenylate cyclase to elevate intracellular cyclic adenosine monophosphate (cAMP) levels

(E) Hemolysis resulting from sequestration of cholesterol in membranes

89. A 22-year-old woman reports the gradual onset and relentless progression of severe pain in the lower left quadrant of her abdomen. She also reported nausea with vomiting and fever. A pelvic examination determined that there was marked tenderness both upon direct palpation and on manipulation of the cervix. A greenish-yellow discharge from the cervical os was noted, but a direct Gram stain of the discharge revealed no potential etiologic agents. Despite this finding, the patient was started on antibiotic therapy. Twenty-four hours later, laboratory culture of the discharge yielded growth of oxidase-positive, gram-negative diplococci on Thayer-Martin medium. A diagnosis of gonococcal salpingitis was made. One week post-therapy, the patient's symptoms were relieved and laboratory culture of her cervix revealed no pathogenic organisms. What is the patient's prognosis?

(A) The patient may not be cured and will require constant monitoring of her cervical flora for the next 6 months

(B) The patient may not be cured and is therefore encouraged to abstain from sexual intercourse or observe safe-sex practices for the next 6 months

(C) The patient is cured and requires no further monitoring

(D) The patient is cured but faces an increased risk of subsequent episodes of pelvic inflammatory disease, infertility, and ectopic pregnancy

90. Which of the following structures contains Hassall's corpuscles?

(A) Thyroid gland
(B) Parathyroid gland
(C) Pineal gland
(D) Thymus
(E) Spleen

91. Synthesis of glycogen from fructose in a person with essential fructosuria requires the activity of which one of the following enzymes?

(A) Transketolase
(B) Aldolase B
(C) Hexokinase
(D) Fructokinase
(E) Glucokinase

92. Renal osteodystrophy is a condition that may follow chronic renal failure. Features of this condition include osteitis fibrosa cystica admixed with osteomalacia. The pathogenesis of this condition is characterized by all of the following EXCEPT

(A) phosphate retention and hyperphosphatemia
(B) low levels of 1,25-dihydroxyvitamin D_3 (calcitriol)
(C) elevated levels of calcitonin
(D) hyperparathyroidism
(E) hypocalcemia

93. A 65-year-old woman is seen before cataract surgery. She has had no previous surgery except for a dental extraction, after which she bled for 10 days and required a 2-unit blood transfusion. One sibling died from postoperative hemorrhage during childhood, and there is a history of bleeding in a number of relatives, both male and female. Her partial thromboplastin time (PTT) is markedly prolonged, and the bleeding time is within normal limits. The most likely diagnosis is

(A) factor VIII deficiency
(B) factor XI deficiency
(C) factor XII deficiency
(D) Fletcher factor deficiency
(E) von Willebrand's disease

94. Enteric pathogens vary with respect to their ability to invade the intestinal mucosa. After infection, which one of the following enteric pathogens is most likely to invade the intestinal submucosa and then disseminate throughout the body?

(A) *Vibrio cholerae*

(B) *Salmonella typhi*

(C) *Shigella dysenteriae*

(D) Nontyphoid *Salmonella*

(E) *Campylobacter jejuni*

Questions 95–96

A 45-year-old woman is admitted to the hospital with an unremitting sore throat. She has undergone radical mastectomy for breast carcinoma and recently underwent adjuvant chemotherapy. Two weeks before, she received a seven-day course of amoxicillin–clavulanic acid (Augmentin) for a recurrent urinary tract infection. Examination of her palate reveals several patches of white, creamy, curd-like friable lesions on the tongue and other mucosal surfaces.

95. This patient most likely has which type of fungal infection?

(A) Sporotrichosis

(B) Dermatomycosis

(C) Candidiasis

(D) Cryptococcosis

96. All of the following therapies would be effective for this fungal infection EXCEPT

(A) ketoconazole

(B) oral fluconazole

(C) topical nystatin

(D) oral griseofulvin

(E) clotrimazole

Question 97

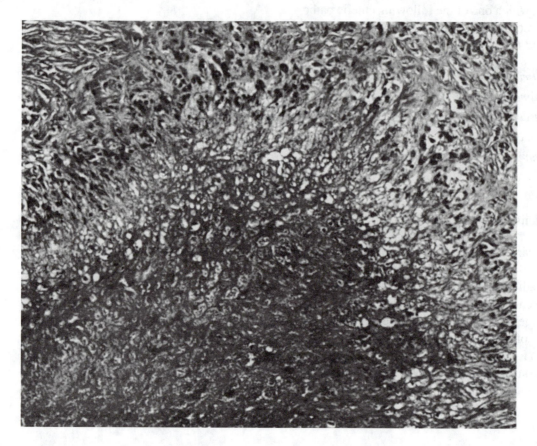

97. An elderly woman had a synovial biopsy and total knee replacement for degenerative joint disease. Sections of the synovium revealed the findings shown in the above photomicrograph, indicating a history of which one of the following conditions?

(A) Colchicine therapy for gout

(B) Repeated fractures

(C) Rheumatoid arthritis

(D) Trauma and foreign body within the joint space

98. Pictured below is a portion of large bowel resected from a middle-aged woman who had repeated bouts of crampy abdominal pain. It would be concluded from the histology that the gross appearance of the bowel would show all of the following features EXCEPT

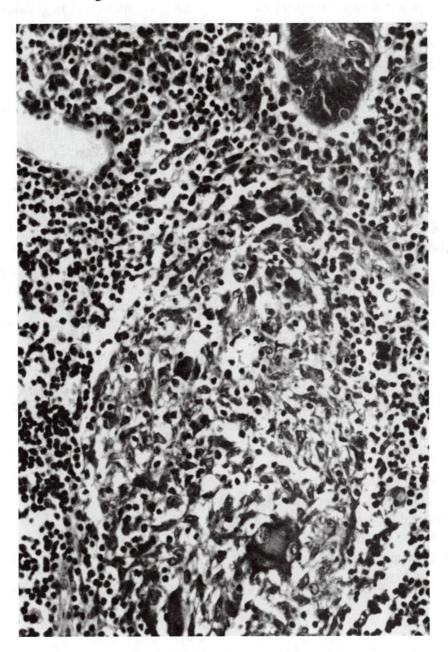

(A) segmental lesions

(B) ''creeping fat''

(C) a thickened wall

(D) pseudopolyps

(E) long, snake-like lesions

99. All of the following statements about RNA are true EXCEPT

(A) RNA occurs only in a single-stranded form
(B) RNA can act to catalyze certain reactions, much like an enzyme
(C) RNA can act as primary genetic material
(D) a molecule of RNA differs from DNA in the number of hydroxyl groups present on the sugar moieties
(E) none of the above

100. Cimetidine is the prototype of a histamine receptor antagonist that

(A) causes sedation
(B) is useful for motion sickness
(C) enhances hepatic drug-metabolizing enzymes
(D) reduces gastric acid secretion
(E) is useful in the treatment of certain allergies

101. All of the following statements about the peptide bond are true EXCEPT the

(A) peptide bond is planar
(B) peptide bond has restricted rotation
(C) α-carbon atoms are in a *trans* configuration
(D) peptide bond atoms do not participate in the secondary structure of proteins
(E) peptide bond has no charge associated with it

102. Ca^{2+} is required for various processes, such as neurotransmission and muscle contraction. However, an elevated level of Ca^{2+} can be cytotoxic to cells. All of the following mechanisms are used by cells to regulate intracellular Ca^{2+} concentration EXCEPT

(A) chelation of Ca^{2+} by ethylenediaminetetra-acetic acid (EDTA)
(B) adenosine triphosphate (ATP)-independent Na^+–Ca^{2+} exchange
(C) ATP-dependent Ca^{2+} pumping
(D) sequestration of Ca^{2+} by binding proteins
(E) sequestration of Ca^{2+} in the endoplasmic reticulum

103. In a family with a disease that has an autosomal dominant inheritance pattern, seven children have been born, four of whom have the disease and three of whom do not. One parent is affected and one is not. What is the probability of the next child born having the disease?

(A) 100%
(B) 50%
(C) 25%
(D) Zero
(E) Cannot be determined

104. The inhibition observed in the Lineweaver-Burk plot below is subject to which one of the following actions? It

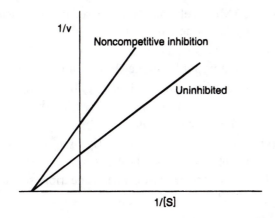

(A) can be reversed by a high concentration of substrate

(B) results from compounds that are transition-state analogs

(C) occurs through the interaction of the inhibitor at the active site

(D) results in a decrease in the V_{max} of the reaction

(E) is characterized by an increase in the K_m for the substrate

105. All of the following statements about the protein kinase C signal transduction pathway are true EXCEPT

(A) after activation, protein kinase C is degraded to protein kinase M

(B) protein kinase C phosphorylates tyrosines on proteins

(C) protein kinase C requires Ca^{2+} for full activation

(D) protein kinase C requires lipids for full activation

(E) protein kinase C is translocated to the plasma membrane

106. A patient is on a ventilator. The patient's anatomic dead space is 150 ml, and the ventilator's dead space is 250 ml. The ventilatory rate is set at 20 per minute. What should the output (tidal volume) of the ventilator be adjusted to so that alveolar minute ventilation is 4 L/min?

(A) 150 ml

(B) 250 ml

(C) 400 ml

(D) 600 ml

(E) 1000 ml

107. Each statement below concerning fenestrated capillaries is true EXCEPT

(A) fenestrations are 60 nm to 100 nm in diameter

(B) they are present in the choroid plexus

(C) they may be partially surrounded by pericytes

(D) they are present in endocrine glands

(E) they have a slit diaphragm that forms a filtration barrier in the renal glomerulus

108. Pathogenic bacteria enter the body by various routes, and entry mechanisms are critical for understanding the pathogenesis and transmissibility of each agent. Which one of the following is a correct association between a pathogen and its common entry mechanism?

(A) *Neisseria meningitidis*—sexually transmitted entry

(B) *Corynebacterium diphtheriae*—food-borne entry

(C) *Rickettsia rickettsii*—entry by contamination of wound with soil

(D) *Clostridium tetani*—inhalation entry

(E) *Borrelia burgdorferi*—arthropod vector-borne entry

Questions 109–111

A 70-year-old man is brought to the hospital, and a neurologist is called for a consultation. The residents caring for the patient tell the physician that he has spastic paralysis on one side of his body but has no sensory deficit

109. On examination, the physician finds that the patient can move neither the right side of his face nor his left extremities. He has right-sided ptosis of the eyelid, and the right eye deviates laterally. The right eye also does not respond to light or exhibit accommodation. What is the most likely site of the patient's lesion?

(A) The midbrain
(B) The pons
(C) The medulla
(D) None of the above

110. The lesion is most likely a cerebral vascular accident, resulting in occlusion of which one of the following arteries?

(A) Basilar artery
(B) Middle cerebral artery
(C) Posterior cerebral artery
(D) Superior cerebellar artery

111. After examining the patient, the physician is most likely to propose which of the following syndromes in his evaluation?

(A) Millard-Gubler syndrome
(B) Weber's syndrome
(C) Brown-Séquard syndrome
(D) None of the above

112. Each statement below concerning cyclic adenosine monophosphate (cAMP) is true EXCEPT

(A) cAMP levels may be increased or decreased by hormone stimulation
(B) it is the second messenger for the action of parathyroid hormone (PTH) on the kidney
(C) it activates protein kinase C by binding to the regulatory subunit and causing dissociation of the catalytic subunit
(D) it is degraded intracellularly by a family of phosphodiesterase isoenzymes
(E) it is synthesized from adenosine triphosphate (ATP)

113. Which one of the following statements about glycogen storage disease type Ia is true?

(A) Liver glycogen is decreased
(B) Renal glycogen is increased
(C) Phosphorylase A is deficient
(D) Debranching enzyme is deficient
(E) None of the above

114. Tay-Sachs disease is marked by all of the following EXCEPT

(A) it is more common among Ashkenazi Jews than other population groups
(B) it is a lysosomal storage disease
(C) it is characterized by an absence of hexosaminidase A
(D) it is characterized by an accumulation of GM_2 gangliosides
(E) it is characterized by an absence of β-galactosidase

115. Which of the following statements regarding coronary artery blood flow in a healthy person is true?

(A) During systole, coronary artery blood flow is uniform from subendocardial to epicardial regions of the left ventricle

(B) Myocardial oxygen extraction, not coronary artery blood flow, increases during exercise

(C) Coronary artery blood flow is directly proportional to arterial blood pressure over a range of pressures within 20–30 mm Hg of normal

(D) Coronary artery blood flow is proportional to myocardial oxygen demands

(E) Coronary artery blood flow is maximal during systole

116. All of the following facts about NAD^+, $NADP^+$, FMN, and FAD nucleotide cofactors in metabolism are true EXCEPT

(A) they are water soluble

(B) they are very tightly bound to flavoproteins

(C) they undergo reversible oxidation and reduction

(D) they are utilized by many dehydrogenase enzymes

117. Which one of the following is NOT part of processing of messenger RNA (mRNA) primary transcripts in eukaryotic cells?

(A) Splicing

(B) Methylation

(C) Addition of a 5U cap

(D) Addition of a polyadenylate (poly A) tail to the 3U end

118. All of the following are proteins that regulate transcription initiation EXCEPT

(A) specificity factors

(B) repressors

(C) activators

(D) promoters

119. An action potential recorded from a microelectrode inserted in a nerve fiber is illustrated in the figure below. All of the following statements describe changes that take place during the action potential recorded by this electrode EXCEPT

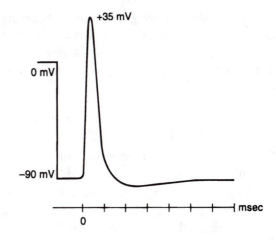

(A) at the peak of the action potential, the number of open Na^+ channels greatly exceeds the number of open K^+ channels

(B) depolarization is caused by an abrupt increase in Na^+ conductance

(C) repolarization is primarily caused by an increase in K^+ conductance

(D) repolarization is caused by activation of the Ca^{2+}–Na^+ channel

(E) chloride channel permeability does not change during an action potential

120. A 35-year-old man presents with loss of pain sensation in the skin of the forearm and lateral border of the leg. He also exhibits loss of tendon reflexes and complains of severe stabbing pains of the legs. This condition could have been prevented by

(A) avoiding the bullet that damaged his cingulate gyrus 13 years ago
(B) early penicillin treatment
(C) avoiding exposure to varicella zoster virus infection
(D) early administration of acyclovir

121. All of the following statements concerning the major determinants of glomerular filtration rate (GFR), which are renal blood flow (RBF) and glomerular hydrostatic pressures, are correct EXCEPT

(A) constriction of the afferent arteriole decreases both RBF and GFR
(B) an increase in RBF, even with little change in glomerular pressure, increases GFR
(C) in a normal kidney, an increase in systemic arterial pressure from 100 to 150 mm Hg increases GFR severalfold
(D) constriction of the efferent arteriole decreases RBF and slightly increases GFR

122. At which of these blood neutrophil levels do patients acquire a significant risk of opportunistic infection?

(A) $<1000/\mu l$
(B) $1000–1500/\mu l$
(C) $1500–2000/\mu l$
(D) $2000–2500/\mu l$
(E) $2500–3000/\mu l$

123. A physician interested in evaluating the effects of a drug on the synthesis of RNA has decided to measure RNA production in cells after treatment with the drug by radiolabeling RNA. Which of the following radiolabeled bases should this physician use?

(A) Tritiated thymine [(^{3}H)-thymine]
(B) Tritiated guanine [(^{3}H)-guanine]
(C) Tritiated adenine [(^{3}H)-adenine]
(D) Tritiated uracil [(^{3}H)-uracil]
(E) Tritiated cytosine [(^{3}H)-cytosine]

124. Of the following statements, which best describes integral membrane proteins? They

(A) have at least one α-helical domain of approximately 20 amino acids, which spans the bilayer
(B) are stabilized within the bilayer by a combination of hydrogen bonds and electrostatic interactions
(C) may be solubilized by altering the pH or the ionic strength
(D) are frequently glycoproteins in which the carbohydrate is on the cytosolic side of the membrane
(E) may display transverse movement in the lipid bilayer

125. For a patient trying to prevent intercourse-related urinary tract infections, which of the following antibiotics would be the most effective and economical when administered only once after coitus?

(A) Cephalexin
(B) Nitrofurantoin
(C) Trimethoprim–sulfamethoxazole
(D) Ciprofloxacin
(E) Penicillin G

126. For which one of the following organisms do opsonic antibodies play a major role in acquired immunity to infection?

(A) *Neisseria meningitidis*, group A
(B) *Vibrio cholerae*
(C) *Clostridium botulinum*
(D) *Shigella flexneri*

127. If end diastolic volume is approximately 115 ml in the volume–pressure curve of the left ventricle below, which of the following statements is most accurate?

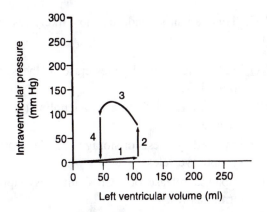

(A) The ejection fraction is approximately 30%
(B) Aortic diastolic pressure is approximately 80 mm Hg
(C) Isovolumic contraction is during the section labeled *3*
(D) Stroke volume is approximately 45 ml
(E) Left ventricular end diastolic pressure is approximately 100 mm Hg

Questions 128–129

A 45-year-old man has complained of increasing abdominal girth, fever, and malaise for the previous 4 months; he has denied having a cough. Physical examination shows a markedly enlarged spleen but no lymphadenopathy. Laboratory evaluation shows a normal chest x-ray, hemoglobin concentration of 15 g/dl, a white blood cell count of 45,000 cells/μl with no blasts seen on the blood smear, and a platelet count of 750,000/μl.

128. The most likely diagnosis is

(A) malignant lymphoma
(B) acute leukemia
(C) chronic myeloproliferative disorder
(D) pulmonary tuberculosis
(E) myelodysplastic disorder

129. The laboratory evaluation for the differential diagnosis of this problem might include all of the following tests EXCEPT

(A) measurement of leukocyte alkaline phosphatase levels
(B) chromosomal evaluation
(C) bone marrow aspiration and biopsy
(D) flow cytometric analysis
(E) determination of red blood cell mass

130. Which one of the following is not a eukaryotic regulatory sequence element found upstream of the messenger RNA (mRNA) initiation site?

(A) α helix
(B) TATA box
(C) GC box
(D) CAAT box
(E) Enhancers

131. Chronic Chagas disease should be considered in patients from Central and South America presenting with which set of the following signs and symptoms?

(A) Periodic fever and chills
(B) Cardiac conduction defects
(C) Multiple mucocutaneous lesions
(D) Persistent diarrhea
(E) Pneumonia

Questions 132–134

A 27-year-old woman presents with muscle weakness, including eyelid ptosis, slurred speech, and difficulty swallowing. The history shows that the woman is being treated for a gram-negative infection with gentamicin. The following tests have been ordered: thyroid function studies, serum creatine kinase, an electromyogram, and a muscle biopsy.

132. The attending physician chides the resident on the case for not ordering edrophonium, which produces a dramatic improvement in the patient's muscle strength when administered intravenously. All of the other tests that were ordered returned with normal values. The resident's working diagnosis is

(A) Duchenne muscular dystrophy (DMD)
(B) monoadenylate deaminase deficiency
(C) myasthenia gravis
(D) hyperthyroidism
(E) toxic drug myopathy

133. This patient's condition most likely results from

(A) inadequate acetylcholinesterase in the synaptic cleft
(B) production of defective acetylcholine (ACh) receptors
(C) impaired synthesis or storage of ACh in presynaptic vesicles
(D) impaired release of ACh from presynaptic terminals
(E) blockade and increased turnover of ACh receptors

134. Aminoglycoside antibiotics create and exacerbate muscle weakness through

(A) inhibition of presynaptic release of ACh
(B) antagonism of the action of acetylcholinesterase
(C) potentiation of the action of acetylcholinesterase
(D) increasing the turnover of ACh receptors
(E) slowing conduction of the action potential

135. All of the following events occur in receptor-mediated endocytosis for uptake of cholesterol into cells EXCEPT

(A) receptor binding at the cell surface
(B) low-density lipoprotein (LDL) receptor degradation
(C) hydrolysis of cholesteryl esters
(D) degradation of apoB-100
(E) endosomal/lysosomal fusion

136. All of the following are components of chromatin EXCEPT

(A) protein
(B) RNA
(C) carbohydrate
(D) DNA

137. Which one of the following protein segments is characterized by its ability to bind to phosphotyrosine-containing peptides?

(A) A helix-loop-helix domain
(B) A leucine zipper
(C) An Src homology 2 (SH2) domain
(D) An Src homology 3 (SH3) domain
(E) A basic region
(F) A pleckstin motif

138. Cholera toxin can affect cells by blocking the guanosine triphosphatase (GTPase) activity of their G_s proteins. On a cellular level, which one of the following would be helpful in reducing the harmful effects of cholera toxin?

(A) Increasing the amount of intracellular cyclic adenosine monophosphate (cAMP)
(B) Inhibiting the activity of the adenylate cyclase in the cell
(C) Inhibiting the G_i proteins within the cell
(D) Adding ligand for the G_s protein-linked receptor
(E) Increasing the amount of protein kinase A (PKA) in the cell

139. Which one of the following statements about the desensitization of receptors is accurate?

(A) Homologous desensitization of nicotinic receptors requires several minutes of repeated stimuli
(B) Desensitization of adrenergic receptors can occur only by reducing the expression of the receptor gene
(C) Desensitization does not change the affinity of a receptor for a ligand, only the activity
(D) Receptor desensitization can be affected by the phosphorylation state of the receptor
(E) Desensitization of one type of receptor cannot be mediated by the actions of another receptor pathway
(F) Desensitization occurs only for nicotinic receptors, not adrenergic receptors

140. A hospitalized patient is found to have a urinary tract infection owing to *Serratia*. A course of antimicrobial therapy with an aminoglycoside is planned. However, the patient has mild renal impairment. The best means to determine the appropriate drug dosage is

(A) body surface area
(B) serum creatinine
(C) serum blood urea nitrogen
(D) creatinine clearance
(E) peak and trough drug levels

141. All of the following match important vasodilators with corresponding tissues EXCEPT

(A) adenosine–heart
(B) carbon dioxide–brain
(C) low oxygen–lung
(D) increased body temperature–skin

142. Surgical instruments are boiled for 10 minutes in a saline solution containing *Escherichia coli*, *Mycobacterium tuberculosis*, and *Bacillus cereus*. Which one of the following organisms is most likely to survive this procedure?

(A) *E. coli*
(B) *M. tuberculosis*
(C) *B. cereus*

143. A length–tension diagram for a single sarcomere is illustrated below. Tension that develops is maximal between points *B* and *C* because

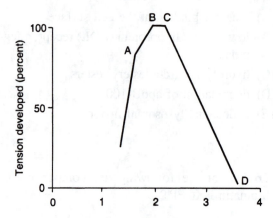

(A) there is maximal overlap between the actin filaments and the cross-bridges of the myosin filaments
(B) the actin filament has pulled all the way out to the end of the myosin filament
(C) the Z disks of the sarcomere touch the ends of the myosin filament
(D) the myosin filament is at its minimal length
(E) actin filaments are overlapping for maximal interaction with myosin

Questions 144–145

The left ventricular and aortic pressure tracings below were recorded during cardiac catheterization of a 62-year-old patient who complains of chest pain and dizziness on exertion.

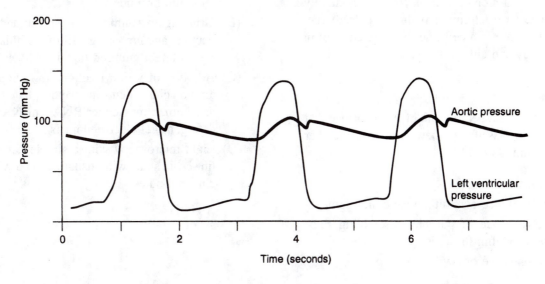

144. The left ventricular and aortic pressure tracings indicate that this patient has

(A) pulmonary stenosis
(B) aortic stenosis
(C) mitral stenosis
(D) aortic insufficiency
(E) mitral insufficiency

145. The most likely change in heart sound in this patient would be

(A) systolic murmur
(B) diastolic murmur
(C) presystolic murmur
(D) mid-diastolic murmur

146. All of the following enzymes may be targets of a new drug that inhibits cellular synthesis of DNA EXCEPT

(A) DNA-dependent DNA polymerase
(B) topoisomerase II
(C) RNA-dependent DNA polymerase
(D) RNA polymerase
(E) DNA ligase

Questions 147–148

A research laboratory has been asked to study a new viral disease, which the researchers think is caused by an arenavirus. They need a relatively simple test to determine if this is indeed true. They have found a cell line (by pure chance) in which they can culture the virus.

147. The most specific trait of Arenaviridae that would help classify the new virus as a member of this family would be

(A) an insect vector
(B) the presence of multiple genomic segments
(C) the presence of particles resembling ribosomes within the virions
(D) the presence of a viral envelope

148. What is the best method to test for the presence of this trait?

(A) Gel electrophoresis; the gel is stained with ethidium bromide
(B) Grinding up a number of the presumed insect vectors, and preparing a filtrate of this material to infect cultured human cells
(C) Addition of virion fractions to radiolabeled amino acids, adenosine triphosphate (ATP), and human messenger RNA (mRNA); then detergent gel electrophoresis
(D) Light microscopy with a simple hematoxylin–eosin stain, with visualization of viral inclusion bodies

149. The tumor pictured in the photomicrograph below arises from which one of the following types of cells?

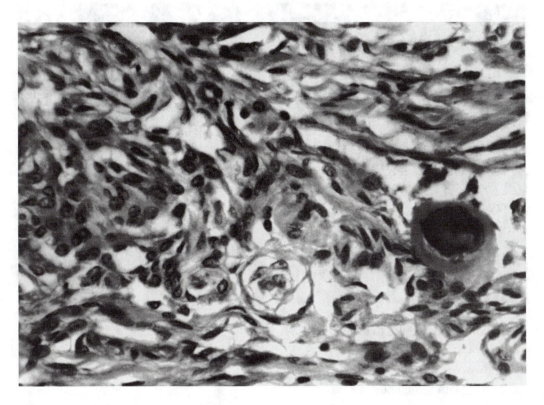

(A) Cerebellar astrocytes

(B) Leptomeningeal cells

(C) Neurons

(D) Oligodendrocytes

(E) Schwann cells

150. A 55-year-old man with a history of chronic alcoholism presents with complaints of fatigue and weakness. His laboratory values are as follows:

Hgb/Hct	11.5/34.0
MCV	110
MCH	38.0
RDW	19.5
WBC	$6.0 \times 10^9/L$

Differential:

Polys	80%	$4.8 \times 10^9/L$
Bands	7%	$0.42 \times 10^9/L$
Lymphs	10%	$0.6 \times 10^9/L$
Monos	5%	$0.3 \times 10^9/L$

Microscopic examination of a peripheral blood smear shows poikilocytosis and hypersegmented neutrophils. This patient most likely has

(A) anemia caused by vitamin B deficiency

(B) anemia caused by iron deficiency

(C) anemia following hemorrhage

(D) sickle cell anemia

(E) β thalassemia minor

(F) severe β thalassemia

151. The hepatic neoplasm pictured below has which one of the following characteristics?

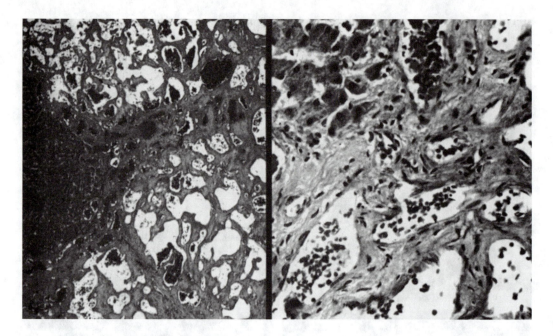

(A) An association with exposure to the carcinogen Thorotrast

(B) Highly aggressive behavior

(C) An association with thrombocytopenia

(D) Foci of hemorrhage and necrosis

Questions 152–155

(A) Inguinal and pubic regions
(B) Perineum, posterior thigh, and leg
(C) Both
(D) Neither

For each organ listed below, select the region to which pain in that organ is usually referred.

152. Ovary

153. Uterus

154. Epididymis

155. Testis

Questions 156–158

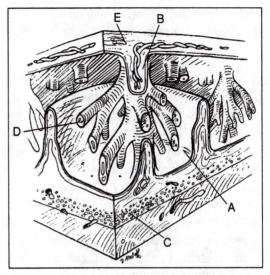

For each morphologic or functional description of a component of the placenta listed below, choose the appropriate lettered structure in the accompanying diagram.

156. This structure is the decidual plate and is penetrated by maternal blood vessels

157. This structure is the intervillous space and contains maternal red blood cells

158. This structure is the chorionic plate and receives the insertion of the umbilical cord

159. The most common cause of cystic fibrosis is the $\triangle$F508 mutation in the cystic fibrosis transmembrane conductance regulator (CFTR) gene. Which one of the following statements concerning potential strategies to fix this defect is correct?

(A) The entire gene or protein should be replaced, because this mutation eliminates a key amino acid within the adenosine triphosphatase (ATPase) domain of the CFTR gene

(B) This mutation causes the chloride channel to be constitutively active, so it could be corrected if the regulatory region could be repaired

(C) This mutation causes the chloride channel to remain closed due to an abnormal fold of the protein, so it could be corrected if the blockage was removed

(D) This mutant protein would be able to function normally, if it could be inserted in the membrane

(E) Patients with this disease could be cured, if the expression of the mutated gene could be increased to normal levels

(F) This mutation causes abnormal splicing of the messenger RNA (mRNA), leading to a greatly truncated protein; therefore, correction of the splicing defect or replacement of the entire gene or protein is required

160. A prepubertal, phenotypic female is referred to a geneticist because a recent karyotyping that was performed for an unrelated reason showed this patient to be 46,XY. Which one of the following statements could be correct?

(A) The patient could have a 17,20-lyase mutation that leads to increased production of testosterone

(B) The patient could have a deletion of the transmembrane domain of the androgen receptor, leading to androgen insensitivity

(C) The patient could have a deletion of the DNA-binding domain of the androgen receptor, leading to androgen insensitivity

(D) Because testosterone does not require a receptor, the defect must be in the synthesis pathway of testosterone

(E) The karyotype must have been performed incorrectly because it is impossible for someone to be 46,XY and phenotypically female

Questions 161–165

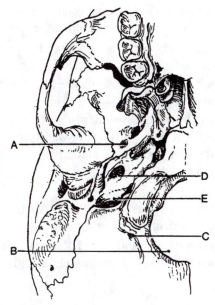

For each artery or vein comprising the vasculature of the cranium, select the lettered foramen or fissure through which it courses, shown on the illustration of the inferior aspect of the cranium.

161. Middle meningeal artery

162. Internal carotid artery

163. Internal jugular vein

164. Emissary vein

165. Vertebral artery

166. A 46-year-old man has symptoms of vomiting and mid-epigastric pain 45 minutes after having two slices of pepperoni pizza and a couple of draft beers. The pain is constant (not crampy) and radiates to the back. Vomiting does not seem to improve the patient's symptoms. The abdomen was diffusely tender with guarding but without rebound tenderness. The patient was not jaundiced. Laboratory values showed an elevated serum amylase level. All of the following statements are true EXCEPT

(A) 80% of cases of acute pancreatitis can be attributed to alcohol and gallstones
(B) elevated serum amylase is specific for the diagnosis of acute pancreatitis
(C) serum lipase remains elevated longer than serum amylase in acute pancreatitis
(D) Ranson's criteria can be useful in determining the risk of serious complications
(E) the patient may have hypocalcemia
(F) the following laboratory tests should be included in this patient's work-up: blood glucose, serum lactate dehydrogenase (LDH), and blood urea nitrogen (BUN)

167. A 12-year-old boy is jaundiced and has an enlarged liver on palpation. Laboratory values show elevated alanine aminotransferase (ALT), aspartate aminotransferase (AST), and direct bilirubin. In addition, the physician noticed Kayser-Fleischer rings on a slit-lamp examination. A diagnosis of Wilson's disease is suspected. All of the following statements are true EXCEPT

(A) the primary defect is a mutation in ceruloplasmin

(B) the patient likely has increased levels of serum free copper and liver copper, and increased urinary copper with d-penicillamine challenge

(C) Wilson's disease is inherited in an autosomal recessive pattern

(D) patients can demonstrate decreased serum ceruloplasmin

(E) in normal subjects, more than 90% of serum copper circulates bound to ceruloplasmin

168. A 40-year-old man with short bowel syndrome due to a resection for Crohn's disease is experiencing large volume diarrhea during the past few weeks. His symptoms are vesicular rash, alopecia, skin ulcers, depression, confusion with regard to time and place, and inability to discriminate tastes. He is deficient in which one of the following nutrients?

(A) Vitamin B$_2$ (riboflavin)

(B) Niacin

(C) Folic acid

(D) Zinc

(E) Iron

(F) Vitamin C

(G) Selenium

169. All of the following associations between signs and disorders are correct EXCEPT

(A) Mallory bodies, α-fetoprotein, des-carboxy-prothrombin—hepatocellular carcinoma

(B) antimitochondrial antibodies, elevated alkaline phosphatase, and γ-glutamyl transpeptidase, middle-aged women—primary biliary cirrhosis

(C) anti–liver-kidney microsomal antibody-1 (anti-LKM1), positive for hepatitis C virus infection, women—autoimmune hepatitis type 3

(D) aspartate aminotransferase (AST)/alanine aminotransferase (ALT) > 2 (ALT < 500)—alcoholic liver disease

(E) ulcerative colitis, cholangiocarcinoma, men—primary sclerosing cholangitis

170. Which one of the following can be used as an antiemetic agent for patients with motion sickness?

(A) Apomorphine, a dopamine agonist

(B) Chlorpromazine, a dopamine antagonist

(C) Promethazine, an antihistamine agent

(D) Pilocarpine, a muscarinic agonist

(E) Ondansetron, a 5-HT$_3$ serotonin receptor antagonist

Questions 171–174

(A) Sleep spindles

(B) Sleep-onset rapid eye movement (REM)

(C) Delta waves

(D) Increased percentage of REM

(E) Normal REM sleep

For each clinical state listed below, select the description of sleep architecture most closely associated with it.

171. Narcolepsy

172. Major depression

173. Nocturnal penile tumescence

174. Night terrors

175. All of the following can be causes of conjugated hyperbilirubinemia EXCEPT

(A) Wilson's disease

(B) Crigler-Najjar syndrome type I

(C) primary biliary cirrhosis

(D) viral hepatitis

(E) Rotor syndrome

(F) gallstones

(G) alcoholic liver disease

176. A 25-year-old woman presents with a 3-week history of periumbilical pain, diarrhea, fever, and weight loss. She reports of having these symptoms once before, and that there was evidence of perianal involvement. Stool culture for bacteria, ova, and parasites is negative. The radiologic barium films of the small bowel and colon demonstrate a "string sign" in the terminal ileum. The endoscopic evaluation, with biopsy of the affected areas reports transmural inflammation. All of the following statements are true EXCEPT

(A) noncaseating granulomas are found in the biopsy specimen

(B) fistulae and sinus tracts are visible on radiographs

(C) smoking is thought to be protective against this disease

(D) this disease occurs anywhere along the gastrointestinal tract, but favors the terminal ileum

(E) endoscopic examination shows "cobblestone" mucosa

177. All of the following statements about gastric acid secretion and peptic ulcer disease (PUD) are true EXCEPT

(A) the mechanism of disease in PUD is an imbalance between protective and aggressive factors (acid)

(B) intake of ethanol, caffeine, tobacco, salicylates, and nonsteroidal anti-inflammatory drugs are risk factors for PUD

(C) hereditary factors play a role in PUD

(D) *Helicobacter pylori* in the duodenum play a role in PUD

(E) histamine and gastrin lead to acid secretion by the parietal cell

(F) acetylcholine leads to acid secretion by the parietal cell

178. A 36-year-old man complains of low-volume bloody diarrhea, crampy abdominal pain, and a fever. Microscopic examination of his stool shows fecal leukocytes. A likely cause of this man's symptoms is

(A) cholera
(B) Zollinger-Ellison syndrome
(C) laxative ingestion
(D) mannitol ingestion
(E) shigella

179. A young female patient with anorexia nervosa is determined to be in late starvation (> 3 weeks). All of the following results would be expected EXCEPT

(A) decreased levels of follicle-stimulating hormone and luteinizing hormone
(B) ketone body production
(C) decreased cardiac output
(D) increased protein breakdown
(E) increased risk of respiratory infections
(F) decreased resting energy expenditure

180. A patient's symptoms lead a physician to think that the patient may have a point mutation in a portion of a gene for which the physician has polymerase chain reaction (PCR) primers. The physician amplifies this region of the patient's DNA using PCR and then performs a single-strand conformational polymorphism (SSCP) analysis on his DNA. Which one of the following statements about the interpretation of this test is correct?

(A) If the patient is heterozygous for a dominant mutation, the physician would see two bands
(B) If the physician sees four bands, the patient has multiple mutations
(C) If the physician sees two bands, the patient is either homozygous normal or homozygous for the mutation
(D) If the physician sees four bands, the patient has a point mutation that is causing his disease
(E) If the patient does not have a point mutation within the amplified region, the physician would see only one band
(F) SSCP would not be useful in this situation

ANSWER KEY

1-D	31-A	61-D	91-C	121-C
2-A	32-C	62-B	92-C	122-A
3-C	33-C	63-D	93-B	123-D
4-A	34-C	64-A	94-B	124-A
5-F	35-B	65-B	95-C	125-E
6-C	36-A	66-A	96-D	126-A
7-A	37-D	67-D	97-C	127-B
8-D	38-A	68-C	98-D	128-C
9-E	39-E	69-A	99-A	129-D
10-B	40-C	70-D	100-D	130-A
11-E	41-A	71-C	101-D	131-B
12-B	42-A	72-C	102-A	132-C
13-B	43-D	73-D	103-B	133-E
14-D	44-C	74-E	104-D	134-A
15-C	45-B	75-C	105-B	135-B
16-C	46-A	76-D	106-D	136-C
17-A	47-C	77-D	107-E	137-C
18-C	48-E	78-B	108-E	138-B
19-C	49-A	79-A	109-A	139-D
20-B	50-E	80-A	110-C	140-E
21-D	51-B	81-B	111-B	141-C
22-C	52-E	82-D	112-C	142-C
23-D	53-A	83-C	113-B	143-A
24-D	54-B	84-A	114-E	144-B
25-A	55-A	85-D	115-D	145-A
26-D	56-C	86-D	116-B	146-C
27-C	57-D	87-B	117-B	147-C
28-A	58-C	88-C	118-D	148-C
29-B	59-E	89-D	119-D	149-B
30-B	60-A	90-D	120-B	150-A

151-C	157-A	163-E	169-C	175-B
152-A	158-E	164-C	170-C	176-C
153-C	159-D	165-B	171-B	177-D
154-B	160-C	166-B	172-D	178-E
155-A	161-A	167-A	173-E	179-D
156-C	162-D	168-D	174-C	180-C

ANSWERS AND EXPLANATIONS

1. The answer is D. *(Pathology; Barrett's esophagus)*
Barrett's esophagus is a result of protracted reflux, due to lower esophageal sphincter incompetence, with the attendant increased exposure to acid, pepsin, and bile acids. Esophageal inflammation and ulceration occur, followed by re-epithelialization and ingrowth of immature pluripotent stem cells. Rather than squamous epithelium, the new epithelium is columnar-lined with gastric or duodenal-type cells, which better tolerate prolonged acid exposure. Inflammation would only be absent in the case of postmortem ulceration and autolysis; such changes may be accompanied by ''leopard spotting''—brown–black esophageal spots that form from acid digestion of hemoglobin.

2. The answer is A. *(Pharmacology; plasma protein binding of drugs)*
Many drugs bind to plasma proteins, which limits glomerular filtration in the kidneys because the drugs are not freely diffusible. Drug–protein interactions that are common generally occur between a wide variety of drugs and albumin or α_1-acid glycoprotein, but not immunoglobulins. Covalent interactions are rare, but when they occur it is generally with reactive antineoplastic drugs. Renal tubular secretion is generally not limited by plasma protein binding of drugs because secretion reduces free plasma drug concentration, which is quickly followed by dissociation of the drug from plasma proteins.

3–4. The answers are: 3-C, 4-A. *(Pharmacology; suicide management)*
Safely removing any pill fragments from the stomach by nasogastric tube is the first step in the management of the patient described in the question because amitriptyline is an anticholinergic that retards gastrointestinal absorption, increasing the likelihood that pill fragments remain. The patient may ultimately need psychiatric hospitalization; because she is unresponsive, there is no urgency in pursuing this. An electroencephalogram would not add any useful information at this time, and seizures, if they occurred, would most likely be related to the toxicity of amitriptyline and a lowering of the seizure threshold.

Tricyclic antidepressants have antiarrhythmic effects, like quinidine. The changes on electrocardiogram, especially with increased or toxic serum levels, include a prolonged P-R interval, prolonged QRS duration, and a prolonged QT interval. In therapeutic dose ranges, tricyclics may suppress premature ventricular contraction.

5. The answer is F. *(Pathology; T-cell acute lymphoblastic leukemia)*
Patients with T-cell acute lymphoblastic leukemia are often teens or young adults and are predominantly male. In more than 50% of patients, the leukemic population in the thymus forms a mediastinal mass. Patients usually have a high white blood cell count, often higher than 5×10^{10}/L. Detection of terminal deoxynucleotidyl transferase (TdT), a nuclear protein, is seen in more than 95% of patients with acute lymphoblastic leukemia (ALL) and 15% of patients with acute myeloblastic leukemia (AML). AML is positive for Sudan black stain and myeloperoxidase, whereas ALL is negative for both.

6. The answer is C. *(Histology; membrane structure and function)*
The plasma membrane consists of amphipathic lipids (predominantly phospholipids and cholesterol) and amphipathic proteins. The hydrophilic portions of these molecules face the external and internal aqueous environments. The hydrophobic portions are in the internal portion of the bilayer. Phospholipids prevent free diffusion of ions and water-soluble molecules, thereby imparting selective permeability properties to the lipid bilayer. Proteins may be restricted to the external portion of the bilayer or span it entirely. In addition, the membrane is fluid, allowing lateral diffusion of even large proteins.

7. The answer is A. *(Biochemistry; polymerase chain reaction)*
A polymerase chain reaction is used to amplify sequences of DNA from a single copy to over 1 million copies. The template DNA is initially denatured in the presence of excess primers, which are short (15–25

base pairs) oligonucleotides homologous to sequences on the template DNA. Because the DNA is denatured and renatured many times by multiple heating and cooling cycles, limiting amounts of primers prevents large-scale amplification of the parent strand. The temperatures at which a polymerase chain reaction is carried out are generally in the range from 55°C–95°C. Heat-resistant DNA polymerase, such as the Taq polymerase, is resistant to heat denaturation.

8. The answer is D. *(Biochemistry; RNA structure and function)*
The primary transcript for messenger RNA (mRNA) is formed in the nucleus, where the elongation proceeds from the 5′ to the 3′ end. Most eukaryotic mRNAs are distinctive in that the 5′ ends are capped by the addition of a methylated guanylic acid residue and the 3′ ends have a polyadenylate tail of 100 to 200 adenosine nucleotides. Most precursor forms of mRNA contain intervening sequences, which are removed by a process known as splicing. The binding of steroid hormones with their receptors to specific genes results in the increased synthesis of the mRNA encoded in those genes.

9. The answer is E. *(Pathology; gastric carcinoma)*
Paget's disease of the breast is a carcinoma involving the nipple and subjacent ductal elements, and Paget's disease of the bone is an idiopathic disease characterized by a high turnover of bone. Neither form is associated with gastric carcinoma. The Leser-Trélat sign is the development of seborrheic keratosis, acanthosis nigricans, or amyloidosis in a patient with gastrointestinal malignancy. Erythema nodosum is seen occasionally with gastrointestinal malignancy.

10. The answer is B. *(Anatomy; epidermis)*
The order of epidermal maturation is stratum basale, stratum spinosum, stratum granulosum, stratum lucidum, and stratum corneum. The stratum basale is the germinal layer of the epidermis. Cells migrate and differentiate from this layer at a rate equal to desquamation of keratin from the outermost layer. The stratum spinosum is superficial to the stratum basale, and its cells are in the process of growth and early keratin synthesis. The stratum granulosum is characterized by the presence of intracellular granules, which contribute to the keratinization process. The stratum lucidum is a homogeneous layer between the stratum granulosum and the stratum corneum that is present only in thick skin. The stratum corneum is the most superficial layer of the epidermis and is mainly composed of keratin.

11. The answer is E. *(Microbiology; recurrent urinary tract infections)*
Longitudinal studies have shown that bacteriuria in women susceptible to urinary tract infections is preceded by colonization of the vaginal introitus with the responsible organism from the rectal flora.

12. The answer is B. *(Pathology; Gaucher's disease)*
Type II Gaucher's disease is the infantile acute cerebral pattern and is characterized by a virtual absence of glucocerebrosidase, with an accumulation of large quantities of β-glucosylceramide in macrophages and hepatocytes. Type I, or the classic form, is the adult type, in which storage of glucocerebrosides is limited to the mononuclear phagocytes. Patients with type I have reduced but detectable levels of glucocerebrosidase. Both type I and type II are autosomal recessive. Niemann-Pick disease is characterized by the accumulation of sphingomyelin, which is due to a deficiency in sphingomyelinase. Tay-Sachs disease, in which ganglioside accumulates, results from lack of *N*-acetylhexosaminidase. The defective enzyme in Krabbe's disease is galactosylceramidase.

13–15. The answers are: 13-B, 14-D, 15-C. *(Histology; epididymis)*
The micrograph shows the epididymis. The epididymis is a highly convoluted tubular organ that conveys sperm and fluid from the testis to the ductus (vas) deferens. Its luminal epithelium is a pseudostratified

columnar epithelium with numerous tall apical stereocilia. These cells secrete poorly characterized substances, which are added to the seminal fluid, and remove other poorly characterized substances from the fluids that drain from the seminiferous tubules in the testis. Apoptosis, or programmed cell death, occurs in the testis as in the thymus.

16. The answer is C. *(Pathophysiology; anthrax)*
A malignant pustule is a clinical manifestation of cutaneous anthrax. It occurs at the site of inoculation and is characterized by a black eschar at its base surrounded by an inflamed ring. Enteritis necroticans, caused by *Clostridium perfringens*, and pseudomembranous colitis, caused by *Clostridium difficile*, are diseases of the gastrointestinal tract that may be characterized by ulcerative lesions in the intestinal mucosa. Lockjaw is a lay name for tetanus; it refers to the muscle and neural spasms caused by the neurotoxin tetanospasmin. Woolsorter's disease is pulmonary anthrax—a diffuse, lethal, progressive pneumonia caused by the inhalation of spores of *Bacillus anthracis*.

17. The answer is A. *(Histopathology; seminomas)*
Seminomas comprise 30%–40% of testicular tumors and are divided into classic and spermatocytic forms. Classic seminomas, as in this case, are composed of nests of tumor cells with abundant clear cytoplasm with vesicular nuclei and angulated nucleoli (*left*). The nests are separated by fibrous strands that contain inflammatory cells, usually lymphocytes and plasma cells (*right*). Mumps orchitis involves large numbers of giant cells; it is an inflammatory reaction, not a neoplasm, and the condition is seen in young individuals. Teratomas contain aberrant ectopic tissues (e.g., brain, cartilage, and epithelial-lined cysts), whereas chorio-carcinomas have syncytiotrophoblastic giant cells and cytotrophoblasts in close apposition.

18. The answer is C. *(Hematology; platelet homeostasis)*
Examination of the peripheral blood smear is essential when evaluating a patient for thrombocytopenia. Unreported abnormalities of the red cells may offer a clue to the etiology, or occasionally one may find a discrepancy between the number of platelets seen on the smear and that found by the automated count. This occurs in pseudothrombocytopenia, where clumping of platelets in a specific anticoagulant [usually ethylenediaminetetraacetic acid (EDTA)] results in marked underestimation of the count.

19. The answer is C. *(Immunology; DiGeorge syndrome)*
Patients with diseases that cause a deficiency in T cells are extremely prone to viral, fungal, and protozoal infections. The patient described in the question presents with severe oral thrush, which is caused by a *Candida* species, and hypocalcemia. These findings are consistent with a diagnosis of DiGeorge syndrome, which results from a defect in the embryonic development of the third and fourth pharyngeal pouches. Both the thymus and parathyroid glands fail to develop, resulting in hypocalcemia. The white blood cell count can be within normal limits, but virtually all of the circulating leukocytes are B cells and plasma cells.

20. The answer is B. *(Pathology; T-cell acute myeloblastic leukemia)*
Patients with acute leukemia often develop metabolic abnormalities. Hyponatremia and hypokalemia are common in patients with acute leukemia because renal tubule abnormalities can be induced by lysozyme or other products of the leukemic cells. Patients with acute lymphoblastic leukemia (ALL) and acute myeloblastic leukemia (AML) also present with pancytopenia. Detection of terminal deoxynucleotidyl transferase (TdT), a nuclear protein, is seen in more than 95% of patients with ALL and 15% of patients with AML. AML is positive for Sudan black stain and myeloperoxidase, whereas ALL is negative for both. The presence of Auer rods (i.e., abnormal primary granules) in the cytoplasm of leukemic cells is diagnostic of AML.

21. The answer is D. *(Pathology; chronic lymphoblastic leukemia)*
Chronic lymphoblastic leukemia (CLL) is found more frequently in males than in females. CLL is uncommon before the age of 40 and is usually seen in patients older than 50. It is the most common form of chronic leukemia in the United States, and it is rare in Asians. CLL represents a clonal expansion of neoplastic B lymphocytes in more than 95% of cases. These cells commonly have trisomy 12 alone or with additional chromosomal abnormalities. Most patients with CLL develop some degree of hypogammaglobulinemia.

22. The answer is C. *(Physiology; fluid balance)*
Infusion of a hypertonic solution instantaneously adds both volume and milliosmoles to the extracellular (and total body) water space. Because the solution is hypertonic, the osmolality increases in the extracellular space (but remains unchanged in the intracellular space), thereby causing osmosis of water out of the cells and into the extracellular compartment. At equilibrium, the extracellular volume is expanded, and its osmolality is increased. In contrast, the intracellular volume is decreased, resulting in an increase in intracellular osmolality.

23. The answer is D. *(Immunology; vaccines as applied to AIDS)*
Of the vaccination procedures listed, the one most likely to be tested by the Food and Drug Administration (FDA) is the procedure that uses a human monoclonal antibody that reacts with the intact CD4 (T4) receptor. Antibodies that react with CD4 should "look like" the portion of human immunodeficiency virus (HIV) that reacts with the CD4 receptor. Therefore, the vaccinated person should make an antibody to the human monoclonal antibody, which may be protective against HIV.

24. The answer is D. *(Immunology; immunologic response)*
The necessary characteristics that a given compound must possess to be immunogenic include a high molecular weight, chemical complexity, and recognition as being foreign. Compounds with a molecular weight greater than 6000 daltons are generally immunogenic, and those with a molecular weight less than 1000 daltons generally are not. Compounds between 1000 and 6000 daltons may or may not be immunogenic, depending upon the degree of foreignness or chemical complexity.

  Haptens are small, low–molecular-weight compounds that become immunogenic when coupled to a high–molecular-weight carrier, such as a conjugate of dinitrophenol and albumin. Whereas a large homopolymer of lysine would not be immunogenic because of a lack of chemical complexity, a smaller polymer containing different molecules would be immunogenic.

25. The answer is A. *(Biochemistry; glycolysis)*
The primary step in the regulation of glycolysis is the conversion of fructose 6-phosphate to fructose 1,6-bisphosphate. The enzyme, 1-phosphofructokinase, is an allosteric enzyme that is inhibited by adenosine triphosphate (ATP) and citrate and is activated by fructose 2,6-bisphosphate. The concentration of fructose 2,6-bisphosphate is, in turn, regulated by glucagon. Acetyl coenzyme A (acetyl CoA) is not an allosteric effector of any of the glycolytic enzymes. Glucose 6-phosphate is an inhibitor of hexokinase.

26. The answer is D. *(Physiology; renal sodium transport)*
Almost 75% of Na^+ is reabsorbed in the proximal tubular epithelium by several processes, including active transport at the basolateral surface, leading to electrogenic potential with additional passive movement; and cotransport of Na^+ at the luminal surface with glucose or amino acids. An additional 22% is reabsorbed by the active transport process in the ascending thick limb of the loop of Henle. The remaining small percentage of Na^+ that reaches the distal tubular epithelium is reabsorbed by a highly regulated aldosterone-sensitive process involving exchange with K^+.

27. The answer is C. *(Pathology; papillary carcinoma)*
The photomicrograph is of a papillary carcinoma of the thyroid gland, and there is a demonstrated association of this type of tumor with previous radiation therapy to the neck. The tumor cells grow on thin fibrovascular stalks and form papillae. The cells have large overlapping nuclei; the nucleoplasm has marked chromatin, which gives the nuclei a clear, "Orphan Annie eye" appearance. Papillary carcinomas also may have stromal calcification, forming concentric laminated concretions called psammoma bodies (*top center*). These carcinomas metastasize through the lymphatics to cervical lymph nodes, but, in general, they are indolent tumors.

28. The answer is A. *(Pathology; pathogenic mechanisms of respiratory pathogens)*
Pertussis and diphtheria are caused by *Bordetella pertussis* and *Corynebacterium diphtheriae*, respectively. Both of these pathogens are extracellular bacteria, which adhere to the respiratory tract and produce exotoxins that contribute to pathogenesis. Because *B. pertussis* is gram-negative, it produces endotoxin, unlike gram-positive *C. diphtheriae*. The neurologic problems associated with the DTP (diphtheria-tetanus-pertussis) vaccine are caused by the pertussis component of the vaccine (which uses whole killed cells).

29–31. The answers are: 29-B, 30-B, 31-A. *(Pharmacology; geriatric depression; migraine headache)*
The patient described in the question is suffering from depression. Monoamine oxidase inhibitor antidepressants (e.g., phenelzine) have a safe cardiac profile (except for some initial orthostatic hypotension) and essentially no anticholinergic activity, making them a good choice in the elderly who are vulnerable to constipation, memory impairment, and urinary retention. Lithium carbonate has a prophylactic role for recurrent depression but not acute depression. The neuroleptic chlorpromazine is not indicated because the patient is exhibiting no psychotic symptoms. Benzodiazepines (e.g., clonazepam) help with anxiety, which this patient does not have, and can sedate, increase cognitive deficits, and increase depression in the elderly.

A negative neurologic examination and lack of sleep disruption from the headache make a brain tumor a less likely diagnosis. In elderly individuals, temporal arteritis is an important cause of head pain and blindness that necessitates prompt diagnosis and treatment with a corticosteroid. Computed tomography scan, cerebrospinal fluid examination, or an electroencephalogram would not aid in diagnosing temporal arteritis.

Lithium is useful for cluster headaches. Ergotamine may interrupt migraine headaches, while methysergide, propranolol, and amitriptyline have prophylactic value.

32. The answer is C. *(Histology; T-cell maturation)*
Maturation of a stem cell to a resting T cell occurs earliest in the cortex. The medullary region is where the variable (V), diverse (D), and joining (J) regions of the T-cell receptor undergo rearrangement. The maturation process is independent of antigen and dependent on contact with thymic epithelial cells for purposes of proliferation and differentiation.

33. The answer is C. *(Pathology; Zellweger syndrome)*
In Zellweger syndrome, the amount of cytosolic catalase is elevated, phytanic acid accumulates in central nervous system (CNS) tissues, the plasma ratio of $C26:0/C22:0$ fatty acids is elevated, and there is a deficiency of platelet activating factor (PAF). Zellweger syndrome results from the absence of or a grossly reduced number of peroxisomes. Peroxisomes are cellular microbodies where oxidation of a very long chain of fatty acids (C26–C40) is initiated, phytanic acid is oxidized, and plasmalogens (such as PAF) are synthesized.

34. The answer is C. *(Pharmacology; gonorrheal and chlamydial coinfections)*
Of all cases presenting clinically as gonorrhea, 45% have coexisting chlamydial infections. Therefore, the correct treatment for gonorrhea is the administration of both penicillin for *Neisseria gonorrhoeae* and tetracycline for *Chlamydia trachomatis*. Amoxicillin is an oral penicillin; probenecid increases its blood level by blocking its excretion.

35. The answer is B. *(Microbiology; meningitis)*
Cryptococcus neoformans is responsible for meningitis in this case. The india ink microscopic staining technique demonstrated the presence of yeast cells producing a capsule (the capsule appears as a clear halo), and the only encapsulated yeast among the options is *C. neoformans*. This organism is an important fungal cause of meningitis, and it often infects AIDS patients.

36. The answer is A. *(Pharmacology; action of aspirin and acetaminophen)*
Aspirin is an effective antipyretic and analgesic drug. Aspirin is also the prototype of a group of nonsteroidal anti-inflammatory agents. Aspirin is associated with a risk of Reye's syndrome in pediatric patients treated for various viral diseases. Aspirin inhibits the cyclooxygenase, not the lipoxygenase, pathway.

37. The answer is D. *(Pharmacology; angiotensin-converting enzyme inhibitors)*
Captopril is the prototype of a group of angiotensin-converting enzyme (ACE) inhibitors. These agents lower blood pressure in poorly understood ways, but a critical role for inhibition of ACE (with loss of production of angiotensin II) seems apparent. ACE inhibitors do not affect renin per se, nor do they have any activity toward angiotensin II receptors.

38. The answer is A. *(Pharmacology; insulin-dependent diabetes mellitus type I therapy)*
Sulfonylureas and other oral hypoglycemics are contraindicated in insulin-dependent diabetes mellitus (IDDM). Insulin therapy to maintain blood glucose levels within a physiologic range is a symptomatic approach to the treatment of IDDM. Blood glucose levels are routinely monitored, and insulin is adjusted to maintain the blood glucose levels. A frequent side effect is hypoglycemia, which is best treated by ingestion of carbohydrates. Some patients who still maintain a normal response to glucagon benefit by injection of glucagon for this crisis as well. Although recombinant forms of insulin have reduced insulin insensitivity caused by an immune response, this problem still persists. Apparently the source of the hormone (animal versus human) is not the only determinant of antigenicity.

39. The answer is E. *(Physiology; allosteric enzymes)*
Allosteric enzymes have sites distinct from the active site where regulatory ligands bind and alter either the V_{max} or the K_m for the substrate. The substrate saturation curves do not obey Michaelis-Menten kinetics and frequently show sigmoidicity, which is indicative of positive cooperativity between active sites. Enzymes that obey Michaelis-Menten kinetics require an 81-fold increase in substrate concentration to achieve an increase from 10% to 90% of the V_{max}. Allosteric enzymes that display positive cooperativity require a smaller increase in substrate concentration to achieve the same increase in V_{max}. The allosteric sites may be located either on the same subunit as the catalytic site or on a separate regulatory subunit. Enzymes with these regulatory properties frequently catalyze reactions that are either rate-limiting or occupy a pivotal point in a metabolic pathway.

40. The answer is C. *(Anatomy; knee)*
The medial collateral ligament prevents abduction of the leg at the knee. It extends from the medial femoral epicondyle to the shaft of the tibia. The oblique popliteal ligament resists lateral rotation during the final degrees of extension. The posterior cruciate ligament prevents posterior displacement of the tibia. The anterior cruciate ligament helps lock the knee joint on full extension.

41. The answer is A. *(Anatomy; female reproductive system)*
Blood flows to the fallopian tubes through branches of the uterine vessels carried in the surrounding mesentery, which is called the mesosalpinx. The ovarian veins drain blood from the ovaries. The right ovarian vein

drains into the inferior vena cava; the left ovarian vein drains into the left renal vein. Lymph from the cervix eventually drains into the internal and external iliac and obturator nodes. Visceral afferent nerves from the uterus follow two pathways: Fibers from the cervix follow the splanchnic nerves (nervi erigentes); however, the body of the uterus and uterine tubes send fibers in parallel to the sympathetic nerves.

42. The answer is A. *(Histopathology; papillomavirus)*
This cervical tissue shows the squamous epithelial changes seen with human papillomavirus (HPV) infection, an epidemic affecting primarily young women. The viral infection causes crenation of nuclei and hyperconvolution, which is accompanied by perinuclear clearing of the cytoplasm. This change has been called condylomatous or koilocytic change and is caused by HPV infection. Some subtypes of HPV predispose the cervical squamous epithelium to dysplasia, and, therefore, these patients are sometimes treated with ablative surgery.

43. The answer is D. *(Pharmacology; antibiotics)*
Tetracycline inhibits protein synthesis in bacteria after it is selectively transported inside the cell by an active transport system. Tetracycline is selectively toxic not only because its transport system is peculiar to prokaryotes but also because it binds to 30S subunits of bacterial ribosomes. In bacteria (as well as in eukaryotic mitochondria), it prevents the binding of charged transfer RNA (tRNA) to the A site on the ribosomal complex, thereby inhibiting peptide bond synthesis. Thus, it is bacteriostatic, not bactericidal. Resistance can develop secondarily to altered influx or efflux of the drug in prokaryotes. It remains in the gastrointestinal tract and causes its most serious side effects there, either by direct irritation or secondary to modifications in gut flora. This can lead to life-threatening colitis. Tetracycline is hardly ever used in children because it accumulates in developing teeth and bones, causing stains and bone deformities.

44. The answer is C. *(Physiology; gluconeogenesis)*
Gluconeogenesis utilizes the enzymes in glycolysis that catalyze reversible reactions. The enzymes that catalyze irreversible steps in glycolysis are hexokinase, 1-phosphofructokinase, and pyruvate kinase. To circumvent the three irreversible reactions, the de novo synthesis of glucose requires four enzymes that are unique to gluconeogenesis: pyruvate carboxylase, phosphoenolpyruvate carboxykinase, fructose 2,6-bisphosphatase, and glucose 6-phosphatase.

45–47. The answers are: 45-B, 46-A, 47-C. *(Pharmacology; properties of anesthetic gases)*
Minimum alveolar concentration (MAC) is that concentration of anesthetic at 1 atm that produces immobility in 50% of patients exposed to a noxious stimulus.

If an anesthetic has a high blood:gas partition coefficient, it is very soluble in blood and is eliminated from the bloodstream into the alveolar air relatively slowly. This tends to prolong recovery time.

Relative potency of anesthetics is directly proportional to their lipid solubility. Among the commonly used agents, nitrous oxide has a very low oil:gas partition coefficient. In contrast, nitrous oxide has a rapid onset of action because of a low blood:gas partition coefficient. Nitrous oxide is neither explosive nor highly metabolized.

48. The answer is E. *(Pharmacology; dopamine receptor antagonism; tardive dyskinesia)*
Metoclopramide is a potent dopamine receptor antagonist that can cause tardive dyskinesia in nonpsychiatric patients. Tardive dyskinesia frequently involves the orobuccal area. Dystonia is a sustained muscle spasm that occurs as an early complication of treatment with an antidopaminergic drug. Wilson's and Huntington's diseases cause chorea, but there is no history to suggest these diseases.

49. The answer is A. *(Pathology; hairy cell leukemia)*
Hairy cell leukemia is caused by expansion of neoplastic B lymphocytes, which often produce monoclonal

immunoglobulin. The disorder is usually seen in patients older than the age of 40 years, and there is a definite male preponderance. These leukemic cells have cytoplasmic (hairy) projections, that can be seen on a blood smear by phase microscopy. These cells also stain positively for tartrate-resistant acid phosphatase (TRAP).

50. The answer is E. *(Pathology; chronic myelogenous leukemia)*
Leukocytosis is the most prominent laboratory finding in patients with chronic myelogenous leukemia (CML). Accompanying the leukocytosis of CML is a marked elevation of serum vitamin B_{12} levels, as well as an increased serum vitamin B_{12}-binding capacity. Elevated levels in the serum of patients with CML are caused by the turnover of the increased granulocytic mass. CML is characterized by marked splenomegaly and the production of increased numbers of granulocytes, particularly neutrophils. The sexes are affected equally. More than 95% of patients with CML have a unique and characteristic chromosome marker in metaphases of marrow—the Philadelphia (Ph) chromosome.

51. The answer is B. *(Biochemistry; titration of glycine, isoelectric point, pK_a)*
Titration of the diprotic form of glycine involves the net removal of one proton from one molecule of glycine. When observing a titration curve for glycine, the addition of base results in two stages on the curve with two pK_a values (pK_a represents the negative logarithm of the acid ionization constant). At very low pH values, the fully protonated form of glycine predominates (^+H_3N—CH_2—COOH). The midpoint of the first stage of the curve, the pH = pK_1 of the ionizing group (COOH), is equal to 2.4. At very high pH values, a proton is removed from the ionizable group $^+NH_3$ so that the predominate form of glycine is H_2N—CH_2—COO$^-$. The midpoint of this section of the curve is 9.6 where the pH = pK_2. The isoelectric point (pI) is the midpoint between the two stages in the titration curve and represents the fully ionized, dipolar form of glycine with no net electric charge. Because glycine has no ionizable group in its side chain, pI is determined by the equation pI = $1/2(pK_1 + pK_2)$.

52. The answer is E. *(Biochemistry; blood glucose and insulin)*
When blood glucose levels fall below normal levels, insulin release is decreased, and there is a secretion of glucagon. Glucagon then induces several effects on the liver. Liver glycogen breakdown is increased by activating glycogen phosphorylase and inactivating glycogen synthase. Increased levels of glucagon also inhibit glucose breakdown by glycolysis in the liver and increase glucose synthesis by glyconeogenesis. All of these effects allow the liver to export glucose to the blood to raise blood glucose levels back to normal.

53. The answer is A. *(Biochemistry; enzyme inhibitors)*
There are two major classes of enzyme inhibitors, reversible and irreversible. Irreversible inhibitors combine with or destroy a functional group on an enzyme that is essential for its activity. The three types of reversible inhibitors are competitive, noncompetitive, and uncompetitive. A competitive inhibitor follows steady-state kinetics in which it competes with substrate for the active site of the enzyme. A noncompetitive inhibitor binds to a site outside of the substrate binding site so that it does not compete for substrate binding and can inhibit enzyme function with or without substrate present. An uncompetitive inhibitor also binds to a distinct site outside of the substrate binding site but inhibits enzyme function only when substrate is bound to the enzyme.

54. The answer is B. *(Pharmacology; gout)*
Colchicine is the anti-inflammatory drug of choice for gout. Allopurinol inhibits xanthine oxidase, the enzyme that converts hypoxanthine to xanthine, and xanthine to uric acid. Thus, allopurinol decreases urate production and is efficacious for the treatment of gout.

55. The answer is A. *(Embryology; cardiovascular system)*

Both branches of the fourth aortic arch remain intact during fetal development. In adults, the left fourth aortic arch forms the aortic arch, and the right fourth aortic arch forms the proximal segment of the right subclavian artery. During development, the first and second aortic arches all but disappear. In adults, they form the maxillary, hyoid, and stapedial arteries. The third aortic arch forms the common carotid artery. The fifth aortic arch disappears. The sixth aortic arch forms the proximal segment of the right pulmonary artery and the ductus arteriosus.

56. The answer is C. *(Immunology; etiology of autoimmune disease)*
Forbidden clones provide a supply of cells that can recognize self-antigens and will serve as cells to stimulate both humoral and cell-mediated immune responses, leading to autoimmunity. B-cell deficiency—primarily a lack of circulating B cells—is a major cause of hypogammaglobulinemia. Type I hypersensitivity (anaphylactic hypersensitivity) is mediated by humoral antibodies, which result from a normal immune response to exogenous antigens. The deletion of forbidden clones leads to tolerance to autoantigens—the opposite of autoimmunity.

57. The answer is D. *(Pharmacology; empiric antibacterial therapy in an immunocompromised host)*
The most likely diagnosis of this patient's condition is septic shock secondary to bacteremia. Chemotherapy for cancer is a common cause of neutropenia with subsequent fever and infection. The risk is high when the white blood cell count is less than $500/\mu l$. In addition, cold, clammy skin is indicative of peripheral vascular shutdown. Lactic acid buildup will lead to metabolic acidosis and compensatory rapid breathing. Patients with neutropenic fever must be treated with double broad-spectrum antibacterial agents for gram-negative rods, including *Pseudomonas*. The combination of piperacillin, a broad-spectrum beta-lactam, and gentamicin, an aminoglycoside that has broad gram-negative activity, is a good choice. In addition, penicillin–aminoglycoside combinations may be synergistic because of the different mechanisms of action of these agents: Penicillins are cell wall synthesis inhibitors, and aminoglycosides inhibit protein synthesis. Single-agent therapy with gentamicin or amikacin would not be as effective for resistant organisms. Both chloramphenicol and gentamicin are protein synthesis inhibitors and would not be expected to work synergistically.

58–60. The answers are: 58-C, 59-E, 60-A. *(Behavioral Science; medical ethics)*
If the physician's sole concern is not to harm the patient with unnecessary worry, the guiding principle is nonmaleficence. If her sole concern is to be able to benefit the patient with urography (which is impossible if the patient refuses because of concerns about the risks), the guiding principle is beneficence. Both are possible. Justice is irrelevant, and gratitude (e.g., for the patient's patronage) is, at most, marginally relevant.

If the physician decides to do what others of her profession do in like circumstances, she is acting without appeal to the independent ethical principles of beneficence and nonmaleficence. Depending on what the professional practice standard dictates, the disclosure decision might prove to be respectful of autonomy or strongly paternalistic, but the decision would still be guided by professional practice. Weak paternalism is entirely irrelevant because the patient is competent.

If the physician is guided by respect for the patient's preferences, she is acting with respect for her patient's autonomy. If the patient would want disclosure, it is possible that such disclosure could fail to benefit him or could even harm him, so neither beneficence nor maleficence is guiding the physician's thinking. Clearly, the basis for her thinking is independent of the usual practice of her profession.

61. The answer is D. *(Ultraviolet damage to DNA)*
Ultraviolet (UV) light causes cross-linking of thymidine base pairs in DNA and cross-links thymidine to cytosine (forming pyrimidine–pyrimidine dimers). In bacteria such as *Escherichia coli*, these lesions are repaired by a system of proteins called the SOS system, which includes the RecA protein, which is involved in the recombination of normal DNA and the repair of damaged DNA, and thus it would not be advantageous

to decrease its activity. Also, it would be foolish to overlap the genes concerned, because one pyrimidine base pair could potentially impair all the genes involved. Removal of introns would also be disadvantageous, because introns are thought to act as buffers of inactive DNA so that a mutation can occur without disrupting the gene. Genes produced with low thymidine content, however, may be less susceptible to damage by UV radiation because fewer pyrimidine base pairs would be involved.

62. The answer is B. *(Histopathology; neuroblastoma)*
Neuroblastomas arise from neural crest cells of the adrenal medulla. The tumors are usually large and soft, with a red–gray cut surface. They may be calcified, with areas of hemorrhage and necrosis. The tumor cells have hyperchromatic nuclei and indistinct eosinophilic cytoplasm. The nuclei are arranged in a spoke-like pattern around a characteristic central mass of neuritic cell processes, called Homer-Wright pseudorosettes, as seen in the illustration. Like pheochromocytomas, neuroblastomas produce catecholamines, but, unlike pheochromocytomas, they do not cause systemic hypertension.

63. The answer is D. *(Genetics; Turner syndrome)*
The patient presented in the question is a classic example of a child with Turner syndrome (i.e., short stature, webbed neck, cubitus valgus), which is best diagnosed through chromosome analysis. The genotype of this patient is most likely to be 45,X. None of the other tests listed in the question would contribute to the diagnosis of Turner syndrome.

64. The answer is A. *(Biochemistry; Michaelis-Menten equation)*
The Michaelis-Menten equation defines the rate equation for a one-substrate, enzyme-catalyzed reaction. The equation is $V_0 = V_{max} [S]/K_m + [S]$, where V_0 = initial velocity, V_{max} = maximum initial velocity, $[S]$ = initial substrate concentration, and K_m = Michaelis-Menten. This equation was derived to explain the rate of a reaction catalyzed by an enzyme that is affected by a continuously changing substrate concentration as substrate is converted to product. Based on this equation, at low levels of $[S]$, $K_m >> [S]$ so that $[S]$ in the denominator of the equation is insignificant. This changes the equation to $V_0 = V_{max} [S]/K_m$, so that V_0 is linearly dependent on $[S]$. When $[S] >> K_m$, the equation is now changed to $V_0 = V_{max}$ because K_m becomes insignificant and the term $[S]$ cancels out. When V_0 is exactly one-half of V_{max}, $K_m = [S]$. $V_0 = 0$ when the equation is now $V_0 = 0$ and not V_{max}.

65. The answer is B. *(Biochemistry; amino acid catabolism)*
The amount of alanine released from skeletal muscle is greater than the amount that can be accounted for in muscle protein. The catabolism of many amino acids in muscle involves the transamination of α-amino groups from amino acids to pyruvate, producing alanine. Thus, the carbon skeleton of much of the alanine released from muscle is derived from glucose via the glycolytic pathway.

66. The answer is A. *(Microbiology; malaria)*
Of the major diseases with geographic relevance, malaria is one of the few that can be rapidly life-threatening. The other diseases listed (i.e., chronic Chagas disease, amebic dysentery, mucocutaneous leishmaniasis, and giardiasis) are either chronically debilitating or subpatent in nature. Amebic dysentery and giardiasis are not life-threatening conditions, and it is not necessary to determine the causative species for treatment of either. No effective treatment exists for chronic Chagas disease, so rapid diagnosis is not essential. Although determination of the species of *Leishmania* is useful in distinguishing cutaneous and mucocutaneous leishmaniasis in terms of treatment, both are long-term infections and are not life-threatening.

67–68. The answers are: 67-D, 68-C. *(Pharmacology; volume of distribution; half-life of elimination)*
The volume of distribution (V_d) is approximately 10 L. V_d is defined as V_d = dose/Cp, where Cp is the

plasma concentration at zero time. In this case, the Cp can be estimated easily because the log plasma concentration versus time plot is linear; it is approximately 100 μg/ml. Thus,

$$V_d = \frac{(20 \text{ mg/kg}) (50 \text{ kg})}{0.1 \text{ mg/ml}}$$
$$= \quad 10,000 \text{ ml}$$
$$= \quad 10 \text{ L}$$

The half-life of elimination of this drug is approximately 4 hours. The half-life of elimination can be determined graphically from the slope of the linear plot. First, note the time when a given concentration (e.g., 50 μg/ml) was detected (5 hours). Next, determine the time when half of the original value (25 μg/ml) was detected (9 hours). Then, calculate the half-life of elimination: 9 − 5 = 4 hours.

69. The answer is A. *(Biochemistry; protein post-translational modifications)*
After proteins are synthesized (translated), many are glycosylated in the lumen of the endoplasmic reticulum and the Golgi complex. Oligosaccharides are attached to proteins by *N*-glycosylation of asparagine side chains or by *O*-glycosylation of serine and threonine side chains. The transfer of oligosaccharides is mediated by an activated lipid carrier, dolichol phosphate.

70. The answer is D. *(Pharmacology; properties of tricyclic antidepressants)*
Tricyclic antidepressants, such as imipramine, inhibit neuronal uptake of norepinephrine, serotonin, and other central nervous system (CNS) amines. Potentiation of local concentrations of these amines may underlie the ability of these agents to reverse symptoms of depression after chronic administration over several weeks. The parent and metabolite compounds of many of these drugs can directly or indirectly affect cardiac function (including α-adrenergic receptor blockade) and, thus, may cause orthostatic hypotension and cardiac dysrhythmias. Indeed, suicide with these agents is quite common, and the cause of death is related to cardiac toxicity. The drugs do not appear to affect dopamine receptors significantly in the concentrations used clinically. Some agents are more selective for serotonin uptake (e.g., fluoxetine, which is not a tricyclic antidepressant) than for norepinephrine uptake (e.g., desipramine, which is a tricyclic antidepressant).

71–72. The answers are: 71-C, 72-C. *(Genetics; cystic fibrosis)*
The frequency of the cystic fibrosis gene is 1/40, the square root of the incidence. Remembering the Hardy-Weinberg law, the gene frequency is equal to the square root of the incidence (q^2). If the incidence = q^2 = 1/1600, then the square root of the incidence, the gene frequency (q), = 1/40.

The proportion of normal siblings of individuals with cystic fibrosis who would be expected to be carriers is 2/3. Due to the recessive pattern of inheritance of cystic fibrosis, each offspring has a 1 in 4 chance of inheriting the disease. This leaves a chance that 2 of the 3 individuals will be heterozygotes, or carriers, for the cystic fibrosis gene. A simple punnet square will reveal that of the possible genotypes one can have in the offspring (of those individuals carrying a recessive disorder), 1 in 4 will have the double dose, or be homozygous for the recessive gene. Two individuals will have a single dose of the recessive gene and be carriers, and one will be normal. Because cystic fibrosis carriers are not clinically affected, there would be 3 normal individuals possible in the offspring. Two of those three will be carriers, hence the 2/3 proportion.

73. The answer is D. *(Immunology; transplants)*
Rejection that occurs a few minutes to a few hours after transplantation is termed hyperacute rejection. It is the result of preformed circulating antibodies to the graft that were made as a result of previous transplantations, blood transfusions, or pregnancies. It usually transpires minutes after the donor kidney is anastomosed, although it can proceed over a period of a few days. The antibodies activate the complement sytem, with ensuing swelling, interstitial hemorrhage, and thrombotic occlusion followed by outright infarction of the kidney. The only therapy is removal of the transplanted tissue.

74. The answer is E. *(Behavioral science; defense mechanisms)*
Borderline patients tend to view things as extremes of black and white, with little ability to perceive the gray zones. In splitting, negative feelings are split off and attributed to one person (or thing), while positive feelings are attributed to another, without the realization that people have both good and bad features. Borderline patients may also project, deny, displace, and manipulate, but the example in the question is of splitting.

75. The answer is C. *(Physiology; regulation of arterial blood pressure)*
A rise in arterial blood pressure within the carotid sinus or an increase in pressure secondary to mechanical massage leads to activation of baroreceptors, which subsequently causes inhibition of the central vasoconstrictor center with activation of the central vagal center. The net short-term effect is a decrease in blood pressure, heart rate, and cardiac output. Ultimately, baroreceptors adapt to the stimulus and are unimportant in the long-term regulation of blood pressure. Clamping of the carotid arteries (in a vagotomized animal) will decrease baroreceptor firing and remove inhibitory pathways from the central nervous system (CNS), leading to increases in pressure and heart rate.

76. The answer is D. *(Pharmacology; properties of lidocaine)*
Local anesthetics block Na^+ channels and decrease conductance of Na^+, thereby inhibiting depolarization and normal conduction of action potentials. Small, myelinated nerve fibers are most sensitive, and differential sensitivity explains preferential blockade for pain sensation as opposed to other sensory modalities. Lidocaine is highly lipid-soluble and may cause convulsions in the central nervous system (CNS) if sufficient amounts are delivered to the brain. By affecting Na^+ channels in cardiovascular tissue, dysrhythmia and decreased contractility may ensue. The ester anesthetics, such as procaine, are substrates for plasma cholinesterases, whereas lidocaine is more slowly metabolized in the liver. Local anesthetics, such as lidocaine, are often used in spinal anesthesia to produce more widespread blockage of neurotransmission.

77. The answer is D. *(Histology; cytoskeleton)*
In muscle cells, actin and myosin filaments cause muscle contraction by a process known as the "sliding filament hypothesis." In nonmuscle cells, actin is involved with endocytosis, exocytosis, cell locomotion, and cytokinesis. The acrosome reaction in sperm of invertebrates allows fusion with an egg and polymerization of actin. The mitotic spindle is composed of the microtubule protein tubulin, not actin.

78. The answer is B. *(Histology; mitochondria)*
Mitochondria are organelles unlike the others within the cell. They contain a ring of DNA that codes for some of the proteins they require; the other proteins are encoded by the nuclear genes. Mitochondria also use a slightly altered genetic code than that used by other mammalian genes: Mitochondria have only 22 transfer RNA (tRNA) molecules (as opposed to 32 in the nucleus), so that 1 tRNA molecule must cover more codons. Some codons are also different (e.g., UGA, a termination codon normally, is a tryptophan codon to mitochondrial tRNA). Finally genes encoding the proteins overlap one another, perhaps reflecting the fact that the genome is so small (16,500 base pairs).

79. The answer is A. *(Microbiology; presentation of cutaneous erythema)*
The etiologic agent of erysipeloid is *Erysipelothrix rhusiopathiae*, a bacterium widely distributed in the environment. Human erysipeloid is clinically described as a slowly spreading cutaneous erythema. Cutaneous edema is characteristic, and the disease is very painful. Cutaneous diphtheria is characterized by a necrotic lesion sometimes associated with insect bites; the bite apparently provides the break in the skin through which toxigenic *Corynebacterium diphtheriae* enters the tissue. Cutaneous nocardiosis is characterized by draining sinus tracts discharging purulent exudate-containing granules. Pontiac fever and listeriosis do not have cutaneous manifestations.

80. The answer is A. (Genetics; gene duplications)
There are as many as 100 to 1000 gene families that contain similar sequences. β-Tubulins and β-like globins are perfect examples of duplicated gene families. There are at least two nonfunctional regions in the human β-like globin gene cluster that have sequences similar to functional β-like genes. Analysis of their DNA sequences shows that they retain their intron/exon structure, but some sequence drift has resulted in sequences that block transcription or terminate protein translation. Some gene duplications, such as those for ribosomal and transfer RNA (rRNA and tRNA), along with genes coding for histones, are necessary to meet the demands of the cell for messenger RNA (mRNA) transcripts. Although there is no accepted model for duplication, it is thought to involve unequal crossover during meiosis.

81. The answer is B. (Genetics; Hardy-Weinberg law)
The frequency of carriers of Tay-Sachs disease can be calculated from the Hardy-Weinberg law, in which the carrier frequency is equal to 2 pq: q is calculated by taking the square root of the incidence, which gives the frequency of the gene, 1 in 60, and p is equal to $1 - q$, or $60/60 - 1/60$, which gives 59/60. As can be seen here, in most cases of rare diseases, p becomes equal to 1, and the carrier frequency then becomes 2q, or $2 \times 1/60$, which gives a carrier frequency of 1/30.

82. The answer is D. (Biochemistry; lipids and arachidonic acid metabolism)
Leukotrienes are compounds formed as the result of the action of lipoxygenase on arachidonic acid. Platelet activating factor (PAF) is an ether phospholipid. Eosinophil chemotactic factor (ECF) is a set of peptides that produces a chemotactic gradient to attract eosinophils. Thromboxanes (TXA_2), like prostaglandins, are synthesized through the action of cyclooxygenase, a reaction that is inhibited by acetylsalicylic acid.

83–84. The answers are: 83-C, 84-A. (Physiology; neuroanatomy; hypoxic injury)
The first of the motor functions to become deficient during hypoxic injury to the brain would be the ability to move the arms. This is due to the fact that the most distal ends of the anterior and middle cerebral arteries anastomose in the cerebral hemispheres over the location on the motor gyrus controlling the arms. The neurons in this anastomosing zone are very sensitive to hypoxic injury.

The hippocampus is well known for its sensitivity to hypoxic injury. Because this area of the brain is involved in immediate memory recall, the patient will not remember where he is nor will he remember his physicians. He will have trouble in the future functioning independently because of this lesion. Recognition of family members would involve distant, or remote, memory, which is not involved with hippocampal functioning. The patient would also be able to perform cognitive functions, such as addition and reading.

85. The answer is D. (Pharmacology; surgical prophylactic antibacterial therapy; drug resistance)
Ampicillin is an extended-spectrum penicillin, which has greater action against some gram-negative organisms compared with penicillin G and early generation semisynthetic penicillins such as methicillin. However, ampicillin is susceptible to beta-lactamases and may not be effective when administered prophylactically against beta-lactamase–containing *Staphylococcus aureus*. Cefazolin is a prototypical first-generation cephalosporin, which has good activity against staphylococcal infections and is relatively impervious to beta-lactamases. Methicillin is prototypical of beta-lactamase–resistant penicillins. Vancomycin is a cell wall synthesis inhibitor with exclusive gram-positive antibacterial activity, owing to its large molecular size, which does not allow it to enter gram-negative bacteria through porins. Vancomycin is not susceptible to beta-lactamases. Imipenem is a beta-lactam antibiotic, which is resistant to beta-lactamases.

86. The answer is D. (Immunology; hypersensitivity reactions)
ABO or Rh incompatibility, the cause of erythroblastosis fetalis, is the result of blood group differences between the mother and the child. Normally, in cases of Rh-incompatible mating, human anti-D globulin

(RhoGAM), an anti-Rh antibody, would be given to the mother shortly after the birth of her first Rh-positive child. This would clear the child's Rh-positive red cells from the mother's circulation before she can be immunized. In the case described in the question, the mother has blood type O negative with normal isohemagglutinin titers, so the preexisting ABO compatibility should clear her system of any "leaked" fetal blood cells. Administration of RhoGAM to an Rh-positive child will cause hemolytic anemia in that child.

87. The answer is B. *(Physiology; gas exchange)*
Anemia reduces the oxygen-carrying capacity of the blood but does not affect arterial oxygen tension. Thus, oxygen delivery is decreased and venous oxygen will have a lower partial pressure at rest and during exercise in the anemic subject. The anemic subject is patient *B* because his oxygen content is reduced for every level of Po_2.

88. The answer is C. *(Physiology; toxins; neurotransmission)*
The woman is suffering from botulism, which is caused by the neurotoxin botulin. The action of botulin involves inhibition of acetylcholine (ACh) release from peripheral nerve endings at the neuromuscular junction. Other bacterial toxins have actions described in (A), (B), (D), and (E) [i.e., diphtheria toxin, tetanus toxin, cholera toxin, and streptolysin O, respectively].

89. The answer is D. *(Pathology; gonococcal salpingitis)*
For all practical purposes, the patient is cured. However, women who suffered from gonorrhea are at risk for future complications, such as subsequent episodes of pelvic inflammatory disease, infertility, and ectopic pregnancy.

90. The answer is D. *(Histology; Hassall's corpuscles)*
Hassall's (thymic) corpuscles are found in the thymus. They are concentrically laminated structures of unknown function that appear during fetal development and increase in number with age. They are thought to be degenerated medullary epithelial cells and display varying degrees of keratinization or calcification.

91. The answer is C. *(Biochemistry; fructosuria; glycogen synthesis)*
Essential fructosuria results from a deficiency in fructokinase, which is found only in the liver and catalyzes the first step in the assimilation of fructose by the liver. Under normal conditions, almost all of the fructose is converted to fructose 1-phosphate and is metabolized in the liver. Hexokinase, which is present in all extrahepatic tissues, can convert fructose to fructose 6-phosphate; however, the K_m of hexokinase for fructose is sufficiently high that this reaction does not occur to any significant extent. When, as a consequence of a deficiency in fructokinase, the accumulation of fructose is high enough, it is converted to fructose 6-phosphate in extrahepatic tissues and metabolized by the glycolytic pathway. Glucokinase, which is found in the liver, is specific for glucose and cannot catalyze the phosphorylation of fructose. Aldolase B is specific for fructose 1-phosphate. Transketolase is a part of the nonoxidative phase of the pentose phosphate pathway.

92. The answer is C. *(Physiology; pathogenesis of renal osteodystrophy)*
Normally, approximately 90% of serum phosphate is not protein-bound and, thus, is filterable at the glomerulus. Of the filtered phosphate, approximately 75% is actively reabsorbed, mainly by cotransport with sodium in the proximal tubule. In chronic renal failure, hyperphosphatemia occurs as the glomerular filtration rate declines. Hyperphosphatemia produces a secondary hyperparathyroidism as excess phosphate ties up the free serum calcium, in essence leading to hypocalcemia. 1,25-Dihydroxyvitamin D_3 levels are reduced directly by the inability of the damaged kidney to convert the 25-hydroxyvitamin D_3 produced by the liver from inactive vitamin D_3 to 1,25-dihydroxyvitamin D_3 and indirectly by the ability of high serum phosphate levels to directly inhibit renal 25-hydroxyvitamin D_3 hydroxylase activity.

93. The answer is B. *(Hematology; differential diagnosis of coagulation disorders)*
Factor XI deficiency is autosomally transmitted and can result in serious postoperative bleeding, although it may be mild enough to cause no spontaneous symptoms. Neither factor XII nor Fletcher factor deficiencies result in a bleeding disorder, and inherited factor VIII deficiency occurs only in males. Severe von Willebrand's disease could result in a positive family history and significant bleeding, but rarely is the factor VIII: C low enough to prolong the partial thromboplastin time (PTT), especially when the bleeding time is normal.

94. The answer is B. *(Microbiology; enteric infections)*
Salmonella typhi is a highly invasive pathogen that is readily disseminated throughout the body. In typhoid fever, this organism invades through the intestinal mucosa and spreads through the body via the lymphatic system. In nontyphoid *Salmonella* infections, the bacteria invade the intestinal submucosa but usually do not spread into other regions of the body. *Campylobacter jejuni* and *Shigella dysenteriae* invade the intestinal mucosa but usually do not penetrate the submucosa or spread throughout the body. *Vibrio cholerae* is noninvasive.

95–96. The answers are: 95-C, 96-D. *(Microbiology; etiology of fungal infections; antifungal therapy)*
The clinical signs and history are consistent with oropharyngeal candidiasis (thrush). This patient is most likely immunocompromised because of her adjuvant chemotherapy. In addition, antibacterial therapy for urinary tract infection predisposes her to develop a fungal infection because of depletion of floral bacteria. Opportunistic, endogenous *Candida* infections in the mouth are common under these conditions. Sporotrichosis is an endogenous systemic infection. Cryptococcosis is also a systemic infection. Dermatophytes usually appear on hair, nails, and skin.

Griseofulvin is effective for dermatophyte infections of nails and hair; it concentrates in the stratum corneum and outer epidermis and stops fungal growth in these tissues. Ketoconazole, fluconazole, and clotrimazole are ergosterol synthesis inhibitors, which are fungistatic or fungicidal (at high concentrations) for *Candida*. Nystatin, a polyene, binds to membrane ergosterol and affects membrane permeability and integrity. Nystatin, like the more commonly used polyene amphotericin B, is fungicidal. Nystatin is effective only in topical preparations for candidiasis, whereas amphotericin B is commonly used systemically. Clotrimazole is effective topically against candidiasis.

97. The answer is C. *(Histology; histopathology of rheumatoid arthritis)*
The synovium pictured in the photomicrograph shows the classic features of a rheumatoid nodule in a patient with rheumatoid arthritis, a disease that affects primarily women. Rheumatoid arthritis initially affects the small joints of the hands and feet and then the larger joints of the knees and elbows. The synovium becomes infiltrated by lymphocytes and plasma cells with lymphoid follicle formation. In some cases, central fibrinoid necrosis occurs with an intense palisade of histiocytes and giant cells forming around the necrotic material, as in this case. Rheumatoid nodules occur in the skin and subcutis, particularly on extensor surfaces, but may also occur in unusual sites such as the lungs, heart, and spleen.

98. The answer is D. *(Pathology; macroscopic features of Crohn's disease)*
The photomicrograph shows chronic inflammation of the bowel, typical of Crohn's disease, or terminal ileitis. This transmural inflammation accounts for the thickened bowel wall. If the process extends into pericolic fat, thick, edematous ''creeping fat'' and fistulae would be seen. The presence of a small granuloma at the base of the colonic gland is helpful in confirming the diagnosis of Crohn's disease. Pseudopolyps occur in ulcerative colitis and are a means of differentiating ulcerative colitis from Crohn's disease.

99. The answer is A. *(Cell biology; functions of nucleic acids)*
RNA differs from DNA by the number of hydroxyl groups present on the sugar moieties and in the kind of pyrimidine bases used; RNA has uracil substituted for thymidine. Because these differences are fairly minor,

RNA can take on the same configurations as DNA; that is, it can be linear, circular, double-stranded, or single-stranded. Molecules of transfer RNA (tRNA) are a perfect example of RNA that has base-paired with itself to form double strands. RNA acts catalytically in certain messenger RNA (mRNA) splicing reactions and is the primary genetic material for a number of viruses.

100. The answer is D. *(Pharmacology; histamine receptor antagonists)*
Cimetidine and ranitidine are H_2-receptor blockers whose main clinical use is in the treatment of ulcers and other peptic disorders. They block the effects of histamine on gastric acid secretion. H_2 antagonists inhibit, not enhance, cytochrome P450 enzymes of the liver. H_1 antagonists (e.g., diphenhydramine, chlorpheniramine) are useful in treating allergies. They also have central effects that are useful in preventing motion sickness; however, they can also cause unwanted sedation.

101. The answer is D. *(Biochemistry; peptide bonds)*
The chemistry of the peptide bond imposes restrictions on higher orders of protein structure. The secondary structure of proteins is stabilized by hydrogen bonds that are formed between the amide hydrogen and carbonyl oxygen of the peptide bond. Because the atoms of the peptide bond lie in a plane, the only rotations that are permissible are around the $C\alpha$—C and the N—$C\alpha$ bonds. There is no formal charge associated with the peptide bond; the electrons of the carbonyl oxygen and the lone pair of electrons on the nitrogen atom are delocalized.

102. The answer is A. *(Physiology; calcium homeostasis)*
Ethylenediaminetetraacetic acid (EDTA) is a chelator of Ca^{2+} but is not normally found within cells and, thus, is not a mechanism by which cells regulate Ca^{2+} concentration. Two important transmembrane proteins in Ca^{2+} homeostasis are the Ca^{2+} adenosine triphosphate (ATPase) pump and the Na^+–Ca^{2+} transport chain. Ca^{2+} binds to a number of intracellular proteins, such as calsequestrin, and these proteins are found in high concentration in the endoplasmic reticulum.

103. The answer is B. *(Genetics; autosomal dominant inheritance)*
Every child has a 50% chance of inheriting a condition with an autosomal dominant mode of inheritance. This does not mean that in a family with eight children, four will necessarily be affected and four unaffected, although this is statistically the most likely possibility. It is also possible that all children will be affected or all will be unaffected, although these possibilities are unlikely.

104. The answer is D. *(Biochemistry; enzyme inhibition)*
The data in the Lineweaver-Burk plot are diagnostic of noncompetitive inhibition. The intercept on the $1/[S]$ axis indicates that the inhibitor has no effect on the K_m for the substrate. The increase in the $1/v$ intercept observed in the presence of the inhibitor indicates a decrease in the V_{max} of the reaction. Noncompetitive inhibitors interact at a site other than the active site. They usually bear no structural resemblance to either the substrate or the transition-state analogs, and their effects cannot be reversed by high concentrations of substrates. Competitive inhibitors, however, interact at the active site, are structurally related to transition-state analogs, and can be reversed by high concentrations of substrate.

105. The answer is B. *(Biochemistry; serine and threonine kinases)*
Protein kinase C is a member of a class of kinases that phosphorylates only serine and threonine, not tyrosines. Protein kinase C is activated by lipids and Ca^{2+}; when activation occurs, protein kinase C moves from the cytoplasm to the plasma membrane via the process called translocation. It is degraded by a calcium-activated protease to form the lipid- and Ca^{2+}-independent protein kinase M.

106. The answer is D. *(Physiology; alveolar ventilation)*
Alveolar ventilation is the product of respiratory rate $\times$ (tidal volume $-$ dead space). In this situation total dead space (400 ml) is the sum of the patient's anatomic dead space (150 ml) and the ventilator's dead space (250 ml). Thus, if the total output of the ventilator is adjusted to 600 ml, then 200 ml of the alveolar volume will be delivered 20 times per minute, and total minute alveolar ventilation will be 4 L/min.

107. The answer is E. *(Anatomy; microcirculation)*
Fenestrated capillaries have circular pores (fenestrae), which are 60 nm to 100 nm in diameter and may be partially surrounded by pericytes. The fenestrae often are spanned by a slit diaphragm, which is filamentous and, thus, does not possess a unit membrane structure. Fenestrated capillaries are present in areas where there is a great deal of molecular exchange with blood (e.g., kidneys, small intestine, endocrine glands, choroid plexus). Although glomerular capillaries are fenestrated, they lack a slit diaphragm; a thick basement membrane forms the filtration barrier.

108. The answer is E. *(Microbiology; pathogenesis of infectious microorganisms)*
Borrelia burgdorferi is spread by ticks and is the cause of Lyme disease. *Rickettsia rickettsii* also is usually spread by ticks. *Clostridium tetani* enters the body through wounds. *Neisseria meningitidis* and *Corynebacterium diphtheriae* both enter via the respiratory tract.

109–111. The answers are: 109-A, 110-C, 111-B. *(Neuroanatomy; neurologic lesions and syndromes)*
The deficits described in the question indicate destruction of cranial nerve (CN) III motor function and total autonomic function of the eye, combined with a spastic paralysis of the contralateral body, indicating upper motor neuron destruction (as opposed to flaccid paralysis, indicating lower motor neuron disease). CN III fibers leave the brain at the level of the midbrain to continue to the ipsilateral eye. CN III is responsible for moving the eye nasally and vertically in both directions; therefore, loss of CN III function results in lateral deviation of the eye. CN III also carries autonomic fibers that originate in the Edinger-Westphal nucleus and are responsible for constriction of the pupil to light and for accommodation. Riding with the oculomotor nerve are sympathetic fibers responsible for dilation of the pupil. The destruction of all of these functions together indicates a lesion of the midbrain where it intersects with the corticospinal tract.

The artery that supplies this intersection of midbrain and corticospinal tract is the posterior cerebral artery. The basilar artery supplies the pons. The middle cerebral artery supplies most of the cerebral hemisphere of either side.

Weber's syndrome is a lesion of the crus cerebri, through which the corticospinal tract passes, as well as a lesion of tissue through which the oculomotor nerve passes. Millard-Gubler syndrome is similar to Weber's syndrome, but the lesion is lower and involves the pons, causing CN VI and CN VII palsy as well as upper motor neuron paralysis of the contralateral body. Brown-Séquard syndrome is a lesion of the spinal cord, involving upper motor neuron damage and weakness of one leg, with contralateral pain and temperature sensitivity of the other.

112. The answer is C. *(Physiology; signal transduction; protein kinases)*
Protein kinase C is activated by Ca^{2+} and diacylglycerol, not by cyclic adenosine monophosphate (cAMP). Cyclic AMP is synthesized from adenosine triphosphate (ATP) in a reaction that is catalyzed by adenylate cyclase. The activity of adenylate cyclase may be either increased or decreased in response to hormone stimulation. Cyclic AMP is the second messenger for the effect of parathyroid hormone (PTH) on the kidney; cAMP also activates protein kinase A. The binding of cAMP to the regulatory subunit results in the dissociation of the regulatory and catalytic subunits and a concomitant increase in protein kinase activity. The degradation of cAMP is mediated by a family of phosphodiesterases, which catalyze the hydrolysis to $5'$-AMP.

113. The answer is B. *(Physiology; glycogen storage diseases)*
Glycogen storage disease type Ia, or von Gierke's disease, is caused by defective glucose-6-phosphatase activity and is characterized by hepatomegaly, renomegaly, and hypoglycemia. The liver shows intracyto-plasmic accumulation of glycogen and a small amount of lipid along with some intranuclear glycogen. The kidney has intracytoplasmic accumulations of glycogen in the cortical tubular epithelial cells. The intestine also shows increased concentrations of glycogen.

114. The answer is E. *(Biochemistry; Tay-Sachs disease)*
Tay-Sachs disease has a reported 1 in 30 carrier rate among Ashkenazi Jews, which is about 10 times higher than in other population groups. It is a lysosomal storage disease caused by mutations in the gene coding for hexosaminidase A, leading to a virtual absence of this enzyme. Deficiency of hexosaminidase A results in an accumulation of GM_2 gangliosides, which normally make up 1%–3% of total brain gangliosides but comprise over 90% in individuals with Tay-Sachs disease. Lack of the enzyme β-galactosidase is an autosomal recessive disorder; however, unlike Tay-Sachs disease, it results in lysosomal storage of GM_1 gangliosides.

115. The answer is D. *(Physiology; coronary artery blood flow)*
Coronary blood flow closely matches myocardial work (or oxygen consumption). Myocardial oxygen extrac-tion is near maximal at rest and does not increase appreciably, even during exercise. Coronary blood flow is maximal during diastole, in which ventricular compression of the capillaries is minimal. In addition, there is significant heterogeneity across the ventricular wall during systole, such that subendocardial blood flow is reduced, and blood flow is shifted to the epicardial vessels. Autoregulation is normally observed in the myocardium, such that blood flow does not change over a large range of perfusion pressures.

116. The answer is B. *(Biochemistry; oxidation reactions, cofactors)*
In many oxidation reactions, hydrogen atoms are transferred from a substrate to a hydrogen exceptor. This process involves the use of electron carriers such as the following nucleotides: oxidized nicotinamide adenine dinucleotide (NAD^+), oxidized nicotinamide adenine dinucleotide phosphate ($NADP^+$), flavin mononucleotide (FMN), and flavin adenine dinucleotide (FAD). These cofactors are water soluble and involved with several reversible oxidation–reduction reactions. NAD^+ and $NADP^+$ are freely diffusible in that they move from one dehydrogenase to the next. They are transformed to their reduced form after accepting one proton and two electrons. FAD and FMN are tightly bound to flavoproteins, which catalyze oxidation–reduction reactions using these flavonucleotides as cofactors. Because they can accept either one or two electrons, flavoproteins containing FAD and FMN prosthetic groups are involved in a wide variety of reactions.

117. The answer is B. *(Biochemistry; transcription)*
When DNA is transcribed by RNA polymerase into messenger RNA (mRNA), the primary transcript contains the coding sequences or exons for one gene. However, these coding sequences are disrupted by noncoding sequences termed introns. Introns are removed from the primary transcript by a process known as splicing. The splicing reactions cleave out the introns and join the exons together to form a continuous coding sequence for a functional polypeptide. At the 5U terminal of the primary transcript, a 7-methylguanosine link is added before transcription is complete, forming a 5U cap. This cap serves two functions in that it binds the mature mRNA to the ribosome for translation and it protects the mRNA from degradation. The polyadenylate tail consists of 20–250 adenylate residues, which are added to the 3U end of the mRNA by the enzyme polyadeny-late polymerase. This tail protects mRNA from enzymatic degradation. Methylation is not a part of mRNA processing, but it is a process that occurs on many adenine and cytosine residues on DNA molecules.

118. The answer is D. *(Biochemistry; transcription)*
The initiation of transcription occurs when RNA polymerase recognizes and binds to specific promoter sequences on the DNA molecule found very close to the RNA synthesis start site. Therefore, to regulate

transcription initiation, the interaction between an RNA polymerase protein and its promoter DNA sequence must be controlled. Three types of proteins regulate transcription initiation, including specificity factors, repressors, and activators. Specificity factors regulate the specificity of an RNA polymerase for a given promoter or set of promoters. A repressor binds to a specific DNA region and induces negative regulation by blocking RNA polymerase binding or movement along DNA strands. An activator offers positive regulation by binding to sites adjacent to the promoter region on DNA and enhancing RNA polymerase binding and activity.

119. The answer is D. *(Physiology; membrane physiology and excitation)*
The resting membrane potential is $-$ 90 mV, which is primarily due to diffusion potentials caused by K^+ (and Na^+) and the electrogenic Na^+–$K+$ pump. Stimulation at time zero [e.g., as occurs with acetylcholine (ACh)] activates a Na^+ channel, thereby greatly increasing Na^+ conductance and leading to depolarization. At the peak of the action potential, the number of open Na^+ channels is 10 times greater than the number of open K^+ channels. Within a short period of time, voltage-gated Na^+ is inactivated, and a K^+ channel opens, greatly increasing the conductance to K^+ and, hence, repolarization. The Ca^{2+}–Na^+ channel (if present) is slow to be activated and normally would depolarize the membrane. Chloride channel permeability does not change during an action potential and, thus, functions passively in this process.

120. The answer is B. *(Pathology; neurologic disease)*
The patient described in the question most likely has tabes dorsalis, a disease that results from an untreated syphilis infection. The causative agent is *Treponema pallidum*, and the antibiotic of choice is penicillin. This disease results in the selective destruction of neurons in the spinal cord near the dorsal root of the spinal nerves, which causes the symptoms described in the question. Varicella zoster virus (VZV) causes shingles, a disease resulting from the activation of the virus in dorsal root ganglia of the spinal nerves, and chickenpox, a vesicular disease that usually affects children. Acyclovir is an antiviral agent that interferes with VZV as well as herpes simplex virus replication and, therefore, is not useful here.

121. The answer is C. *(Physiology; glomerular filtration rate)*
Blood enters the glomerulus via an afferent arteriole and leaves via an efferent arteriole. A decrease in renal blood flow (RBF) or a decrease in glomerular hydrostatic pressure tends to decrease the glomerular filtration rate (GFR). Accordingly, constriction of the afferent arteriole generally has this effect. An increase in RBF that increases hydrostatic pressure increases GFR. This effect of RBF persists even without an increase in hydrostatic pressure because of a subtle oncotic effect. Although raising systemic pressure would theoretically increase hydrostatic pressure and GFR, the effect is greatly minimized by normal autoregulation in the kidney. Thus, RBF and hydrostatic pressure are maintained by afferent arteriolar constriction in the presence of this increase over normal systemic pressures. Constriction of the efferent arteriole increases hydrostatic pressure (and GFR), but this effect is also offset by the above-mentioned decrease in RBF; thus, only a modest increase in GFR is normally observed.

122. The answer is A. *(Hematology; neutropenia and infection)*
Neutropenia is defined as an absolute neutrophil count of less than 1500/μl. Although there is a modest risk of acquired infection beginning at this level, patients with neutrophil counts of less than 1000/μl for any length of time are at significant risk of acquired infection and patients with counts below 500/μl are at extreme risk. The percentages of formed elements determined by peripheral blood count are of limited value; they must be multiplied by the total white cell count to arrive at absolute numbers of circulating granulocytes, monocytes, and lymphocytes. Leukocyte percentages determined by a 100-cell manual differential count have extremely broad 95% confidence intervals that may yield broad apparent shifts in absolute numbers. New cell counters with machine analysis of percentages of neutrophils, monocytes, and lymphocytes (even eosinophils and basophils) offer a better estimate of absolute number.

123. The answer is D. *(Biochemistry; DNA and RNA composition)*
DNA is composed of the purines adenine and guanine and the pyrimidines thymine and cytosine. RNA is composed of the same bases with the exception that thymine is replaced by uracil. Therefore, DNA or RNA can be selectively labeled by using tritiated thymine [(^{3}H)-thymine] or tritiated uracil [(^{3}H)-uracil], respectively.

124. The answer is A. *(Biochemistry; integral membrane proteins)*
Integral membrane proteins are stabilized by hydrophobic interactions between the lipid bilayer and the amino acid side chains. Detergents are required for solubilization. Approximately 20 amino acids in an α-helical conformation are required to span the width of the bilayer. These proteins display compositional asymmetry, with the carbohydrate moieties always being on the side of the membrane away from the cytoplasm. They may display lateral, but not transverse, movement within the membrane.

125. The answer is E. *(Pharmacology; urinary tract infection therapy)*
Penicillin G is the treatment of choice. It is inexpensive, and it is a broad-spectrum antibiotic effective in the treatment of urinary tract infections. The serum levels are so low that it is unlikely to alter the natural bacterial flora of the host.

126. The answer is A. *(Immunology; opsonic antibodies)*
Opsonic antibodies are important for acquiring immunity to infection by group A *Neisseria meningitidis* because they permit recognition and destruction of *N. meningitidis* at the onset of infection. *Vibrio cholerae*, *Clostridium botulinum*, and *Shigella flexneri* exert their pathogenic effects via toxins. Opsonic antibodies are not known to protect against the action of *V. cholerae*, *C. botulinum*, or *S. flexneri*.

127. The answer is B. *(Physiology; mechanics of the heart)*
At the end of the period of isovolumic contraction (2), the pressure inside the ventricle has risen to equal the pressure in the aorta at end diastole (80 mm Hg). At this point, ventricular pressures push the aortic valve open, and blood begins to pour out of the left ventricle (3) while it continues to contract. The fraction of end diastolic volume (115 ml) that was ejected was 60% because stroke volume was 115 − 45 = 70 ml. After isovolumic relaxation, left ventricular end diastolic pressure was near atmospheric pressure.

128–129. The answers are: 128-C, 129-D. *(Pathology; chronic myeloproliferative disorder)*
An elevated platelet count and a low white blood cell count are suggestive of chronic myeloproliferative disorder. Malignant lymphoma can be eliminated as a possible diagnosis because of the lack of lymphadenopathy, and acute leukemia can be eliminated because of the lack of blasts on the blood smear. No cough and the normal chest x-ray eliminate pulmonary tuberculosis, which is often associated with myeloproliferative disorders.

Because the cytochemical stains indicate a myeloid disorder, flow cytometric analysis to determine the surface phenotype of peripheral blood and bone marrow cells is not necessary. The leukocyte alkaline phosphatase score is low in chronic myelogenous leukemia (CML) and, therefore, might be useful for differential diagnosis. Since 90% of the patients with CML have a chromosomal translocation resulting in the Philadelphia chromosome, chromosomal evaluation is appropriate. Bone marrow aspiration and biopsy distinguish CML from other chronic myeloproliferative disorders, such as polycythemia vera and agnogenic myeloid metaplasia. Determination of the red blood cell mass distinguishes between polycythemia vera and CML, because the red blood cell mass is high in the former but not in the latter.

130. The answer is A. *(Biochemistry; eukaryotic transcription, regulatory sequences)*
RNA transcription initiation in eukaryotic cells is highly dependent on positive regulatory elements. RNA polymerases have very little, if any, affinity on their own for their corresponding promoters. Therefore,

transcription initiation depends on several activator proteins that recognize specific regulatory elements upstream of the mRNA initiation site. The TATA box is found 25–30 base pairs upstream of the initiation site with the sequence TATAAAA. This site is recognized by the transcription factor TFIID required for RNA polymerase binding to DNA. The GC box (GGGCGG) is located several hundred base pairs from the initiation site and regulates transcription initiation by binding the transcription factor SP1. CCAAT boxes (GCCAAT) are also located several hundred base pairs upstream from the mRNA initiation site and are bound by the transcription activator CTF1. An additional regulatory element in eukaryotic cells, known as an enhancer, has a more complex structure and exerts its regulatory effects regardless of its position relative to the mRNA initiation site. An α helix is a common secondary protein structure not directly associated with nucleic acids or mRNA initiation sites.

131. The answer is B. *(Pathology; Chagas disease)*
Patients with chronic Chagas disease present with cardiac conduction defects. The other signs and symptoms listed are classic for several diseases that are endemic in Central and South America, including malaria, visceral and cutaneous leishmaniasis, and amebiasis. Chronic Chagas disease (chronic trypanosomiasis) results from gradual tissue destruction of the heart, most likely caused by damage to myofibrils and the autonomic innervation of the heart. This results in the conduction defects and megacardia that are hallmarks of the disease. Parasitemia at this point is subpatent; parasites are difficult to detect in either the blood or tissues. Periodic fever and chills are indicative of malaria. Cutaneous and mucocutaneous lesions are seen in leishmaniasis. Persistent diarrhea and pneumonia can be the result of a number of infectious agents endemic in this region, although these symptoms are not seen in either acute or chronic Chagas disease.

132–134. The answers are: 132-C, 133-E, 134-A. *(Pathology; myasthenia gravis)*
Edrophonium is a short-acting acetylcholinesterase inhibitor, which increases synaptic acetylcholine (ACh) levels. An increase in muscle strength on administration of edrophonium is diagnostic of myasthenia gravis.

Myasthenia gravis is a neuromuscular disorder with muscle weakness caused by blockade of ACh receptors by autoantibodies to the ACh receptors. The antibody–receptor complex is incapable of responding to ACh and is also rapidly internalized and degraded.

Aminoglycosides inhibit prejunctional release of ACh and also block postsynaptic sensitivity to ACh. Patients with myasthenia gravis are particularly susceptible to neuromuscular blockade by aminoglycosides.

135. The answer is B. *(Biochemistry; cholesterol uptake into cells)*
Cholesterol is carried through the bloodstream as plasma lipoproteins. Low-density lipoprotein (LDL) is abundant in cholesterol, cholesteryl esters, and apoB-100 (the major apoprotein). LDL carries cholesterol through the blood plasma until apoB-100 is recognized by specific LDL receptors on the cell surface. Receptor binding initiates receptor-mediated endocytosis, which brings the LDL particle and the receptor into the cell via an endosome. The endosome then fuses with a lysosome, causing enzymatic hydrolysis of cholesteryl esters and degradation of apoB-100. This releases cholesterol, fatty acid, and amino acids into the cytosol. The LDL receptor escapes degradation and returns to the cell surface to begin the process again.

136. The answer is C. *(Biochemistry; chromatin)*
Chromatin contains the chromosomal material in nondividing eukaryotic cells. Upon cell division, chromatin condenses into a specific number of chromosomes. Chromatin is made up of equal portions of protein and DNA plus a small amount of RNA. The protein portions consist of histone proteins, which are tightly associated with DNA, and nonhistone proteins, which regulate gene expression. The DNA in chromatin is wrapped tightly around five classes of histones to form distinct structural units called nucleosomes. This forms an arrangement known as ''beads on a string.'' These nucleosome structures are compacted further into 30-nm fibers before arrangements into one loop (50×106 base pairs), one rosette (6 loops), one coil (30 rosettes), and two chromatids (2×10 coils).

137. The answer is C. *(Molecular biology; motifs of DNA binding and protein–protein interaction)*
Motifs are structural elements that, when combined, form the core of a domain, which are the functional structural units of a polypeptide. An Src homology 2 (SH2) domain has approximately 100 amino acids, two β-pleated sheets, and two α-helices. SH2 domains are also known to bind specifically to phosphotyrosine-containing peptides. Src homology 3 (SH3) domains, helix-loop-helix domains, and leucine zippers are also involved in protein–protein interactions, but they have different binding requirements. SH3 domains bind proline-rich sequences, whereas helix-loop-helix domains and leucine zippers are involved in forming dimers (usually of transcription factors). Basic regions of a protein are often found to bind DNA. Pleckstin motifs are known to bind phospholipids.

138. The answer is B. *(Molecular biology; G proteins)*
G_s (s for stimulatory) proteins function by activating adenylate cyclase to produce more cyclic adenosine monophosphate (cAMP). The G_s proteins are able to activate adenylate cyclase when bound to GTP. Thus, the guanosine triphosphatase (GTPase) activity of the G_s proteins is a mechanism that allows the protein to "turn itself off." The cholera toxin that blocks the GTPase activity leads to a constitutively active G_s protein; therefore, the levels of cAMP within the cell increase, and the cAMP acts as a second messenger. Thus, whereas increasing the amount of intracellular cAMP would make the situation worse, inhibition of adenylate cyclase would act to counteract the effects of cholera toxin. Because protein kinase A is activated by cAMP, increasing the concentration of PKA would not be protective. cAMP can act directly on certain ion channels. Therefore, even a reduction of the amount of PKA may not eliminate the effects of the toxin. Additional ligand for the G_s protein-linked receptor would increase the activation of the G_s proteins. G_i proteins (i for inhibitory) act to reduce the activity of adenylate cyclase; therefore, inhibition of these proteins would also make the situation worse. However, activation of G_i proteins may be helpful.

139. The answer is D. *(Molecular biology; desensitization)*
Desensitization can occur in a number of ways including homologous pathways, in which only one type of receptor is involved, and heterologous pathways, in which one type of receptor is desensitized through the activity of another type of receptor. For nicotinic receptors, desensitization may take less than 1 second, whereas desensitization is slower for adrenergic receptors. However, adrenergic receptors have mechanisms that act to desensitize them in ways other than regulation of transcription. These methods include phosphorylation of the receptor by cyclic adenosine monophosphate (cAMP)-dependent kinases or β-adrenergic receptor kinase. Nicotinic desensitization can also be affected by phosphorylation, because addition of a phosphate group may speed the desensitization process. Although desensitization may change the affinity of the receptor for its ligand (either increase or decrease), this is usually not the mechanism of desensitization. It is the decrease in receptor function, not ligand binding, that is the actual method of desensitization.

140. The answer is E. *(Pharmacology; pharmacokinetics of drugs)*
Nomograms (i.e., body surface area, creatinine clearance) are reliable indicators of appropriate drug dosages in only approximately 50% of patients with renal insufficiency. Actual peak and trough levels are the only way to guarantee a therapeutic level of antimicrobial agents and avoid toxicity.

141. The answer is C. *(Physiology; regulation of peripheral blood flow)*
Compared with other tissue, the lung is relatively unique in having a vasoconstrictor response to hypoxia rather than a vasodilator response. Although the mechanism remains obscure, the rationale seems to be to divert blood flow from poorly ventilated regions of the lung, thus improving the matching of ventilation and perfusion. The vascular bed in the heart, like those in many other organs, dilates to adenosine, and this vasodilator mechanism may be common in its matching of blood flow to local tissue metabolism. The brain has a very well-described and important vasodilator response to carbon dioxide.

142. The answer is C. *(Microbiology; sterilization; disinfection)*
Bacterial endospores are the life-forms most resistant to heat, and they can survive boiling for several minutes. Medically important endospore-formers include members of the genera *Bacillus* and *Clostridium*. Non–spore-formers such as *Escherichia coli* and *Mycobacterium tuberculosis* are more heat-sensitive than spore-formers and are usually killed after several minutes of boiling.

143. The answer is A. *(Biochemistry; effect of actin and myosin filament overlap on muscle contraction)*
It is generally accepted that maximal contraction of muscle fiber will occur when the overlap between actin filaments and the cross-bridges of the myosin filaments is optimal. At point *D*, the actin filament has pulled all the way out to the end of the myosin filament without overlap, and tension is minimal. As the muscle shortens past the optimal length, *C*, actin filaments tend to overlap each other and the myosin filaments decrease in length *A*, contributing to the decline in contraction at shorter than optimal lengths.

144–145. The answers are: 144-B, 145-A. *(Physiology; cardiac dynamics)*
The gradient that occurs between the ventricular and aortic systolic pressures is diagnostic of aortic stenosis. The normal aortic valve provides a negligible resistance, and the aortic pressure is nearly identical to the ventricular pressure during the phase of rapid ventricular ejection. A similar picture is seen if right ventricular and pulmonary pressures are measured in the presence of pulmonary valve stenosis, but the pressures are proportionately reduced because of the low resistance of the pulmonary circulation.

Semilunar valve stenosis represents an impediment to the ejection of blood from the ventricle and results in an ejection-type murmur during systole. An ejection murmur is diamond-shaped (i.e., it is a crescendo–decrescendo sound that has maximal intensity in midsystole, when the pressure gradient is largest).

146. The answer is C. *(Biochemistry; DNA replication; retroviruses)*
RNA-dependent DNA polymerase synthesizes DNA from an RNA template and is essential for the replication of retroviruses, not cells, and is, therefore, not a potential target of the new drug. Topoisomerase II relaxes supercoiled DNA. RNA polymerase synthesizes a primer fragment for DNA-dependent DNA polymerase. DNA ligase anneals the Okazaki fragments on the lagging strand of DNA synthesis.

147–148. The answers are: 147-C, 148-C. *(Microbiology; eukaryotic and viral commonalities)*.
Arenaviruses are multisegmented RNA viruses with inclusion granules in the virions that contain ribosomes derived from their host cells. Although arenaviruses have envelopes, this is a trait shared by many viruses, including herpesviruses and orthomyxoviruses. Likewise, many viruses have multiple genomic segments, including orthomyxoviruses and paramyxoviruses. Only arenaviruses contain ribosomes; in fact, the Latin word ''arena'' means sand. The presence of ribosome-containing granules makes the virus look grainy under the electron microscope.

To determine if the unknown virus is an arenavirus, it is important to locate the characteristic ribosomes. To test for the presence of ribosomes in virions, it would be necessary to supply ribosomal substrates to virion fractions and test the ability of these fractions to translate cellular messenger RNA (mRNA) and radiolabeled amino acids into proteins that could be isolated on a detergent (SDS) gel. Gel electrophoresis and ethidium bromide are useful for separating and staining double-stranded DNA fragments, because ethidium bromide is an intercalating dye for DNA. Light microscopy with a hematoxylin–eosin stain would be useful for viewing viruses with known inclusion-body–forming properties but not useful in determining if an unknown virus is an arenavirus.

149. The answer is B. *(Histology; histopathology of meningiomas)*
The tumor in the photomicrograph is a meningioma, which has a marked predilection for women and arises from the pia–arachnoid cells of the leptomeninges. It is usually well circumscribed and may have a hyperos-

totic reaction of overlying bone associated with it. The tumor cells are arranged in whorls or nests, and they are frequently observed with concentric calcified concretions called psammoma bodies, as shown on the *right* of the photomicrograph.

150. The answer is A. *(Pathology; pathophysiology of anemia)*
The result of a diet deficient in vitamin B_{12} or folate can be macrocytic, normochromic anemia with characteristic hypersegmented neutrophils. Anemia caused by folate or vitamin B_{12} deficiency often also presents with thrombocytopenia and agranulocytopenia. Microcytic, hypochromic erythrocytes are observed in iron deficiency anemia and β thalassemia minor. In addition, basophilic stippling and target cells can be seen in thalassemia minor. In sickle cell crisis, the anemia is normocytic and normochromic, as is the anemia associated with hemorrhage. Severe β thalassemia is uniformly fatal in children.

151. The answer is C. *(Pathology; microscopic features of hemangioma)*
The hepatic neoplasm pictured is a benign cavernous hemangioma. This is the most common mesenchymal tumor of the liver, and, if it reaches an enormous size, it may be associated with a bruit over the liver and thrombocytopenia owing to venous stasis and in situ thrombosis. The neoplasm is composed of dilated vascular spaces lined by flattened, cytologically bland endothelial cells (*at right*). Angiosarcomas of the liver have highly aggressive behavior and usually have foci of hemorrhage and necrosis. They are associated with particular carcinogens, one of which is Thorotrast, a radioactive medium widely used 50 years ago.

152–155. The answers are: 152-A, 153-C, 154-B, 155-A. *(Anatomy; pelvic innervation).*
Afferent nerves from the pelvic viscera travel along autonomic pathways. Afferent nerves from the ovary, testis, upper to middle ureter, uterine tubes, urinary bladder, and uterine body travel along the least splanchnic nerve to the lower thoracic segment and along the lumbar splanchnic nerves to the upper lumbar segments of the spinal cord; thus, pain is referred to the inguinal and pubic regions as well as the lateral and anterior aspects of the thigh. Afferents from the epididymis, uterine cervix, and distal ureter travel along the pelvic splanchnic nerves to the midsacral spinal segments; thus, pain is referred to the perineum, posterior thigh, and leg.

156–158. The answers are: 156-C, 157-A, 158-E. *(Anatomy; placental)*
The placenta consists of a decidual plate (*C*) facing the endometrium and a chorionic plate (*E*) facing the fetus. The decidual plate and chorionic plate are fused at the margins of the discoid placenta. These two plates are interconnected by cytotrophoblastic cell columns (*B*). Large numbers of chorionic villi (*D*) project away from them into the intervillous space (*A*). Maternal blood vessels end on the decidual plate and pour maternal blood into the intervillous space. Maternal blood directly bathes the chorionic villi. Thus, the human placenta is said to be a hemochorial placenta.

159. The answer is D. *(Genetics; cystic fibrosis, molecular medicine, gene therapy)*
Although replacing the entire gene or protein provides a cure for the disease, the ΔF508 mutation is not within an adenosine triphosphatase (ATPase) domain of the cystic fibrosis transmembrane conductance regulator (CFTR) gene. This mutation is within the NBF1 domain and leads to degradation of the mutant protein within the endoplasmic reticulum, because of its being folded improperly and inability to traffic to the plasma membrane. However, if this protein could be inserted into the membrane, it would function normally. The patency of the chloride channel is unaffected by the ΔF508 mutation except for its inability to reach the membrane. As for altering the regulation of the channel activity, increasing expression of this mutant protein would not be helpful because the CFTR would be unable to reach the membrane and perform its normal function. Splicing of the CFTR is also unaffected by this mutation.

160. The answer is C. *(Genetics; testosterone and its receptor)*
17,20-Lyase is an enzyme involved in the production of testosterone. Deficiency of this enzyme does not affect adrenal cortex function. It can cause a 46,XY person to be phenotypically female, if the deficiency is severe enough to reduce sufficiently the production of testosterone. Androgen insensitivity can also cause a 46,XY individual to be phenotypically female. This syndrome is caused by mutations in the androgen receptor. Like other steroid hormone receptors, it contains a steroid-binding domain and a DNA-binding domain; however, it does not contain a transmembrane domain, as the steroid hormones are able to diffuse through the plasma membrane to bind with the receptor intracellularly.

161–165. The answers are: 161-A, 162-D, 163-E, 164-C, 165-B. *(Anatomy; cranial vasculature)*
The foramen spinosum transmits the middle meningeal artery (*A*), a branch of the maxillary artery. The carotid canal (*D*) transmits the internal carotid artery, whereas the jugular foramen (*E*) contains the internal jugular vein in addition to the glossopharyngeal, vagus, and spinal accessory nerves. Each posterior condylar canal (*C*) transmits a large emissary vein. The vertebral arteries enter the cranial cavity through the foramen magnum (*B*) along with the spinal accessory nerve; the spinal cord also transmits the foramen magnum.

166. The answer is B. *(Physiology; acute pancreatitis)*
An elevated serum amylase level is a useful test result for evaluating a patient with suspected acute pancreatitis, but it is not specific for acute pancreatitis. Serum amylase can be elevated in other conditions (e.g., acute cholecystitis, dissecting abdominal aortic aneurysms, mesenteric ischemia or infarction, and common bile duct stones). Lipase also can be elevated in acute pancreatitis. Lipase is more specific for pancreatitis, and levels remain high longer than amylase, making lipase useful for patients who present later. In determining the severity of acute pancreatitis, two classification systems can be used. Ranson's criteria includes 11 clinical signs and laboratory tests that are performed during the first 48 hours after admission to assess the risks of complications. Among these criteria are $> 10\%$ decrease in hematocrit, > 5mg/dl increase in blood urea nitrogen (BUN), serum calcium < 8mg/dl, and partial pressure of oxygen in arterial blood (PaO_2) < 60 mmHg. Glasgow's criteria can be completed on admission. Glucose, lactate dehydrogenase (LDH), and BUN levels are included in both the Ranson and Glasgow scoring systems, so they should be performed in a patient who is thought to have pancreatitis. Approximately 80% of cases of acute pancreatitis are due to alcohol and gallstones. Another 10% of cases are due to metabolic abnormalities (e.g., hyperlipidemia), drugs (e.g., steroids, thiazide diuretics), and trauma. And 10% of cases are idiopathic, with a small role for hereditary pancreatitis (approximately 1%).

167. The answer is A. *(Genetics; Wilson's disease)*
Although Wilson's disease patients often have decreased serum ceruloplasmin, the primary defect is not in ceruloplasmin (chromosome 3). The genetic defect is on chromosome 13, and it is thought to be a deficiency of a P-type adenosine triphosphatase (ATPase). This enzyme is important in the assembly of ceruloplasmin; thus, a defect in this enzyme can yield low serum ceruloplasmin. Normally, more than 90% of plasma copper is bound to ceruloplasmin. Thus, Wilson's disease patients can have increased serum free copper and increased urinary copper (which may increase further upon challenge with d-penicillamine). Liver copper is always elevated in Wilsons disease. Wilson's disease is inherited as an autosomal recessive trait.

168. The answer is D. *(Biochemistry; vitamin/mineral deficiencies)*
Zinc deficiency is characterized by facial and extremity rash, skin ulcers, alopecia, confusion, apathy, depression, dysgeusia, and poor wound healing. Riboflavin deficiency is characterized by angular stomatitis, anemia, cheilosis, geographic tongue, skin desquamation, and seborrheic dermatitis. Niacin deficiency is identified by pellagra or dermatitis, dementia, diarrhea, angular stomatitis, painful tongue, and headache. Folic acid deficiency is recognized by anemia, sore tongue, mouth ulcers, nausea, diarrhea, depression, and fatigue.

Iron deficiency is known by anemia, angular stomatitis, atrophic tongue, and spoon nails (koilonychia). Vitamin C deficiency can present as scurvy with gingivitis, joint and muscle pain, and bleeding abnormalities. Selenium deficiency can result in myositis or even cardiomyopathy. Patients with short bowel syndrome require vitamin and mineral supplements, particularly zinc and the fat-soluble vitamins.

169. The answer is C. *(Physiology; interpretation of laboratory tests in liver disease)*
Autoimmune hepatitis (AIH) type 3 is associated with anti-soluble liver antigen (SLA) antibodies, not anti–liver–kidney microsomal antibody-1 (anti-LKM1). Anti–LKM1 is seen in AIH type 2. Type 3 is the only type of AIH that is *not* associated with hepatitis C infection. In hepatocellular carcinoma, Mallory bodies and α-fetoprotein demonstrate that the tumor is of hepatocellular origin. Des-carboxyprothrombin (DCP) is an abnormal form of prothrombin that is often produced by hepatocellular carcinoma tumor cells. Primary biliary cirrhosis is a disease that results in destruction of intrahepatic bile ducts. It is associated with antimitochondrial antibodies, increased alkaline phosphatase, and γ-glutamyl transpeptidase. Approximately 90% of patients with primary biliary cirrlosis are middle-aged women. Aspartate aminotransferase (AST) and alanine aminotransferase (ALT) are the most accurate markers of hepatocellular necrosis. In patients with alcoholic liver disease, AST/ALT > 2, because ALT is more sensitive to vitamin B_6 deficiency and does not increase to greater than 500 because of this disease. If the AST/ALT ratio is greater than 2, but the ALT is greater than 500, then another diagnosis should be considered. Primary sclerosing cholangitis is a cholestatic liver disease characterized by inflammation and sclerosis of the intrahepatic and extrahepatic bile ducts. Approximately 70% of patients have concomitant inflammatory bowel disease, in particular, ulcerative colitis. The incidence of cholangiocarcinoma in these patients is as high as 10%–15%. Unlike the other immune-mediated liver diseases, 75% of patients with primary sclerosing cholangitis are men.

170. The answer is C. *(Pharmacology; antiemetic agents)*
Dopamine stimulates vomiting and inhibits gut motility. Apomorphine is a dopamine (D_2) agonist that acts at the chemoreceptor trigger zone to induce vomiting. Chlorpromazine is a D_2 receptor antagonist that also blocks α-adrenergic receptors. It is a useful antiemetic agent in cancer chemotherapy, but it is ineffective against motion sickness. Antihistamines and antimuscarinic agents (e.g., promethazine and scopolamine) are effective for prevention of the vomiting caused by motion sickness because they act at the vestibular nuclei and potentially at other sites that are involved in the response of motion sickness. However, they are not effective against other causes of vomiting. Pilocarpine is a muscarinic agonist that can increase gastric secretions and can be used to treat glaucoma; therefore, it would not be useful as an antiemetic. Ondansetron and other serotonin antagonists work centrally and peripherally to reduce vomiting; however, they are ineffective against motion sickness. These agents work mainly at the chemoreceptor trigger zone but also have some prokinetic acitivity.

171–174. The answers are: 171-B, 172-D, 173-E, 174-C. *(Behavioral science; sleep architecture)*
In narcolepsy, sleep attacks are sleep-onset rapid eye movement (REM) periods that intrude into wakefulness. The motor paralysis component of sleep-onset REM periods that is associated with narcolepsy is called cataplexy. REM sleep normally occurs about 90 minutes after sleep onset, but in major depression, it occurs after only 45 minutes. There are also increased amounts of REM throughout the night in depressed individuals. Vaginal lubrication and penile tumescence occur spontaneously during normal REM sleep. Night terrors are characterized by partial awakening in terror from stages III and IV (when delta waves occur) of slow-wave sleep (SWS).

175. The answer is B. *(Physiology; causes of hyperbilirubinemia)*
Wilson's disease, primary biliary cirrhosis, viral hepatitis, gallstones, alcoholic liver disease, and Rotor syndrome do not impair the liver's ability to conjugate bilirubin; however, they can lead to conjugated (or

direct) hyperbilirubinemia. In Crigler-Najjar syndrome type I, there is no functional bilirubin uridine diphosphate-glucuronosyltransferase (the enzyme responsible for conjugation). Thus, Crigler-Najjar syndrome is associated with unconjugated (or indirect) hyperbilirubinemia.

176. The answer is C. *(Pathology; Crohn's disease)*
This patient has Crohn's disease. Crohn's disease is associated with patchy involvement and ''skip'' lesions. Although Crohn's disease occurs anywhere along the gastrointestinal tract, it frequently involves the terminal ileum. Fistulae, sinus tracts, and the ''string sign'' can be seen on radiographs. Microscopic examination may show transmural inflammation, aphthoid ulcers, and noncaseating granulomas. Endoscopy demonstrates ''cobblestone'' mucosa. Crohn's disease is directly associated with smoking. Smoking is thought to be protective against ulcerative colitis but not Crohn's disease.

177. The answer is D. *(Pathology; peptic ulcer disease)*
Helicobacter pylori play a minor role in peptic ulcer disease (PUD); however, they do not reside in the duodenum. *H. pylori* are found in the gastric antrum of more than 95% of patients with duodenal ulcers. Other risk factors for PUD include hereditary traits as well as intake of ethanol, caffeine, tobacco, salicylates, and nonsteroidal anti-inflammatory drugs. Normally, histamine, gastrin, and acetylcholine lead to acid secretion. Peptic ulcers result from an imbalance between protective factors and aggressive factors.

178. The answer is E. *(Pathology; causes of diarrhea)*
Shigella is an invasive bacterium that leads to inflammation, fever, and white blood cells in the stool. None of the other choices lead to tissue invasion and inflammation. Cholera causes severe secretory diarrhea without invasion or fecal leukocytes. Zollinger-Ellison syndrome of acid hypersecretion results from a non–β-cell tumor of the endocrine pancreas. The tumor leads to the production of excess gastrin. Mannitol ingestion would lead to osmotic diarrhea without inflammation. Laxative use would not involve inflammation, and chemical ingredients in laxatives could be detected in the stool.

179. The answer is D. *(Biochemistry; starvation)*
In late starvation, ketone bodies are produced from lipids, so there is less need for gluconeogenesis. Thus, protein breakdown decreases. Other metabolic adaptations are decreased levels of insulin, follicle-stimulating hormone, luteinizing hormone, decreased cardiac output, decreased ventilation, and increased risk of developing respiratory infections. Malnutrition due to starvation causes the body to decrease its resting energy expenditure; however, it may be increased in the setting of malnutrition due to metabolic stress (e.g., severe burns).

180. The answer is C. *(Genetics; single-strand conformational polymorphism analysis, polymerase chain reaction)*
Single-strand conformational polymorphism (SSCP) analysis is a technique that can be used as a screening test for mutations within a region of DNA. It uses the differences in intrastrand binding to separate DNA strands of different sequences. Because complimentary strands take different conformations when using this technique, the physician would see two bands in a homozygote—one for each of the complimentary strands. If the patient is a heterozygote, the physician would see four bands. However, the physician cannot tell whether a point mutation within the examined region is responsible for the disease by analyzing the patient's DNA alone. It is necessary to either sequence the region or compare the banding patterns to both normal and mutant controls. Otherwise, the physician might misdiagnose someone who merely has a silent point mutation, or the physician might rule out a disease for which the patient is actually homozygous. In addition, the possibility of errors being created during polymerase chain reaction amplification does exist.

QUESTIONS

DIRECTIONS: *Single best answer questions* consist of numbered items or incomplete statements followed by answers or by completions of the statement. Select the ONE lettered answer or completion that is BEST in each case.

Matching questions consist of a list of four to twenty-six lettered options (some of which may be in figures) followed by several numbered items. For each numbered item, select the ONE lettered option that is most closely associated with it. Each lettered option may be selected once, more than once, or not at all.

Questions 1–2

A 32-year-old volunteer fireman receives second-degree burns over approximately 30% of his body and third-degree burns over another 40%. Intravenous fluid and electrolyte therapy is initiated on site, and the patient is transported to the burn ward of a large metropolitan hospital. Approximately 2 weeks after thermal injury, the patient becomes septic with *Pseudomonas aeruginosa*.

1. The patient's sepsis possibly developed because of

(A) inability of B cells to produce opsonins
(B) inhibition of chemotactic activity of mononuclear leukocyte
(C) lack of circulating segmented neutrophils in the bloodstream
(D) inhibition of the production of immunoglobulin M
(E) induction of Bruton's agammaglobulinemia by the severe thermal injury

2. The most promising chemotherapeutic agent for treatment of this patient belongs to which of the following categories?

(A) Imidazole antibiotics
(B) Immune modulators
(C) Quinolone antibiotics
(D) Thymosin fractions
(E) Amphotericin B

3. Each of the following types of clinical syndromes are associated with cerebellar disorders EXCEPT

(A) ataxia
(B) nystagmus
(C) parkinsonism
(D) asthenia

Questions 4–5

A 52-year-old man presents with the complaint of blood in his stools. He reports that he has experienced some changes in his bowel habits over the last 18 months and recently has become aware of the sensation that his evacuations are not complete. Proctoscopic examination reveals a large ulcerating mass in the descending colon. Biopsy results confirm the diagnosis of carcinoma of the colon, and the malignant mass is surgically removed. The patient is placed on appropriate chemotherapy and discharged 2 weeks later to be followed in the oncology clinic. Monthly blood specimens taken during the next year reveal the following carcinoembryonic antigen (CEA) levels:

	CEA (ng/ml)
Preoperative sample	50
Postoperative sample (day 1)	65
Month 1	15
Month 2	5
Months 3–9	<2.5
Month 10	10
Month 11	25
Month 12	40

4. The patient's serum CEA levels were assayed periodically because of the usefulness of CEA in

(A) localization of certain tumors in vivo
(B) diagnosing carcinoma of the colon
(C) diagnosing carcinoma of the pancreas
(D) diagnosing carcinoma of the prostate
(E) follow-up for the recurrence of certain malignancies

5. The CEA levels obtained during months 10 to 12 for this patient indicate that

(A) metastases have developed
(B) the initial diagnosis of colon cancer was incorrect
(C) surgical removal of the tumor was complete
(D) a revised diagnosis of carcinoma of the pancreas is warranted
(E) the patient is having an anamnestic response to the tumor

6. A 28-year-old white male presents with unexplained weight loss and lymphadenopathy of 2 months duration. He admits to using intravenous drugs and states that he has shared needles with his girlfriend, whom he has been dating for 5 years. He has also shared needles and had unprotected intercourse with one other woman. The physician suspects that the man may be infected with the human immunodeficiency virus (HIV). Which of the following tests is useful in evaluating this patient for HIV infection?

(A) Enzyme-linked   immunosorbent   assay (ELISA) for anti-HIV antibody
(B) Complete blood count with differential
(C) Restriction fragment length polymorphism (RFLP) search for viral proteins
(D) Absolute number of CD8$^+$ lymphocytes
(E) Western blot for viral antigens

7. Each of the following is classified as a primary generalized seizure EXCEPT

(A) myoclonic
(B) tonic–clonic status
(C) infantile spasms
(D) absence

8. A 20-year-old woman presents with ptosis and diplopia that fatigues with use and recovers with rest. The patient has high levels of antibody against acetylcholine receptors. The best diagnosis among the following diseases is

(A) Lambert-Eaton myasthenic syndrome
(B) porphyria
(C) myasthenia gravis
(D) Guillain-Barré syndrome

9. Which one of the following statements concerning HIV-1 is correct?

(A) The gp 120 envelope protein of the virus binds specifically to the CD8 antigen on T lymphocytes
(B) HIV-1 is a member of the lentivirus group of retroviruses and causes transformation of T lymphocytes in culture
(C) Viral reverse transcriptase causes incorporation of the viral genome into the host DNA; however, the viral DNA is not copied during cell division
(D) Viral reverse transcriptase lacks a proofreading mechanism, which results in the well-documented "microheterogeneity" of envelope proteins
(E) HIV can only be transmitted from one cell to another by direct contact of an infected lymphocyte with a healthy cell

10. All of the following are poorly understood complications of HIV infection EXCEPT

(A) acquired immunodeficiency syndrome (AIDS)-related dementia complex
(B) acute T4-cell leukemia or lymphoma
(C) Kaposi's sarcoma
(D) polyclonal activation of B lymphocytes with resultant hypergammaglobulinemia
(E) aggressive non-Hodgkin's lymphoma

11. A 45-year-old man presents to the emergency room with shortness of breath. He has never traveled before and had just been to the doctor yesterday to prepare for his trip to central Africa. His doctor told him that his health was fine and prescribed him a prophylactic course of primaquine to prevent malaria. During the physical examination, the emergency room physician notes icterus, a jaundiced appearance to the skin, and a lack of color under the tongue. His pulse is 102, his blood pressure is 125/85, and his respiration rate is 19. Which of the following diseases is indicated by the history and physical exam?

(A) Wilson's disease
(B) Polycythemia vera
(C) Disseminated intravascular coagulation
(D) Acute hemolytic anemia
(E) Hereditary spherocytosis

12. A 27-year-old woman who is 2 months post partum presents with weakness that has worsened over several weeks and progressed from the legs to the trunk and then to the arms and face. The weakness is hyporeflexive but there is no significant sensory loss. The best diagnosis is

(A) myasthenia gravis
(B) Lambert-Eaton myasthenic syndrome
(C) Guillain-Barré syndrome
(D) syphilis

13. All of the following statements about non-fluent aphasia are correct EXCEPT

(A) it is produced by lesions in the cortex
(B) naming and repetition are impaired
(C) comprehension is relatively preserved
(D) it is also called Broca's aphasia
(E) speech is polysyllabic and repetitious

14. All of the following are cardinal features of Parkinson's disease EXCEPT

(A) tremor
(B) rigidity
(C) seizures
(D) bradykinesia
(E) postural instability

15 . All of the following statements about generalized tonic–clonic seizures are correct EXCEPT

(A) they cause a generalized increase in muscle tone
(B) they cause a loss of consciousness
(C) they result in postictal lethargy and confusion
(D) they are also called grand mal seizures
(E) they are preceded by an aura of abnormal smells, tastes, or visual sensations

16. An 8-month-old black female was brought to the emergency room with shortness of breath, icterus, and pallor under the tongue. The infant measured below the 5th percentile for her age with respect to height and weight, despite her weighing above the 80th percentile at birth. Examination of the peripheral smear indicates a hypochromic, microcytic anemia with some target cells and some teardrop-shaped erythrocytes. Unconjugated bilirubin is markedly elevated. Hemoglobin electrophoresis reveals increased fetal hemoglobin (Hb F) and double the normal amount of hemoglobin A_2 (Hb A_2); there is very little hemoglobin A (Hb A). There are no other hemoglobin bands. What is the primary diagnosis for this patient?

(A) β-thalassemia major
(B) Iron deficiency
(C) Sickle cell disease
(D) Hereditary spherocytosis
(E) Methemoglobinemia

17. All of the following are part of the criteria for the diagnosis of multiple sclerosis EXCEPT

(A) one central nervous system lesion
(B) two separate attacks of symptoms
(C) symptoms are consistent with a white matter lesion
(D) patients are age 10–50 years
(E) no other disease has similar symptoms

18. All of the following statements about generalized absence seizures are correct EXCEPT

(A) they may consist of staring and altered mental state
(B) they are also called petit mal seizures
(C) they are almost exclusively seen in adults
(D) there is no significant postictal state

19. Which one of the following is NOT a product of the Embden-Meyerhof glycolytic pathway?

(A) Acetaldehyde
(B) Glyderaldehyde-3-phosphate
(C) 2-Phosphoglycerate
(D) Glucose-6-phosphate
(E) Fructose-6-phosphate
(F) Pyruvate

20. Which one of the following statements about the retinoblastoma protein is most likely true?

(A) Hypophosphorylated retinoblastoma protein binds to the transcription factor called E2F and causes a G_1 arrest

(B) Hyperphosphorylated retinoblastoma protein binds to p21 and causes a G_2 arrest

(C) Hyperphosphorylated retinoblastoma binds to E2F and causes a G_2 arrest

(D) Hyperphosphorylated retinoblastoma binds to p21 and causes a G_1 arrest

(E) Retinoblastoma protein is phosphorylated by the cyclin B-cdc2 kinase complex

Questions 21–22

To answer this group of questions, refer to the following diagrammatic representation of the heart in an infant with congenital heart disease.

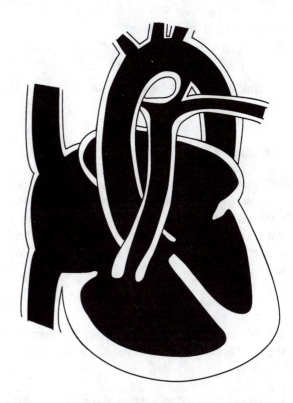

21. Which cyanotic congenital heart disease does this infant have?

(A) Truncus arteriosus

(B) Transposition of the great arteries

(C) Patent ductus arteriosus

(D) Tetralogy of Fallot

(E) Coarctation of the aorta

22. Many congenital heart defects produce non-laminar, jet-stream patterns of blood flow. These turbulent jets frequently leave the infants especially susceptible to

(A) myocardial infarction
(B) rheumatic heart disease
(C) infective endocarditis
(D) valvular calcification
(E) mitral valve prolapse

Questions 23–26

A 2-year-old female is brought to her pediatrician because of progressive muscular weakness and recurrent episodes of hepatic encephalopathy with nausea and vomiting. An inherited defect in metabolism is suspected, and tests reveal low serum carnitine.

23. Which of the following correctly describes the normal function of carnitine in fatty acid metabolism?

(A) A coenzyme that is required for the dehydrogenation of acyl coenzyme A (CoA), forming a double bond between the β- and γ-carbons
(B) A coenzyme that is added to free fatty acids on the outer mitochondrial membrane
(C) A carrier protein that holds the growing acyl chain in fatty acid synthesis
(D) A carrier protein that shuttles long-chain fatty acids into the mitochondrial matrix
(E) A carrier protein that shuttles short-chain fatty acids out of the liver to adipose tissue

24. Which of the following statements concerning the β-oxidation of fatty acids is correct?

(A) Single carboxylic acids are released in successive cycles during the metabolism of fatty acids
(B) All of the energy released is stored in the form of reduced equivalents of nicotinamide–adenine dinucleotide (NADH)
(C) Phosphorylation of a fatty acid and the subsequent generation of acyl CoA are the committed steps in oxidation
(D) Fatty acids are converted into glucose by the formation of pyruvate from acetyl CoA
(E) Elevated levels of malonyl CoA activate the transfer of fatty acyl CoA into the mitochondrial matrix

25. All of the following characterizations of carnitine deficiency are correct EXCEPT

(A) some victims of this autosomal recessive disease respond to oral carnitine therapy
(B) a diet restricted to short- and medium-chain fatty acids may prove useful
(C) pathologic deposition of lipid is frequently seen in muscle biopsies
(D) a form of the disease confined to muscle is less severe and may involve defective transport of carnitine into the cell
(E) a deletion mutation in the gene for carnitine palmitoyltransferase would result in an entirely different phenotype

26. All of the following statements correctly pair a metabolic pathway with its appropriate subcellular location EXCEPT

(A) oxidative phosphorylation occurs in mitochondria
(B) fatty acid synthesis occurs in mitochondria
(C) glycolysis occurs in the cytosol
(D) gluconeogenesis occurs in both the cytosol and the mitochondria
(E) ganglioside degradation occurs in lysosomes

Questions 27–29

A 30-year-old female lawyer presents to her physician's office for an increase in fatigue over the last 2 months. She has been involved in a difficult case at work and has lost five pounds. During the physical exam, the physician notes delayed capillary refill in the nailbeds and a pale appearance of the inner lining of the eyelids. A peripheral smear reveals hypochromic erythrocytes.

27. Which of the following tests would be most useful in confirming the probable diagnosis?

(A) Serum ferritin and total iron-binding capacity (TIBC)
(B) Schilling's test
(C) Glucose 6-phosphate dehydrogenase assay
(D) Hemoglobin electrophoresis
(E) Serum folate and serum cobalamin (vitamin B_{12})

28. Which of the following statements about the causes of acquired anemia is correct?

(A) Cobalamin deficiency is often secondary to chronic liver disease
(B) Methotrexate is frequently associated with hypochromic, microcytic anemias
(C) Women are more susceptible to iron-deficiency anemia because they tend to eat less red meat
(D) Folate deficiency frequently leads to neurologic disease, which may not respond to therapy
(E) Folate deficiency can develop over months in a poorly nourished person

29. Which of the following statements regarding the control of transferrin and ferritin synthesis is correct?

(A) Hepatic synthesis of transferrin and ferritin is principally regulated at the level of messenger RNA (mRNA) transcription by the presence of iron
(B) Hepatic synthesis of transferrin and ferritin is principally regulated by the level of tissue oxygenation and the presence of sufficient heme
(C) Hepatic synthesis of transferrin and ferritin is principally regulated after mRNA transcription by an iron-binding protein that is inactive in the presence of iron
(D) The rate of transferrin turnover in the serum is a function of the presence of iron
(E) The half-life of ferritin mRNA is the site of critical regulation in ferritin synthesis

30. Which of the of following statements correctly pairs a commonly prescribed ulcer medication with its mechanism of action?

(A) Atropine blocks acetylcholine release by the vagus nerve

(B) Ranitidine and cimetidine competitively block the gastrin receptor

(C) Colloidal bismuth inhibits gastrin release

(D) Omeprazole irreversibly inhibits the hydrogen–potassium adenosine triphosphatase

(E) Sucralfate competitively inhibits carbonic anhydrase

Questions 31–34

For each statement below, select the phase of the cell cycle that best corresponds to the property described.

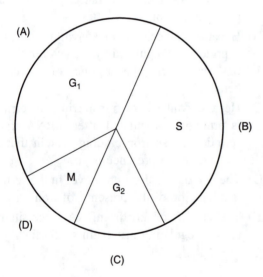

Standard cell cycle

31. Replication of nuclear DNA

32. Interval between completion of nuclear division and beginning of DNA synthesis

33. Process of nuclear division, leading up to the moment of cell division

34. Cytokinesis occurs at the end of this phase of the cell cycle

35. Which of the following statements concerning fatty acid synthesis is correct?

(A) Palmitoyl coenzyme A (CoA) helps regulate the committed step in fatty acid synthesis through feedback inhibition of acetyl CoA carboxylase

(B) Hormone-dependent enzyme phosphorylation, which is important in gluconeogenesis, is not important in fatty acid synthesis

(C) Low levels of citrate increase the synthesis of malonyl CoA by reducing substrate inhibition of acetyl CoA carboxylase

(D) The growing fatty acid chain is elongated by a series of enzymes that exist as separate polypeptides in the mitochondrial matrix

(E) Niacin is the precursor for a coenzyme that is important in the addition of carboxyl groups to the growing fatty acid chain

Questions 36–37

A 40-year-old woman with refractory peptic ulcer disease presents to a gastroenterologist for a complete evaluation. She is a nonsmoker and drinks only infrequently. Endoscopy reveals ectopic ulcers in the esophagus as well as numerous ulcers in the stomach and duodenum. The physician considers a diagnosis of Zollinger-Ellison syndrome.

36. Which of the following problems characterizes the cause of peptic ulcer disease in most patients with Zollinger-Ellison syndrome?

(A) Increased vagal tone in the gastric branch
(B) Increased release of histamine
(C) Increased secretion of gastrin
(D) Increased secretion of pepsin
(E) Decreased mucous production

37. Which of the following statements correctly characterizes the secretion of acid by parietal cells?

(A) Carbonic anhydrase in the parietal cell splits carbonic acid into a bicarbonate ion, which is secreted into the blood, and a hydrogen ion
(B) Hydrogen ions are secreted passively down their gradient into the gut
(C) Cyclic adenosine monophosphate (cAMP) levels are elevated in response to either gastrin or muscarinic receptor stimulation
(D) H_2-histamine receptor activation causes elevation of intracellular calcium levels
(E) Gastrin and acetylcholine stimulate parietal cell acid production but histamine inhibits it

Questions 38–40

A 75-year-old woman with a 35-year history of noninsulin-dependent (type II) diabetes mellitus is admitted to the hospital for mental status changes. The physician considers a diagnosis of chronic renal failure and investigates the possibility of dialysis.

38. All of the following are common characteristics of chronic renal failure EXCEPT

(A) hypokalemia
(B) elevated triglycerides
(C) uremic fetor
(D) normochromic, normocytic anemia
(E) proteinuria

39. Which of the following statements correctly characterizes the role of the kidney in acid–base homeostasis?

(A) Cells of the proximal tubule are the only cells in the body with the complete enzymatic machinery for urea biosynthesis, an important route for excreting acid
(B) Carbonic anhydrase, located on the brush border of tubule cells, splits carbonic acid into a bicarbonate anion and a hydrogen ion; the hydrogen ion is pumped into the cell
(C) Bicarbonate is actively synthesized from pyruvate in the distal tubule cells
(D) Tubule cells actively secrete bicarbonate anion as a potassium salt
(E) The tubule cells secrete ammonia as one of the mechanisms to excrete excess acid

40. An arterial blood gas reveals a pH of 7.26, and her anion gap is 12. Which of the following statements correctly describes her metabolic acidosis due to renal failure?

(A) A large anion gap is indicative of better compensation

(B) The metabolic acidosis is caused by an excess production of ammonia in the tubule cells

(C) The large anion gap indicates that her plasma bicarbonate is elevated

(D) This patient has probably already passed the hyperchloremic phase of her acidosis

(E) Long-standing metabolic acidosis is not related to renal osteodystrophy

41. All of the following are primarily G_1 cyclins EXCEPT

(A) cyclin E

(B) cyclin D_1

(C) cyclin D_2

(D) cyclin D_3

(E) cyclin B

Questions 42–43

A neurologist postulates that the extent of physical disability following a cerebrovascular accident (CVA) is related to personality type. Five hundred such patients were classified according to the severity of their physical deficit (mild or severe) and simultaneously assigned to one of four personality groups (1 = most prone to depression and 4 = least prone to depression), based on a personality assessment questionnaire developed by the investigator. The table below depicts the number of subjects in each category.

Personality Type	Severity of Condition		
	Severe	**Mild**	**Totals**
1	60	40	100
2	60	40	100
3	132	68	200
4	48	52	100
Totals	300	200	500

42. This study is an example of a

(A) prospective cohort study

(B) case–control study

(C) cross-sectional study

(D) experimental study

(E) randomized controlled clinical trial

43. What is the most appropriate statistical test for determining whether a significant association exists between the extent of physical disability and personality type?

(A) Analysis of variance
(B) Independent sample (pooled) *t* test
(C) Paired *t* test
(D) Chi-square test
(E) Correlation/regression analysis

44. All of the following are cyclin-dependent kinase inhibitors EXCEPT

(A) p21
(B) p27 Kip1
(C) p53
(D) p16
(E) p57 Kip2

45. All of the following statements about G_0 arrest are true EXCEPT

(A) G_0 is a specialized, nongrowing state of the cell cycle
(B) the rate of protein synthesis is drastically reduced
(C) the slowly dividing cells can remain in G_0 for weeks or even years
(D) the cells in G_0 have more cyclin-dependent kinases and G_1 cyclins than cells in G_1

Questions 46–47

A 29-year-old man with no prior medical history is transported to the hospital after being involved in a serious motor vehicle accident. The bleeding has been slowed by the paramedics, but the man has lost a substantial amount of blood. His blood pressure on arrival at the hospital is 72/30. Right heart catheterization with a Swan-Ganz catheter is performed. The physician begins volume replenishment with units of packed red blood cells and plasma.

46. Which of the following pharmacologic agents would be most useful in supporting this man's cardiovascular system?

(A) Albuterol
(B) Propranolol
(C) Furosemide
(D) Dobutamine
(E) Tubocurarine

47. The physician estimates that the patient's systemic circulation was compromised for a total of 4 hours. In the intensive care unit 36 hours later, his serum potassium level is 5.7, increased from 4.8 when he was admitted (normal = 3.4–5.0). Which of the following tests would be most useful in confirming the origin of this man's new problem?

(A) Antinuclear antibody screen
(B) Blood urea nitrogen and serum creatinine
(C) Antistreptolysin O (ASO) titer
(D) Complete blood count
(E) Digoxin level

48. All of the following statements are correct descriptions of bias EXCEPT

(A) comparisons are made between groups that differ with respect to determinants of the outcome other than those under study
(B) methods of measurement are consistently dissimilar among groups
(C) two factors or processes are associated, and the effect of one is confused or distorted by the effect of the other
(D) random variation of the primary determinants
(E) a process at any stage of inference tending to produce results that depart systematically from the true values

49. All of the following are examples of confounding bias EXCEPT

(A) diabetes mellitus is a risk factor for atherosclerotic disease
(B) serum triglycerides are a risk factor for coronary heart disease, but not independently of serum cholesterol
(C) the association between exercise and coronary events in a particular study resulted from the fact that smoking cigarettes is a risk factor for coronary heart disease and the exercise group smoked less
(D) an observed association between oral contraceptives and thrombophlebitis is due to the way in which the history of exposure was reported

50. An 8-year-old girl is taken to her pediatrician's office because of blood in her urine and "puffiness." Her mother indicates that the child has also been lethargic for the past 2 or 3 days. The girl has no history of cardiac or renal disease. The mother reveals that her child had a sore throat that kept her from 2 days of school about 12 days ago. The girl's blood pressure is 140/100. Which of the following diseases is suggested by the history and physical findings?

(A) Systemic lupus erythematosus
(B) Acute tubular necrosis
(C) Acute glomerulonephritis
(D) Juvenile onset (insulin-dependent) diabetes mellitus
(E) Hyperaldosteronism

51. All of the following statements regarding definitions of biostatistics terms are true EXCEPT

(A) mean is the sum of values divided by the number of values
(B) median is the point where the number of observations above equals the number below
(C) mode is the most frequently occurring value
(D) standard error is numerically less than the standard deviation
(E) range is the lowest-to-highest value of the average difference of individual values from the mode

52. Which one of the following statements best describes a cohort study?

(A) Prevalence survey of a group of individuals with a particular disease, performed at a single point in time
(B) Compares the frequency of a purported risk factor in a group of cases and a group of controls
(C) Subjects are free of disease at the beginning of the observation, but are then exposed or not exposed to risk factors
(D) Presents in detail a single case or handful of cases

53. Which one of the following equations best describes the odds ratio?

	Cases	Non cases	
Exposed	A	B	A+B
Not exposed	C	D	C+D
	A+C	B+D	

(A) $\dfrac{A/(A+B)}{C/(C+D)}$

(B) $\dfrac{A/D}{B/C}$

(C) $\dfrac{A+B}{C+D}$

(D) $\dfrac{AD}{BC}$

Questions 54–55

A 35-year-old woman presents to the emergency room with severe, stabbing abdominal pain that is constant and radiating from the epigastrium to the back and chest. She is nauseated and says that her abdomen feels bloated as well as painful, and the pain is worse lying down. During the physical exam, the physician notes tachycardia, a low-grade fever, an absence of bowel sounds, guarding, and an exquisitely tender abdomen. The remainder of the physical exam is noncontributory. Further questioning reveals that the patient drank excessive amounts of alcohol last night; she has no prior medical or family history for cardiac disease. A plain radiograph of the abdomen shows no air under the diaphragm.

54. Which of the following processes is most likely in this patient?

(A) Perforated duodenal ulcer
(B) Myocardial infarction
(C) Abdominal aortic aneurysm
(D) Acute pancreatitis
(E) Renal colic

55. All of the following are criteria for diagnosing alcoholism EXCEPT

(A) alcohol-related relationship problems leading to separation or divorce
(B) loss of memory while using alcohol (blackouts)
(C) loss of a job due to alcohol-related problems
(D) alcohol-related disease including delirium tremens, hepatitis, or cardiomyopathy
(E) two or more arrests related to alcohol

56. Which one of the following is a form of parenteral drug administration?

(A) Sublingual
(B) Intramuscular
(C) Oral
(D) Rectal

57. Which one of the following is a general anesthetic given intravenously?

(A) Halothane
(B) Ketamine
(C) Ether
(D) Procaine
(E) Nitrous oxide
(F) Lidocaine

58. The reactivation of acetylcholinesterase is caused by which one of the following cholinergic agonists?

(A) Isoflurophate
(B) Edrophonium
(C) Neostigmine
(D) Acetylcholine
(E) Pilocarpine
(F) Pralidoxime

59. Which of the following statements concerning α_1-antitrypsin deficiency is correct?

(A) Liver disease is always preceded by lung disease
(B) The deficiency may be a common but unrecognized cause of many cases of neonatal hepatitis
(C) Direct restriction fragment length polymorphism (RFLP) analysis of the gene is the only means of definitive diagnosis
(D) Of individuals who are homozygous for the deficiency, panacinar emphysema develops in about 33% of persons surviving into adulthood
(E) There is no interaction between smoking and the protein deficiency

60. Which of the following is appropriate pharmacologic management of routine delirium tremens (i.e., alcohol withdrawal)?

(A) Haloperidol therapy for up to 3 weeks
(B) Phenytoin (Dilantin) tapered over 10 days
(C) Chlordiazepoxide (Librium) tapered over 5 days
(D) Morphine for up to 1 month
(E) Nortriptyline for up to 6 months

Questions 61–63

An 11-year-old boy with a history of episodic dyspnea associated with wheezing has the following spirometric tracings in the pulmonary function laboratory:

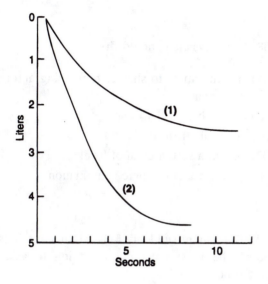

61. Which of the following is the most likely description of curves (*1*) and (*2*)?

(A) Before (*1*) and after (*2*) inhalation of methacholine
(B) Before (*1*) and after (*2*) inhalation of metaproterenol
(C) Before (*1*) and after (*2*) inhalation of cromolyn sodium
(D) Before (*1*) and after (*2*) inhalation of beclomethasone
(E) Curves (*1*) and (*2*) arise from normal variation of forced expiratory maneuvers within a subject

62. A possible pharmacotherapeutic approach to control this boy's symptoms may include which one of the following agents?

(A) Antihistamine
(B) Propranolol
(C) Ibuprofen
(D) Theophylline
(E) Bethanechol

63. Inhalation of an irritant that stimulates nonmyelinated C fibers near epithelial cells lining the airway lumen produces reflex bronchoconstriction via the

(A) sympathetic nerve endings
(B) hypoglossal nerve
(C) phrenic nerve
(D) vagus nerve
(E) intercostal nerve

64. Which one of the following cholinergic antagonists is an antimuscarinic agent?

(A) Nicotine
(B) Tobucurarine
(C) Succinylcholine
(D) Scopolamine
(E) Gallamine
(F) Pancuronium

65. The irreversible inactivation of acetylcholinesterase is caused by which one of the following cholinergic agonists?

(A) Neostigmine
(B) Edrophonium
(C) Isoflurophate
(D) Carbachol
(E) Pilocarpine
(F) Bethanechol

Questions 66–67

A 68-year-old woman suddenly develops a fever of 38.2° C and a severe headache one evening. The following morning she also experiences a stiff neck and uncharacteristic drowsiness. At the emergency room, her temperature is 38.8° C, and there is pain and resistance on flexion of her neck. The patient is noted to be mentally competent although lethargic. A cerebral spinal fluid sample is obtained by lumbar puncture.

66. On the basis of the history and physical examination of this patient, what is the most probable diagnosis?

(A) Viral meningitis
(B) Fungal meningitis
(C) Bacterial meningitis
(D) Viral encephalitis
(E) Brain abscess

67. On the basis of the patient's age, the probable etiologic agent is

(A) *Staphylococcus aureus*
(B) *Haemophilus influenzae*
(C) *Streptococcus pneumoniae*
(D) *Neisseria meningitidis*
(E) none of the above

Questions 68–70

A 48-year-old homeless man appears ataxic and confused in the emergency room. He is unshaven, mildly jaundiced, and has a bleeding scalp wound over the right frontotemporal area.

68. The physician should first

(A) ask the nurse to shower him, using antilice treatment
(B) suture his head wound
(C) order skull films
(D) obtain a serum ethanol level
(E) perform a neurologic examination

69. The patient suddenly falls into unconsciousness. The most emergent condition to assess would be

(A) subdural hematoma
(B) epidural hematoma
(C) delirium tremens
(D) hepatic encephalopathy
(E) AIDS

70. Appropriate treatment of delirium tremens includes all of the following EXCEPT

(A) monitor for generalized seizures
(B) treat with intravenous fluids
(C) monitor vital signs for autonomic arousal
(D) treat with chlordiazepoxide
(E) treat with disulfiram (Antabuse)

Questions 71–74

A previously healthy 60-year-old man collapsed while playing with his grandchildren. Although he quickly regained consciousness and became fully alert, his family called an ambulance. The emergency medical team found no abnormalities on the electrocardiogram or on physical examination. However, the patient was admitted to the coronary care unit of the local hospital. During the evening, the patient was noted to have a fast rhythm with a wide complex on his monitor followed by hypotension and loss of consciousness.

71. After electrical cardioversion with 200 watt-seconds of direct current, possible therapy may include

(A) intravenous propranolol
(B) digitalis
(C) intravenous lidocaine
(D) intravenous diltiazem
(E) epinephrine

72. Blood is drawn from the patient serially over the next 8–48 hours, and serum enzyme studies are consistent with a diagnosis of myocardial infarction. The most likely change noted was

(A) a decrease in aspartate aminotransferase
(B) an elevation in creatine kinase muscle brain isoenzyme (CK-MB)
(C) an increase in lactate dehydrogenase
(D) a decrease in pseudocholinesterase
(E) a decrease in alkaline phosphatase

73. A radionuclide scan (with technetium 99m pyrophosphate) performed in the hospital 48 hours after the initial incident indicates significant damage to the anterior wall of the left ventricle. Subsequent coronary artery angiography most likely shows occlusion of the

(A) right coronary artery
(B) left circumflex artery
(C) coronary sinuses
(D) left anterior descending coronary artery
(E) atrioventricular nodal artery

74. After being discharged from the hospital after successful coronary artery bypass surgery, the patient is placed on low-dose aspirin therapy. The rationale for selecting this therapy includes

(A) lowering the patient's body metabolism
(B) decreasing anxiety
(C) inhibiting endothelial cell prostacyclin metabolism
(D) inhibiting platelet thromboxane A_2 synthesis
(E) decreasing circulating leukotriene D_4

75. Which one of the following fatty acids found in a normal diet is metabolized by the α-hydroxylase pathway?

(A) Linoleic acid
(B) Phytanic acid
(C) Arachidonic acid
(D) Palmitic acid
(E) Decenoic acid

76. Low levels of cellular 3-hydroxy-3-methyl-glutaryl coenzyme A (HMG CoA) reductase activity in humans is most likely to result from

(A) a vegetarian diet
(B) the administration of a bile acid–sequestering resin
(C) familial hypercholesterolemia
(D) a long-term high cholesterol diet

Questions 77–78

A 35-year-old man contracts something resembling the flu, receives no treatment, and is sick for a few days. Three and one-half weeks later, he develops "a feeling of pins and needles" in his fingers and toes. Three days after that he has trouble speaking and eating, and he keeps cutting the right side of his face while shaving because "it is numb." The next day, upon waking, he has trouble with his gait. He goes to the hospital, and he tells the physician that he has never been ill before in his life. He is barely able to lift his arms to a horizontal position, and he cannot walk well. All of his tendon reflexes are absent.

77. Which one of the following diseases is the patient most likely to have?

(A) Myasthenia gravis
(B) Polio
(C) Guillain-Barré syndrome
(D) Raynaud's phenomenon

78. This disease is thought to be caused by

(A) destruction of anterior horn cells due to picornavirus infection
(B) autoantibodies to the acetylcholine (ACh) receptors
(C) damage to spinal nerves
(D) peripheral arteriosclerosis

Questions 79–81

The figure below shows flow–volume curves after inhalation to total lung capacity (TLC) and a forced expiratory maneuver to residual volume (RV) from a normal person and a patient. Absolute volume of gas within the thorax was determined independently in a body plethysmograph. The patient was a middle-aged man with a history of chronic cough with expectoration and complaints of shortness of breath and an increasing inability to exercise. In addition, a chest x-ray revealed an enlarged heart and congested lung fields with increased markings attributable to old infections.

79. From the following flow–volume curve, which of the following statements is correct regarding the patient?

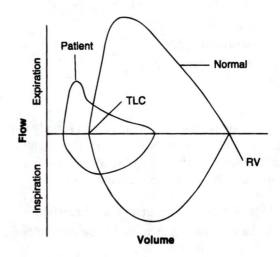

(A) TLC is greatly reduced
(B) RV is reduced
(C) Vital capacity is greatly increased
(D) Flow rate over most of expiration is less than predicted
(E) Elastic recoil of lung is likely to be greater than predicted

80. An arterial blood gas is drawn from the patient and his arterial P_{CO_2} is 50 mm Hg (normal = 40 mm Hg) and P_{O_2} is 55 mm Hg (normal is >90 mm Hg). Which of the following factors is most likely to have contributed to his CO_2 retention?

(A) A low physiological shunt
(B) An increased minute ventilation
(C) A decreased work of breathing
(D) A large increase in physiologic dead space
(E) Diminished ventilatory drive (in relation to their arterial blood gas values)

81. On examination, during inspiration, neck vein distention is noted, and an early diastolic gallop and holosystolic murmur are detected. These symptoms are likely due to

(A) atrial fibrillation
(B) tricuspid regurgitation
(C) a decrease in atrial pressure
(D) atrioventricular blockade
(E) aortic insufficiency

82. Which one of the following adrenergic agonists is both a direct-acting agent and an indirect-acting agent?

(A) Clonidine
(B) Dopamine
(C) Ephedrine
(D) Ritodrine
(E) Amphetamine
(F) Tyramine

83. Which one of the following adrenergic agonists is a catecholamine?

(A) Clonidine
(B) Dopamine
(C) Ephedrine
(D) Albuterol
(E) Amphetamine
(F) Metaproterenol

84. A 28-year-old woman with a family history of skin cancer presented with a rapidly growing (3 to 6 months) asymptomatic lesion on her right scapular area. The lesion was brown with a bluish-red (violaceous) color, and its border was palpably elevated. The lesion described is likely to be a

(A) hemangioma
(B) pigmented basal cell carcinoma
(C) pigmented dermatofibroma
(D) melanoma
(E) subungual hematoma

85. Which one of the following adrenergic blockers is an α-blocker?

(A) Propranolol
(B) Reserpine
(C) Cocaine
(D) Prazosin
(E) Guanethidine
(F) Atenolol

86. Which one of the following drugs is a barbiturate?

(A) Diazepam

(B) Thiopental

(C) Lorazepam

(D) Ethanol

(E) Buspirone

(F) Hydroxyzine

87. Topoisomerase enzymes are important in the replication of DNA because they

(A) anneal Okazaki fragments

(B) relax supercoiled DNA

(C) degrade histone proteins

(D) "proofread" newly synthesized DNA

(E) synthesize the RNA primer fragment

88. Which one of the following central nervous system stimulants is a hallucinogen?

(A) Caffeine

(B) Amphetamine

(C) Theobromine

(D) Nicotine

(E) Doxapram

(F) Tetrahydrocannabinol

(G) Nikethamide

Questions 89–90

A teenager who is below average in both weight and height is seen for complaints of vomiting of bile-stained material, abdominal distention, and pain. Further questioning reveals a periodic history of respiratory infections. Cystic fibrosis is suspected, and the diagnosis confirmed when pilocarpine iontophoresis produces an abnormally high sweat chloride concentration (> 60 mEq/L).

89. The patient is noted to have pancreatic achylia (absence of secretion of pancreatic digestive enzymes). As a result of the achylia, deficiency in absorption of which of the following vitamins may result in prolonged prothrombin times?

(A) Vitamin A

(B) Vitamin B_6

(C) Vitamin C

(D) Vitamin D

(E) Vitamin K

90. A history of frequent respiratory infections is noted in the patient. A recent sputum analysis indicates the presence of *Staphylococcus aureus*, *Haemophilus influenzae*, and *Pseudomonas aeruginosa*. Although the value of antibiotic therapy in cystic fibrosis remains unclear, a conventional approach to such therapy based on sputum culture might include

(A) gentamicin and ceftazidime

(B) nalidixic acid and kanamycin

(C) nitrofurantoin

(D) pentamidine

(E) rifampin and isoniazid

91. In the United States, the most common tumor in males is found in which one of the following organs?

(A) Kidney

(B) Colon

(C) Prostate gland

(D) Liver

(E) Testis

Questions 92–93

A patient is noted to have paroxysmal episodes of hypertension, tremor, weakness, and sweating. Urinary catecholamines and their metabolites are elevated, and a computed tomography (CT) scan of the abdomen detects a mass within the adrenal gland.

92. The tumor most likely involves which one of the following cells?

(A) Zona glomerulosa
(B) Zona fasciculata
(C) Zona reticularis
(D) Chromaffin cells of the medulla

93. If the tumor is deemed inoperable, pharmacotherapy of the above disorder may include which one of the following drugs?

(A) Clonidine
(B) Propranolol
(C) Methyldopa
(D) Phenoxybenzamine

94. Correct statements concerning toxic exposure to organophosphates include which one of the following?

(A) Aminophylline is the agent of first choice in reversing the respiratory symptoms
(B) Atropine and pralidoxime are useful antidotes
(C) Exposure must be inhalational since organophosphates are not well absorbed through the skin
(D) Immediate injection of epinephrine is a useful antidote

95. In general, tolerance to self-antigens exists, even if the antigens are not expressed in the thymus. For example, antigens on the pancreatic islet cells produce insulin. Which of the following statements is a reasonable explanation for this?

(A) Pancreatic antigens are shed and are transported to the thymus via the circulation; at the thymus, they are associated with the major histocompatibility complex (MHC) and induce positive selection of immature T cells
(B) Immature $CD4^+CD8^+$ thymic T cells are transported to the pancreas, where they undergo negative selection; they then return to the thymus for final maturation
(C) Mature T cells circulate to the pancreas, recognize pancreatic antigen in context of self MHC, which stimulates them via the T-cell receptor; however, no interleukin-1 is produced, so T cells are inactivated
(D) T-cell progenitors in the bone marrow circulate to the pancreas before being transported to the thymus; they undergo negative selection at the pancreas and then proceed to the thymus where T-cell differentiation occurs

96. Which of the following structural motifs is important for the transcriptional activation produced by some steroid-bound hormone receptors?

(A) Zinc fingers
(B) EF hands
(C) β-pleated sheets
(D) Immunoglobulin folds
(E) Gly-X-Y repeats

97. The retroviruses have many unique biologic and biochemical features. All of the following are properties of the retroviruses EXCEPT

(A) they are genetically diploid
(B) the particles contain an RNA-dependent DNA polymerase
(C) they require integration into the host genome for proper replication
(D) the RNA has minus polarity
(E) the retroviral group antigens are highly reactive between strains

98. All of the following complications are common in patients with chronic hemolytic anemias EXCEPT

(A) cardiac arrhythmias
(B) emphysema
(C) congestive heart failure
(D) severe infection by encapsulated organisms
(E) chronic liver failure

99. All of the following statements about immunoglobulin classes are correctly paired with a characteristic feature EXCEPT

(A) immunoglobulin A (IgA) is found in mucosal secretions from the breast, gut, and respiratory tract
(B) immunoglobulin G (IgG) crosses the placenta
(C) immunoglobulin M (IgM), frequently found as a pentamer, efficiently activates the complement cascade
(D) immunoglobulin D (IgD) antibodies against IgG are present in high titers in many patients with rheumatoid arthritis
(E) immunoglobulin E (IgE) mediates type I hypersensitivity by activating mast cells and basophils

100. All of the following statements concerning hemoglobin genes and thalassemia are correct EXCEPT

(A) normal individuals inherit four copies of the α-chain, two from each parent
(B) most α-thalassemias involve deletions of α-chain genes due to a nonhomologous crossover
(C) α-thalassemias vary in severity depending on the number of defective α-chain genes
(D) α-thalassemias are sex-linked because the α-chain genes are located on the X-chromosome
(E) α-chain abnormalities can generally be confirmed by the use of restriction endonucleases

101. All of the following statements about multiple endocrine neoplasia (MEN) type IIb are correct EXCEPT

(A) pheochromocytoma and the accompanying sympathomimetic signs are a common presentation
(B) the disorder is hereditary, and the gene has been mapped to chromosome 10
(C) some research suggests that the neoplastic clones may have arisen from abnormal neural crest cells
(D) neuromas of the conjunctival, labial, and buccal mucosa are not unusual
(E) Zollinger-Ellison syndrome is present in about 20% of cases

102. All of the following are characteristics of nephrotic syndrome EXCEPT

(A) proteinuria
(B) hematuria
(C) generalized edema
(D) hyperlipidemia
(E) focal segmental glomerulosclerosis

103. All of the following may result from chronic alcohol abuse EXCEPT

(A) cerebellar degeneration and ataxia
(B) esophagitis and Mallory-Weiss tears
(C) testicular atrophy or amenorrhea
(D) mild-to-moderate hypertension and elevated serum triglycerides
(E) bronchogenic carcinoma

104. Acute pancreatitis is associated with all of the following EXCEPT

(A) alcohol ingestion
(B) biliary tract disease
(C) elevated serum triglycerides
(D) α_1-antitrypsin deficiency
(E) major abdominal surgery or trauma

105. All of the following statements describe the biologic properties of immunoglobulin E (IgE) EXCEPT

(A) it has the shortest half-life of all classes of immunoglobulins
(B) low levels of circulating IgE are due in part to the high-affinity binding of the Fc portion to mast cells and basophils
(C) it can cause agglutination of particulate antigens
(D) it is elevated in cases of certain parasitic infections

106. A patient hospitalized for multiple fractures was placed on a prophylactic antibiotic. Two days prior to discharge, diarrhea developed, requiring intravenous rehydration. The antibiotic was changed to a broad-spectrum cephalosporin, but diarrhea continued and the patient's condition deteriorated. All of the following actions are appropriate EXCEPT

(A) sigmoidoscopic examination
(B) proper isolation of the patient
(C) Gram stain of feces for white blood cells
(D) a request for *Clostridium difficile* toxin test
(E) changing the antibiotic to clindamycin

107. Agnogenic myeloid metaplasia with myelofibrosis is characterized by all of the following features EXCEPT

(A) hypocellular bone marrow
(B) normal levels of leukocyte alkaline phosphatase
(C) teardrop-shaped erythrocytes
(D) hepatomegaly
(E) splenomegaly

108. All of the following characteristics of warfarin are accurate EXCEPT

(A) it is useful in pregnant women because it does not cross the placenta
(B) it affects hepatic synthesis of clotting factors present in blood
(C) it is effective after oral administration
(D) it is primarily used in chronic therapy
(E) therapy can be reversed by administration of vitamin K

109. Each of the following enzymes is essential for protecting red blood cells from the hydrogen peroxide generated in vivo EXCEPT

(A) glutathione peroxidase
(B) 6-phosphogluconate dehydrogenase
(C) catalase
(D) transketolase
(E) glutathione reductase

110. All of the following statements concerning the Arthus reaction are true EXCEPT

(A) it usually requires large amounts of antibody and antigen
(B) it results in localized rupture of vessel walls followed by tissue necrosis
(C) neutrophils and platelets are present at the site of the reaction
(D) it is the most common type III reaction seen in humans

111. Zidovudine (ZDV) [formerly known as azidothymidine (AZT)] has all of the following properties EXCEPT

(A) ZDV reduces the chances of progression to AIDS in asymptomatic HIV-infected subjects
(B) ZDV improves the clinical symptoms of immunologic function, survival period, and quality of life of advanced AIDS patients
(C) ZDV is very toxic to bone marrow
(D) ZDV is effective only in the treatment of patients with advanced AIDS
(E) prolonged treatment with ZDV (1–3 years) results in resistance to this drug

112. All of the following mediators released during mast cell activation cause an increase of vascular permeability EXCEPT

(A) histamine
(B) eosinophil chemotactic factor (ECF)
(C) serotonin
(D) slow-reacting substance of anaphylaxis

113. Major risk factors for the development of chronic obstructive pulmonary disease (COPD) include all of the following EXCEPT

(A) smoking
(B) air pollution
(C) occupational exposure to irritant gases and particles
(D) α_1-antitrypsin deficiency
(E) intravenous drug abuse

114. Characteristics of Duchenne muscular dystrophy (DMD) include all of the following EXCEPT

(A) decreased amounts of dystrophin in affected muscles
(B) hypertrophy of affected muscle groups
(C) autosomal dominant inheritance via mutated chromosome 20
(D) one-third of the cases resulting from spontaneous mutation
(E) sarcomere hypercontraction and contraction band formation

115. A young child develops pharyngitis, a fever, and a rash. β-Hemolytic, gram-positive cocci in chains are isolated from the throat and are found to be catalase-negative. All of the following statements about the virulence factors of this pathogen are true EXCEPT

(A) hemolysis results from production of extracellular hemolysins
(B) the organism produces membrane-bound protein (M protein), which has antiphagocytic properties
(C) the organism produces lipoteichoic acid, which is necessary for attachment to mucosa
(D) the organism is not encapsulated
(E) the rash is produced by a toxin distinct from the hemolysins

116. Cushing's syndrome is a complex array of symptoms that are due to excess glucocorticoid levels. All of the following statements about Cushing's syndrome are correct EXCEPT

(A) the disease may be associated with an adenoma of the pituitary corticotropes
(B) the disease may be secondary to abnormal hypothalamic function with excessive release of corticotropin releasing factor (CRF)
(C) the disease may be due to ectopic adrenocorticotropic hormone (ACTH) synthesis
(D) some aspects of the syndrome may be due to long-term therapy with glucocorticoids
(E) increased long bone length is common in patients prior to puberty

117. All of the following statements about protein synthesis are true EXCEPT

(A) the activated form of an amino acid is called aminoacyl transfer RNA (tRNA)
(B) the addition of aminoacyl tRNA to the growing peptide chain and subsequent translocation is an energy-requiring process
(C) the formation of the peptide bond is catalyzed by peptidyltransferase
(D) synthesis occurs in the mitochondria as well as in the cytoplasm of cells
(E) synthesis can occur in the absence of RNA

118. Each statement below concerning osteoclasts is true EXCEPT that they

(A) are found in Howship's lacuna
(B) resorb bone
(C) are stimulated by calcitonin
(D) are multinucleated
(E) help remodel bone

119. Asymptomatic bacteriuria is noted in a 35-year-old pregnant woman in her second trimester. Five years ago, during her first pregnancy, she presented with acute pyelonephritis, which required hospitalization and parenteral antibacterial therapy. Since then, recurrent sexual intercourse–related urinary tract infections have been prevented by a single dose of nitrofurantoin after coitus. All of the following agents would be contraindicated for this patient during the remainder of her pregnancy for prevention of acute pyelonephritis EXCEPT

(A) trimethoprim/sulfamethoxazole
(B) minocycline
(C) amoxicillin
(D) gentamicin

120. Thymomas are associated with all of the following diseases EXCEPT

(A) myasthenia gravis

(B) systemic lupus erythematosus

(C) hypogammaglobulinemia

(D) Graves' disease

(E) neutrophil agranulocytosis

(F) polymyositis

121. All of the following statements concerning the human immunodeficiency virus (HIV) are true EXCEPT that

(A) the virus can infect T cells, macrophages, and any other cell type with a CD4 receptor

(B) viral infection can spread between cells without the involvement of free virus

(C) the viral infection process involves endocytosis of the HIV particle into the cell

(D) replication of the viral nucleic acid occurs in the nucleus

Questions 122–126

(A) Recall of four items after 5 minutes

(B) Repetition of digits, forward and reversed

(C) Interpretation of proverbs

(D) Serial 7's subtraction

(E) Copying simple shapes and objects

For each area of the brain listed below, select the most appropriate test for functional evaluation. (The patient's language function is assumed to be normal.)

122. Visual cortex; visual association areas of parietal lobe; motor areas of frontal lobe

123. Pontine and midbrain reticular activating system (RAS)

124. Prefrontal cortex

125. Left hippocampus and temporal lobe

126. RAS; left parietal lobe; hippocampus and other cortical and subcortical memory areas

127. For antibiotic therapy, it is useful to understand both the action of the prescribed antibiotic and the pathogenesis of the bacteria responsible for a patient's infection. For example, the aminoglycoside antibiotic gentamicin does not enter mammalian cells and, therefore, is ineffective against intracellular pathogens. Considering only this information, gentamicin is effective against all of the following infections EXCEPT

(A) *Haemophilus influenzae* type B epiglottitis
(B) *Pseudomonas aeruginosa* burn infections
(C) *Klebsiella pneumoniae* respiratory infections
(D) *Escherichia coli* urinary tract infections
(E) *Chlamydia trachomatis* infections

128. All of the following characteristics of a typical virus are true EXCEPT

(A) it contains either RNA or DNA as its genetic material
(B) it can reproduce itself
(C) the nucleic acid is single stranded or double stranded
(D) it contains a protein coat called a capsid

129. Which one of the following statements is true for both prokaryotic and eukaryotic cells?

(A) They both contain extensive internal membranes unconnected to the plasma membrane
(B) They both contain organelles
(C) They both contain a membrane-bound nucleus
(D) They both utilize membrane transporters to allow passage of macromolecules
(E) Most of the cellular DNA is in the form of a single circular molecule

130. All of the following statements about β_1-adrenergic receptors are true EXCEPT

(A) they promote increased heart rate and contractility on binding agonists
(B) they bind catecholamines
(C) they induce relaxation of smooth muscle in bronchial passages on binding agonists
(D) the rank order of affinities for agonists is isoproterenol > norepinephrine > epinephrine
(E) they induce elevation of cyclic adenosine monophosphate (cAMP) levels by activation of adenylate cyclase

131. The essential transcriptional binding factor that binds directly to the TATA box initiating RNA polymerase II transcription in mammalian cells is

(A) TFIID
(B) TFIIE
(C) TFIIB
(D) TFIIS

Questions 132–136

(A) Behavioral–psychoeducational approaches
(B) Structural–strategic approaches
(C) Intergenerational–experiential approaches
(D) Sociobiological approaches

Match each treatment technique with the school of family therapy most associated with that technique.

132. Clarification of transgenerational relationship patterns

133. Clarification of relationship patterns within the nuclear family

134. Training in social learning theory

135. Cognitive reframing

136. Elaboration of the family's identity

137. During mitosis, all of the following events occur at telophase EXCEPT

(A) duplication of each original centriole is completed
(B) spindles disappear
(C) new membranes form around the daughter nuclei
(D) the two sister chromatids separate into independent chromosomes
(E) cytokinesis is nearly complete
(F) the nucleolus becomes visible again

138. All of the following statements about the termination of messenger RNA (mRNA) translation are true EXCEPT

(A) it is recognized by the stop signal codon UAG
(B) it requires the aid of termination factors
(C) the complete polypeptide is released
(D) it is followed by dissociation of the two ribosomal subunits
(E) it does not require guanosine triphosphate (GTP) hydrolysis

139. An α-helix protein conformation is an example of which one of the following structures?

(A) Primary structure
(B) Secondary structure
(C) Tertiary structure
(D) Quaternary structure

Questions 140–144

A 15-year-old boy develops insulin-dependent diabetes mellitus (IDDM). His parents want to know the risk of their other children developing diabetes. The pedigree below was developed for the family. Match each of the affected son's siblings in the pedigree to the best estimate of risk.

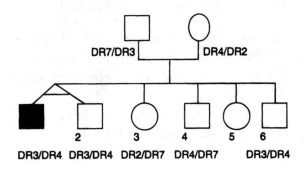

(A) 2%
(B) 5%
(C) 20%
(D) 50%
(E) 100%

140. The proband's monozygous twin (II-2)

141. The proband's sister with human leukocyte antigen (HLA) DR2/DR7 (II-3)

142. The proband's brother with HLA DR4/DR7 (II-4)

143. The proband's sister for whom no HLA typing is available (II-5)

144. The proband's brother with HLA DR3/DR4 (II-6)

Questions 145–149

(A) Arsenic

(B) Lead

(C) Tin

(D) Cadmium

(E) Mercury

Match each of the following clinical or pathological descriptions with the appropriate heavy metal.

145. Intense exposure to the vapor causes acute interstitial pneumonitis

146. Inorganic form commonly used in insecticides and rodenticides; gas is produced in smelting and refining of metals and causes severe hemolysis and hematuria

147. Produced epidemic levels of disease in preschool children; with chronic exposure, it causes cognitive impairment, language dysfunction, and, when severe, mental retardation

148. Chronic exposure to vapors leads to neurologic symptoms including insomnia, excitability, and memory loss

149. Uncouples oxidation and phosphorylation in glycolysis by forming an unstable acyl intermediate

Questions 150–154

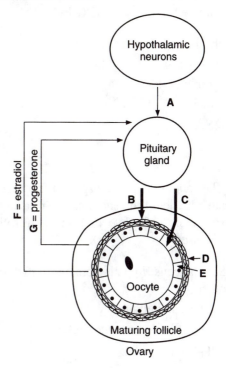

Match each of the following descriptions of cell signalling with the hormones or cells identified in the figure.

150. Responds to luteinizing hormone (LH) with increased synthesis of androstenedione and testosterone, which are used as substrates for estradiol synthesis

151. Increases pituitary responsiveness to gonadotropin-releasing hormone (GnRH) during the follicular phase in preparation for the LH surge

152. Elicits the correct response only when secreted in a pulsatile manner; precocious sexual development can be arrested by constant infusion of a synthetic analogue

153. Causes ovulation at midcycle

154. Estradiol and inhibin act together to decrease the pituitary gland's synthesis of this hormone

155. All of the following substances are associated with cell membranes EXCEPT

(A) phospholipid
(B) cholesterol
(C) carbohydrates
(D) proteins
(E) DNA

156. Phospholipids are transported from the cytoplasmic leaflet of the endoplasmic reticulum to the exoplasmic leaflet by which one of the following processes?

(A) Spontaneous flipping from one leaflet to another
(B) Membrane budding
(C) Phospholipid exchange proteins
(D) Flippase protein

157. The serum electrolytes for a patient who is being treated for lung cancer are notable for an elevated calcium level. All of the following would support the malignancy as being the cause of the hypercalcemia EXCEPT

(A) decreased levels of calcitriol
(B) decreased levels of parathyroid hormone (PTH)
(C) decreased levels of PTH-related protein
(D) decreased serum phosphorus
(E) a calcium level that is even higher than that seen in primary hyperparathyroidism

158. Which one of the following statements accurately describes vitamin D?

(A) Conversion to the active form 25-hydroxyvitamin D in the liver depends on stimulation by parathyroid hormone (PTH)

(B) Conversion to the active form 1,25-dihydroxyvitamin D is regulated primarily by substrate availability and occurs in the distal tubules of the kidney
(C) Vitamin D is water soluble
(D) The vitamin D receptor is located on the plasma membrane
(E) A major function of vitamin D is to increase the absorption of calcium and decrease the absorption of phosphorus in the intestine
(F) Vitamin D stimulates the secretion of PTH
(G) Although vitamin D is commonly converted to its active form in the kidney, it can also be activated in macrophages

159. A patient complains of headaches, and the physician notes that she seems nervous and is sweating profusely. On physical examination the physician initially finds that the patient has orthostatic hypotension. When the blood pressure measurement is repeated, the patient is hypertensive. Her history includes medullary carcinoma of the thyroid, for which she had surgery performed several years ago. Which one of the following statements is correct?

(A) The patient likely has multiple endocrine neoplasia (MEN) syndrome type I
(B) The physician should check her cortisol level because she likely has a pheochromocytoma
(C) The patient should take a nonsteroidal anti-inflammatory drug, and no further evaluation is needed
(D) A 24-hour urinary excretion of epinephrine, norepinephrine, and their metabolites would be more useful in this case than the current plasma values of these substances
(E) A computed tomography (CT) scan with intravenous contrast material should be performed immediately
(F) No defects are seen in the adrenal glands on CT scan; therefore, the patient does not have a pheochromocytoma

160. Which one of the following enzyme deficiencies is matched to the correct outcome?

(A) 3-β-Dehydrogenase deficiency—increased cortisol production and decreased androgen production
(B) 21-Hydroxylase deficiency decreased—cortisol production and increased aldosterone deficiency
(C) 17,20-Desmolase deficiency—normal cortisol production and decreased aldosterone production
(D) Aromatase—decreased cortisol production and increased androgen production
(E) 18-Hydroxylase deficiency—decreased cortisol production and increased aldosterone production
(F) 17-α-Hydroxylase deficiency—decreased cortisol production and increased deoxycorticosterone and corticosterone production

161. A 10-year-old boy with type I diabetes mellitus presents with vomiting and abdominal pain. His glucose level was tested after a large meal, and it was elevated. He appears dehydrated and is breathing with "sighing" respirations. Which one of the following statements is correct?

(A) Although hypokalemia is a concern in this patient, the physician does not need to worry about diabetic ketoacidosis because that only occurs in type II diabetes mellitus
(B) This patient took too much insulin
(C) Initial laboratory results indicate that his potassium level is within normal limits; therefore, the physician can proceed with the treatment without risk of causing hypokalemia
(D) If the patient is mildly acidotic, a single bolus of bicarbonate should be given to correct the acid–base imbalance
(E) This patient's current condition could not have been prevented, because it is an inevitable complication of type I diabetes mellitus
(F) Rehydration can be started before the patient is given any insulin

162. People often have difficulty changing their behavior, even when change would benefit their health. Which one of the following is the most effective way to help someone modify his behavior?

(A) Give positive reinforcement continually, whether or not the person is achieving the goal that was set
(B) Give positive reinforcement for coming close to the goal and gradually become stringent
(C) Do not give positive reinforcement until the person has completely reached his goal
(D) Give negative reinforcement to make a person's old behavior less likely to occur
(E) Punish the person's undesired behavior

163. Considering an obese person (250 lbs), a person of average weight (150 lbs), and body mass index (BMI), which one of the following statements is correct?

(A) The obese person has a larger number of intestinal cells
(B) The obese person has a fewer number of fat cells, but the cells are larger
(C) The obese person eats the same proportion of calories from fat, but eats more calories than the average person
(D) The obese person eats the same number of total calories as the average person, but eats a higher percentage of calories from fat
(E) The person of average weight burns more calories running 1 mile in 8 minutes than the obese person burns walking 1 mile in 20 minutes
(F) The person of average weight and the obese person burn the same number of calories as each other in walking a mile, no matter how long it takes them

Questions 164–168

(A) Infant A: O, MN, Rh$^+$
(B) Infant B: A, MN, Rh$^-$
(C) Infant C: A, M, Rh$^+$
(D) Infant D: AB, N, Rh$^+$
(E) Infant E: B, MN, Rh$^+$

A deranged former employee snuck into the hospital nursery and clipped the identification bracelets from five newborn boys. To correct the situation, blood typing has been done on the infants and their parents. Match the following parents to the correct infant.

	Mother			Father		
	Blood Group			**Blood Group**		
Family	**ABO**	**MN**	**Rh**	**ABO**	**MN**	**Rh**
164.	B	N	Rh$^-$	A	MN	Rh$^-$
165.	B	N	Rh$^+$	AB	N	Rh$^-$
166.	AB	MN	Rh$^+$	O	MN	Rh$^+$
167.	O	M	Rh$^+$	A	M	Rh$^+$
168.	A	M	Rh$^+$	A	N	Rh$^+$

Questions 169–172

(A) Diagnosis
(B) Treatment
(C) Remission
(D) Recurrence
(E) Terminal phase

Match each description with the psychosocial stage of cancer it best characterizes.

169. Period of short-term focus, when palliation of pain and patient support are paramount

170. Period during which denial may prevent proper management

171. Anxious waiting may cause emotional pain during this phase

172. Malaise, nausea, and vomiting may foster noncompliance

Questions 173–177

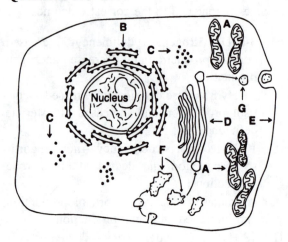

Match each of the following descriptions or events with the appropriate structure or location in the diagrammatic representation of the cell.

173. O-linked glycosylation as well as acylation and sorting of many proteins

174. Translation of hexokinase

175. Ultimate destination for cytosolically synthesized proteins with special amino-terminal sequence signals

176. Ultimate destination for proteins with mannose 6-phosphate signals

177. Translation of proteins with signal sequences

Questions 178–180

(A) Lewy bodies
(B) Hippocampal neurofibrillary tangles
(C) Argentophilic intraneuronal inclusions
(D) Prions
(E) Multinucleated giant cells

Match each of the following diseases that affect the brain with its most characteristic neuropathologic finding.

178. Alzheimer's dementia

179. AIDS

180. Parkinson's disease

ANSWER KEY

1-B	31-B	61-B	91-C	121-C
2-C	32-A	62-D	92-D	122-E
3-C	33-D	63-D	93-D	123-B
4-E	34-D	64-D	94-B	124-C
5-A	35-A	65-C	95-C	125-A
6-A	36-C	66-C	96-A	126-D
7-B	37-A	67-C	97-D	127-E
8-C	38-A	68-E	98-B	128-B
9-D	39-E	69-B	99-D	129-D
10-B	40-D	70-E	100-D	130-C
11-D	41-E	71-C	101-E	131-A
12-C	42-C	72-B	102-B	132-C
13-E	43-D	73-D	103-E	133-B
14-C	44-C	74-D	104-D	134-A
15-E	45-D	75-B	105-C	135-B
16-A	46-D	76-D	106-E	136-C
17-A	47-B	77-C	107-D	137-D
18-C	48-D	78-C	108-A	138-E
19-A	49-D	79-D	109-D	139-B
20-A	50-C	80-E	110-D	140-D
21-D	51-E	81-B	111-D	141-A
22-C	52-C	82-C	112-B	142-B
23-D	53-D	83-B	113-E	143-B
24-C	54-D	84-D	114-C	144-C
25-E	55-B	85-D	115-D	145-E
26-B	56-B	86-B	116-E	146-A
27-A	57-B	87-B	117-E	147-B
28-E	58-F	88-F	118-C	148-E
29-C	59-B	89-E	119-C	149-A
30-D	60-C	90-A	120-D	150-D

151-F	157-C	163-D	169-E	175-A
152-A	158-G	164-B	170-A	176-F
153-B	159-D	165-D	171-C	177-B
154-C	160-F	166-E	172-B	178-B
155-E	161-F	167-C	173-D	179-E
156-D	162-B	168-A	174-C	180-A

ANSWERS AND EXPLANATIONS

1–2. The answers are: 1-B, 2-C. *(Microbiology; sepsis following severe burn)*
Pseudomonas aeruginosa is a major cause of sepsis in burn patients. The bacterium is ubiquitous in the environment and is a member of the indigenous flora of some people. Once it gains entry through the physical barrier of the skin, *P. aeruginosa* causes significant tissue damage. It is capable of invading the epithelium of blood vessels, leading to repeated seeding of the bloodstream.

Patients with burns over more than 20% of their body demonstrate a lack of chemotactic activity of mononuclear leukocytes 15 to 45 days after the thermal injury. Inhibition of activity corresponds to the appearance of a chemotactic inhibitor in the serum. An inability to produce opsonin antibodies and a decrease in the production of immunoglobulin M (IgM) are associated with splenectomy. A decrease in the number of circulating segmented neutrophils occurs during bone marrow failure. Bruton's agammaglobulinemia is a sex-linked genetic dysfunction.

P. aeruginosa and other pseudomonads frequently display multiple drug resistance. The mortality rate in pseudomonas septicemia approaches 80%. A new group of antibiotics, the quinolones, have shown good in vitro activity against *P. aeruginosa*; the number of cases of disease successfully treated with the quinolones is increasing. Imidazole antibiotics and amphotericin B are antifungal agents; the imidazoles are now considered alternatives to amphotericin B therapy in some mycoses. Immune modulators, such as thymosin and interferon, have shown potential in treating infections controlled by the cell-mediated immune system.

3. The answer is C. *(Neurology; cerebellar disorders)*
Parkinsonism is a basal ganglia disorder associated with degeneration in the basal ganglia and the substantia nigra. Ataxia is often caused by cerebellar lesions and presents as an awkwardness of posture and gait with a tendency to fall to the same side as the cerebellar lesion. Asthenia, also associated with cerebellar lesions, presents with muscles tiring more easily than normal. Nystagmus is a repetitive, tremor-like, oscillating movement of the eye that can occur with cerebellar lesions.

4–5. The answers are: 4-E, 5-A. *(Pathology; carcinoembryonic antigen analysis)*
Carcinoembryonic antigen (CEA) is associated with carcinoma of the colon and pancreas; however, because CEA also occurs in nonmalignant conditions (e.g., as a result of cigarette smoking), it is not considered to be diagnostic of, but merely suggestive of, a cancerous condition. Assays for CEA show their greatest promise in monitoring for the recurrence of certain malignancies after surgery or chemotherapy.

The presence of CEA in the serum is correlated with the tumor burden of the host. The higher the level of CEA, the greater is the patient's tumor mass. Following surgical excision of the tumor, the CEA level should drop very low, perhaps even to indiscernible levels. If the CEA level increases again, it suggests that the tumor has metastasized and appropriate therapeutic or surgical intervention is indicated. The patient presented in the questions is gravely ill. Surgical removal of the tumor was incomplete, and metastases have developed, as indicated by the rise in CEA in months 10 to 12. The chemotherapeutic regimen should be reevaluated, and the patient should be thoroughly examined for possible radiologic and surgical treatment.

6. The answer is A. *(Immunology; HIV, AIDS)*
An enzyme-linked immunosorbent assay (ELISA) for anti-HIV antibody is the mainstay in screening for HIV. ELISA is relatively sensitive (as any screening should be), but its low specificity requires confirmation with a Western blot for the anti-HIV antibody. A Western blot for viral proteins is not effective. Although viral proteins do circulate in the serum of infected individuals, the concentration of antigen is not detectable. The absolute number of CD4$^+$ lymphocytes is used to monitor the progress of HIV-infected patients but is not particularly useful as a screening tool. In most cases, any substantial loss of T4 cells occurs many years after infection. Polymerase chain reaction (PCR) techniques, which allow extremely sensitive detection of

a small fragment of viral (or any) DNA sequence, are currently being investigated as a potential tool in screening for HIV infection. A complete blood count with standard differential is not useful in the diagnosis of HIV infection because decreases in the number of white blood cells differentiated by routine light microscopy occur only late in the disease. Furthermore, elevations in the white cell count can be indicative of a host of inflammatory processes, which may or may not be related to HIV.

7. The answer is B. *(Neurology; generalized seizures)*
Status epilepticus is defined as prolonged or repetitive seizures without a period of recovery between attacks. When tonic–clonic seizures are involved (e.g., in tonic–clonic status), this state can be life threatening. Myoclonic seizures are primary generalized seizures that are sudden, brief, single, or repetitive muscle contractions involving one body part or the entire body. Absence (petit mal) seizures are primary generalized seizures that consist of a sudden cessation of ongoing conscious activity or loss of postural control. Infantile spasms are primary generalized seizures that occur in infants between birth and 12 months of age. These seizures consist of several types of brief synchronous contractions of the neck, torso, and both arms (usually in flexion). They can occur in an otherwise normal infant, but they often occur in infants with underlying neurologic disease.

8. The answer is C. *(Neurology; neuromuscular disease)*
Myasthenia gravis, which is rare, has a bimodal age distribution; it occurs in women in their teens and twenties and in men aged 60 years or older. It presents with proximal weakness, especially ptosis and diplopia that fatigues with use and recovers with rest. Myasthenia gravis is an autoimmune disease. Patients with myasthenia gravis produce antibodies that destroy the acetylcholine receptor of the muscles. Although myasthenia gravis and Lambert-Eaton myasthenic syndrome strongly resemble each other clinically, Lambert-Eaton myasthenic syndrome does not involve extraocular muscles. Therefore, patients with Lambert-Eaton syndrome do not have ptosis and diplopia.

9. The answer is D. *(Immunology; HIV, AIDS)*
The HIV-1 virus is a cytopathic member of the lentiviruses; it lyses T lymphocytes in culture whereas its sister virus human T-cell lymphotrophic virus (HTLV) transforms them into an immortal cell line. The two viruses are related by the enzyme reverse transcriptase, which uses the viral RNA genome to synthesize linear DNA. The DNA is incorporated into the cellular genome via recombination and forms a template for normal mammalian replication processes. Once incorporated, the viral DNA is replicated and given to all of the cell's progeny. New strategies for intervention are focused on more effective chronic therapy for infected people and vaccination for uninfected people. Lysis of an infected cell results in a prolific release of viral progeny that are capable of infecting a large number of uninfected T4-helper cells. Direct contact is not required, and research efforts toward binding these free particles with soluble CD4 antigen may prove fruitful. The envelope proteins, including gp 120, are important in the binding, entry, and uncoating of the virus. The gp 120 envelope protein is involved in the recognition of the CD4 antigen. Efforts to develop an effective vaccine have been elusive because the envelope antigens are subject to frequent mutation. This high rate of mutation is probably the result of selection pressure, which favors a viral transcriptase prone to frequent error. Most other DNA-synthesizing enzymes (including all of the DNA synthases in healthy mammalian cells) have extensive proofreading mechanisms, which HIV reverse transcriptase lacks.

10. The answer is B. *(Immunology; HIV, AIDS)*
Fully developed AIDS is associated with lysis and death of CD4$^+$ lymphocytes, the T4-helper cells. The disease is staged, and therapy is indexed by the absolute number of circulating T4 cells. No T4 leukemias or lymphomas have been reported to date. A closely related virus, the HTLV-1, does cause T-cell leukemias and lymphomas; however, this virus is a transforming virus not a cytopathic virus like HIV. AIDS-related

dementia is probably associated with HIV infection of microglia, which are monocytes in the central nervous system. The dementia clinically manifests in 70% of AIDS patients, and neuropathologic lesions are present in 80%–90% of autopsies in AIDS victims. Kaposi's sarcoma is another regular feature of AIDS whose cause remains enigmatic. The polyclonal activation of B lymphocytes and non-Hodgkins (B-cell) lymphomas may be different manifestations of a common problem, but further research is needed to clarify the pathologic process of these two problems familiar to many AIDS patients.

11. The answer is D. *(Hematology; glucose 6-phosphate dehydrogenase deficiency hemolytic anemia)*
Pallor under the tongue, delayed capillary refill in the nailbeds, and, in Caucasian people, general lack of color are indicative of anemia. The acute onset, obvious signs of jaundice, the patient's race, and the recent prescription of primaquine indicate acute hemolytic anemia resulting from glucose 6-phosphate dehydrogenase deficiency. The patient's tachycardia and tachypnea are a reflection of the sympathetic activation produced by inadequate tissue oxygenation. Such sympathetic activation is not unusual, and some patients with more chronic hemolytic anemias develop prominent high-output S_3 flow murmurs as a result of chronic hypoxia. Wilson's disease is a complex of symptoms (primarily liver and pancreatic failure) related to the inappropriate storage of copper; jaundice (but not hemolysis) develops over time in a patient with Wilson's disease. Polycythemia vera is the neoplastic growth of hematopoietic stem cells, which gives rise to an unregulated excess of the cellular components of blood; platelets, erythrocytes, and lymphocytes can be elevated individually or in combination. Disseminated intravascular coagulation occurs when the clotting cascade is inappropriately activated and platelets (not erythrocytes) are depleted to a dangerous low. Hereditary spherocytosis does cause hemolytic anemia, but the disease is not generally triggered but rather is present early in adulthood. The anemia is a chronic, lifelong anemia secondary to a defect in the plasma membrane of the erythrocytes. The name spherocytosis reflects the odd appearance of the erythrocytes in the peripheral smears from these patients.

12. The answer is C. *(Neurology; neuromuscular disease)*
Guillain-Barré syndrome is an acute inflammatory polyridiculopathy in which there is inflammation of the nerve roots and peripheral nerves. It often follows viral infection, surgery, pregnancy, and other immune-altering events. It runs a monophasic course with weakness progressing for several days to weeks, reaching a plateau, then recovering over a period of several weeks to months. Clinically, the diagnosis is confirmed by weakness, often, but not always, in an acsending pattern (from legs to trunk to the arms and face). The weakness is hyporeflexive, but there is no significant sensory loss. Rapidly progressive weakness with absent reflexes and no sensory change is almost always Guillain-Barré syndrome. Myasthenia gravis presents with proximal weakness, especially ptosis and diplopia, that fatigues with use and recovers with rest. Myasthenia gravis and Lambert-Eaton myasthenic syndrome strongly resemble each other clinically, except Lambert-Eaton myasthenic syndrome does not involve extraocular muscles. Syphilis does not present this ascending pattern of weakness.

13. The answer is E. *(Neurology; aphasia)*
The two main types of aphasia are fluent and nonfluent. Nonfluent aphasia is generally produced by lesions in the cortex in the anterior part of the dominant hemisphere around the sylvan fissure and is often referred to by other names (e.g., Broca's aphasia). Patients with nonfluent aphasia have difficulty producing language and either cannot speak or do so only in monosyllabic and short telegraphic phrases. Naming and repetition are also impaired, but comprehension is relatively preserved. Fluent aphasia results in speech that is fluent and even loquacious, but nonsensical.

14. The answer is C. *(Neurology; Parkinson's disease)*
Parkinson's disease is a gradual, progressive, degenerative disease of the basal ganglia (extrapyramidal)

motor system. Seizures are not a feature of Parkinson's disease. There are four cardinal features to Parkinson's disease. One feature is a usually to-and-fro, pronation-supranation resting tremor that diminishes with voluntary movement. Another is rigidity with diffuse increase in muscular tone and sometimes a cog-wheeling property to joints when passively moved. Bradykinesia (slowness of movement) and postural instability are also features.

15. The answer is E. *(Neurology; generalized seizures)*
Generalized tonic–clonic (grand mal) seizures consist of the sudden onset, often without any preceding aura, of jerky tonic and clonic activity of both arms and legs with a generalized increase in muscle tone and loss of consciousness. Tongue biting and incoherence may also be involved. Seizures usually last 1–2 minutes and often resolve with postictal lethargy and confusion.

16. The answer is A. *(Genetics; β-thalassemia)*
Hemoglobin A (Hb A) is the normal hemoglobin tetramer with a subunit stoichiometry of $\alpha_2\beta_2$, and most individuals have a hemoglobin composition with 97% Hb A. Hemoglobin A_2 has a subunit stoichiometry of $\alpha_2\delta_2$ and normally accounts for less than 3% of total hemoglobin. Normal adults usually have less than 1% of their total hemoglobin comprised of the fetal form (i.e., Hb F), which has the subtypes $\alpha_2\gamma_2$. Infants with β-thalassemia major usually present after the sixth month, when the hemoglobin promoters gradually switch from γ subunit production (for Hb F) to β subunit production (for Hb A). White people of Mediterranean descent have the highest carrier frequency, and the heterozygous state is also relatively common in people from central Africa, Asia, and parts of India. Jaundiced skin, icterus, elevated unconjugated bilirubin, and pallor under the tongue are a relatively specific indication of hemolytic anemia. The infant's failure to thrive indicates a chronic course that is now emerging. The peripheral smear indicates a hypochromic anemia but specifically lacks evidence of spherocytosis or sickle cell anemia. Spherocytosis has a much more chronic course that often emerges in the second or third decade of life. Iron deficiency is a possibility, but ineffective erythropoiesis is not the only problem; iron deficiency does not cause hemolysis. The unconjugated bilirubin and teardrop cells indicate active destruction as well as ineffective erythropoiesis; therefore, iron deficiency is not a sufficient explanation. The inherited form of methemoglobinemia causes an anemia that is much less severe than the one described and would probably not be noted except as an incidental finding on routine evaluation.

17. The answer is A. *(Neurology; multiple sclerosis)*
The diagnosis for multiple sclerosis is primarily clinical despite the variability in signs and symptoms. The following are well-proven guidelines for the diagnosis: (1) two separate central nervous system lesions, (2) two separate attacks of symptoms, (3) symptoms are consistent with a white matter (myelin) lesion, (4) objective deficits on examination, (5) age 10–50 years of age, (6) no other disease with similar symptoms.

18. The answer is C. *(Neurology; generalized seizures)*
Generalized absence (petit mal) seizures are seen almost exclusively in children. The seizures usually do not have a significant aura or postictal state, but may consist of a few seconds of staring and altered mental status so brief that it escapes detection by untrained observers. Often children are thought to be daydreaming when they are actually experiencing a seizure.

19. The answer is A. *(Biochemistry; glycolysis)*
Glycolysis is a highly regulated pathway that metabolizes enough glucose to meet the cell's need for adenosine triphosphate (ATP). In the Embden-Meyerhof pathway, each molecule of glucose is converted to two molecules of pyruvate. This process results in the production of four molecules of ATP. However, because of the consumption of two molecules of ATP during earlier steps, there is a net gain of two molecules of ATP. Acetaldehyde is produced during anaerobic metabolism of glucose, which does not require the mitochondria.

20. The answer is A. *(Cell biology; cell cycle)*
The retinoblastoma protein (Rb) is a tumor suppressor gene that binds to several important gene regulatory proteins, but its binding capacity depends on its state of phosphorylation. When Rb is dephosphorylated it binds a set of gene regulatory proteins (e.g., the transcription factor E2F), which causes a G_1 arrest. Phosphorylated Rb releases the E2F and other proteins, allowing them to act. Rb does not bind to the cdk inhibitor p21 nor does it arrest cells in the G_2 of the cell cycle. Rb can be phosphorylated in vivo by several kinases, such as the cyclin-dependent kinase complexes (e.g., cyclin-cdk2, cyclin D-cdk4), but not by the cyclin B-cdc2 kinase complex.

21–22. The answers are: 21-D, 22-C. *(Pathology; tetralogy of Fallot).*
Congenital heart disease occurs in 1% of births and is usefully classified into two categories: cyanotic and noncyanotic. An infant with a cyanotic heart disease generally begins to show signs of oxygen desaturation within hours to days after birth, depending on the severity of the lesion. The cyanosis results from poor oxygenation in the blood and peripheral tissues. Generally speaking, cyanosis indicates a lesion that causes a substantial right-to-left shunt or a lesion in which the lungs are left out of the circulation. Patent ductus arteriosus and coarctation of the aorta are typically noncyanotic lesions at birth, although a patent ductus can lead to cyanosis later. Truncus arteriosus is a cyanotic lesion in which the aorta and pulmonary artery have fused into one large vessel that overrides both chambers; typically there is also a ventricular septal defect to accommodate the combined outflow. The diagram clearly shows two different outflow vessels. Transposition of the great arteries is a cyanotic lesion in which the right ventricle sends its output to the system and the left ventricle sends its output to the lungs. Because the return flows are not switched in the common variety of transposition, the result of transposition is two entirely separate circulations (unless the ductus arteriosus remains patent). The systemic circulation is never oxygenated, and the pulmonary circulation is never deoxygenated.

The abnormal flow patterns associated with most congenital heart defects cause local jet streams; that is local regions of fluid with high-velocity turbulent flow. Unlike the laminar flow that normally predominates, jet streams can be directed at the tissue (especially on the valves), resulting in tiny lesions to the delicate endocardium. The intact endocardium is resistant to most organisms, but the damaged endocardium provides a rough surface that is ideal for bacterial or viral attachment. Infectious endocarditis is an important source of morbidity and mortality in infants with congenital heart disease. Because it involves coronary artery disease in over 90% of cases, myocardial infarction is highly unusual in men younger than 20 and women younger than 30 years, even when the patients have a positive family history for cardiac disease. Mitral valve prolapse is a common finding, occurring in about 7% of adults between the ages of 20 and 40 years. Mitral valve prolapse is unusual in children and is not increased in infants with congenital heart defects, unless they also have connective tissue diseases. In most adult cases, mitral valve prolapse is asymptomatic except for their increased incidence of valvular endocarditis. By definition, rheumatic heart disease always follows a streptococcal infection (usually of the pharynx), and it is thought that the pathophysiology is related to immune dysregulation (not structural abnormalities in the heart). Valvular calcification is generally related to endocardial damage, but calcification is a process of long-term inflammation and calcium deposition.

23–26. The answers are: 23-D, 24-C, 25-E, 26-B. *(Biochemistry; carnitine deficiency; fatty acid oxidation; compartmentalization of metabolism)*
Carnitine deficiency is a relatively rare hereditary disorder with two forms: The form illustrated in this question is systemic, whereas the other variant is confined only to muscle and tends to manifest itself in older people after they exercise strenuously. Carnitine is important for transporting long-chain fatty acids into the mitochondria where β-oxidation occurs. Flavin adenine dinucleotide (FAD) is the coenzyme that is required for the formation of carbon–carbon double bonds in virtually all metabolic pathways. Free fatty acids are acetylated with acetyl coenzyme A (CoA) on the outer surface of mitochondria; then, carnitine is

exchanged for acetyl CoA, and the carnitine-complexed fatty acid is moved into the mitochondria. A different enzyme catalyzes the second exchange, this time freeing the carnitine by replacing it with acetyl CoA. Acyl carrier protein is the pantothenate derivative that holds the growing fatty acid during synthesis. Very low density lipoprotein (VLDL) is the carrier for fatty acids being exported by the liver to adipose tissue.

The discovery that oxidation occurs in cycles that release two carbon units in the form of acetyl CoA was a major advance in understanding fatty acid metabolism. The hydrolysis of pyrophosphate following formation of acyl CoA commits a fatty acid to degradation in the oxidative pathway. Adenosine triphosphate (ATP) molecules are not directly synthesized in the oxidative sequence; rather, energy is stored in reduced equivalents of both NADH and $FADH_2$. Because malonyl CoA is a substrate for fatty acid synthesis, high levels of malonyl CoA inhibit the fatty acid oxidation pathway to prevent a futile cycle of synthesis and oxidation. Understanding that fatty acid degradation cannot result in glucose is absolutely fundamental in understanding how the various metabolic pathways are integrated by the body. Because the body cannot make pyruvate (the building block for glucose) from any of the products of fatty acid or ketone breakdown, the β-oxidative pathway can produce only reducing equivalents and acetyl CoA units.

Oral carnitine replacement therapy should always be tried, but patients are not uniformly responsive. Because short- and medium-chain fatty acids do not require carnitine for their transport into mitochondria, a diet that excludes long-chain fatty acids may provide a great deal of relief. However, designing such a diet is far from trivial, and most patients find it difficult to comply. In the nonsystemic form, muscle biopsies are frequently taken to determine the cause of muscular weakness. The reasons for the lipid accumulation remain obscure. Because carnitine is a carrier that is attached and then immediately cleaved following fatty acid transfer, a deficiency in the enzymes for attachment or for cleavage would mimic a substrate carnitine deficiency almost identically. There are two separate enzymes (one for attachment and one for cleavage) named carnitine palmitoyltransferase I and II, respectively.

In order to allow for integration of different metabolic pathways, some key substrates are found in several different pathways. For some reactions, the energy state of the cell regulates the direction that a substrate like acetyl CoA follows. In other pathways, the entrance of a substrate is mainly regulated by substrate availability; in these cases, if a substrate is available to the enzymatic machinery, it is utilized. Thus, pathway compartmentalization within the cell keeps substrates from being available to the wrong pathway and helps prevent futile cycles of synthesis and degradation. Oxidative phosphorylation and fatty acid oxidation occur in the mitochondria; glycolysis and fatty acid synthesis occur in the cytosol. The pathways for gluconeogenesis and urea synthesis have enzymes in both the cytosol and mitochondria. Gangliosides and other complex lipid–carbohydrate molecules are degraded in the acidic lysosome. Several lysosomal storage disorders have been described in which particular lysosomal enzyme activities are deficient, which results in buildup of substrate.

27–29. The answers are: 27-A, 28-E, 29-C. *(Hematology; differential diagnosis of acquired anemia).*
Nutritional deficiencies, drugs, and several gastrointestinal disorders can give rise to acquired anemias. The principal classification of anemias is based upon the size and color of the circulating red blood cells. Megaloblastic anemias are generally hyperchromic and macrocytic. In the bone marrow, the maturation of the cytoplasm proceeds at a normal rate, whereas cell division is slow, and thus the cells are especially large. The slow cell division is a result of inefficient DNA synthesis. Deficiencies in either folate or cobalamin are a common cause of megaloblastic anemia; both of these nutrients serve essential roles in nucleotide biosynthesis. However, this woman's anemia is not megaloblastic. Schilling's test reveals the exact cause of cobalamin deficiency in a patient with low levels of serum cobalamin by determining the body's secretion of intrinsic factor and measuring the ileum's ability to absorb the intrinsic factor–cobalamin complex. Iron deficiency is a common cause of new onset hypochromic, microcytic anemias, and total iron-binding capacity (TIBC) and serum ferritin provide confirmation. TIBC is a measure of transferrin (the serum's iron transfer protein), which is increased in patients who are iron deficient because the body attempts to trap all available

iron for hematopoiesis. Ferritin, the body's storage form of iron, is usually decreased in patients who are iron deficient and is increased in patients who are iron overloaded. Glucose 6-phosphate dehydrogenase deficiency is generally restricted to people of Asian, African, or Mediterranean descent, and the acute anemia is almost always traceable to a new prescription or infection. In addition, the anemia is hemolytic and is thus accompanied by signs of acute hemolysis (e.g., jaundice, icterus, elevated unconjugated bilirubin). A hemoglobinopathy becoming clinically significant this late in life is unusual; in addition, hemoglobinopathies are not common in white people.

Cobalamin deficiency is probably the most serious cause of anemia, because cobalamin deficiency can also result in irreversible damage to the nervous system. The neurologic complications begin with demyelination and can eventually include damage to the cerebral cortex. Cobalamin deficiency also has a more insidious onset due to the low daily requirement and the relatively large stores of cobalamin in the liver. Thus, patients can cease to absorb new cobalamin and not show symptoms for years. In some cases, the anemia may not present until after the neurologic complications because the anemia emerged too slowly to become symptomatic. Pernicious anemia is the most common cause of cobalamin deficiency. In pernicious anemia, atrophy of the gastric mucosa leads to decreased secretion of intrinsic factor (IF). Because IF is required for ileal absorption of cobalamin, the cobalamin deficiency that results from gastric atrophy can be quite severe. Both ileal resection and Crohn's disease can interfere with sufficient absorption of the cobalamin–IF complex and cause a similar deficiency. Although neither cobalamin nor folate deficiency is directly associated with chronic liver damage, folate deficiency is relatively common in alcoholics who may have associated cirrhosis. The liver's store of folate is relatively small in relation to the daily requirement of folate. Since most alcoholics are malnourished, the stores can be depleted rather quickly (i.e., in months) resulting in a relatively sudden onset of symptomatic folate deficiency. In contrast, cobalamin stores are relatively large in relation to the daily requirement, and a malnourished person is able to use the stored reserve of cobalamin for 1 to 2 years. Women are more susceptible to iron deficiency because they menstruate, which drains their iron stores each month. Even a short period of poor nutrition can result in relatively quick depletion of iron stores, especially in a woman with insufficient starting reserves.

The iron-binding protein of liver illustrates a classic case of coordinated protein synthesis; levels of transferrin and ferritin are regulated in opposite fashions by a single mechanism that is post-transcriptional [i.e., following the synthesis of messenger RNA (mRNA)]. Transferrin mRNA is normally degraded rapidly, but in the presence of the activated (i.e., iron free) iron-binding protein, a 3' stem–loop structure is stabilized, and the mRNA is no longer susceptible to degradation. Ferritin, the storage form of iron, has a 5' stem–loop structure that is recognized by the activated iron-binding protein. When the activated protein is bound to the stem–loop, initiation of ferritin translation is prevented. Therefore, when there is no iron to inactivate the iron-binding protein, the transferrin message is stabilized, and transferrin synthesis increases, while ferritin translation is blocked. When iron binds to the protein and inactivates it, ferritin translation begins proportional to the amount of message, and the transferrin message is rapidly degraded prior to translation.

30. The answer is D. *(Pharmacology; peptic ulcer disease)*
The H$_2$-histamine receptor blockers (e.g., ranitidine and cimetidine) are the mainstay of peptic ulcer disease treatment. They competitively block the receptors and powerfully downregulate parietal cell acid production, thus providing adequate therapy for most patients with peptic ulcer disease. Sucralfate and omeprazole are relatively new drugs whose efficacy is being demonstrated as their use continues to grow. Sucralfate specifically targets the ulcer bed and coats it for up to 12 hours; it shows very little affinity for normal mucosa, and it is not absorbed systemically. Omeprazole is absorbed systemically, although it is not associated with any substantial systemic toxicities. The irreversible mechanism of action of omeprazole makes it especially useful in the treatment of refractory cases due to Zollinger-Ellison syndrome. Colloidal bismuth is another coating agent whose mechanism of action may also involve antibiotic effects against the organism *Helicobacter pylori*, which can be identified in a substantial majority of patients with chronic peptic ulcer disease.

There is evidence to indicate that *H. pylori* may destroy the mucosal lining, and, therefore, make patients susceptible to gastritis as well as to peptic ulcer disease. Atropine blocks the muscarinic receptors on the parietal cells, but it is not as efficacious as the histamine receptor blockers. Furthermore, oral or intravenous atropine is associated with a myriad of systemic side effects and is, therefore, not commonly used for chronic medical conditions. There are no clinically useful gastrin receptor blockers available for prescription in the United States.

31–34. The answers are: 31-B, 32-A, 33-D, 34-D. *(Cell biology; cell cycle)*
The cell cycle is divided into several distinct phases. Replication of the nuclear DNA usually occupies only a portion of interphase, called the S phase of the cell cycle. The interval between the end of DNA synthesis and the beginning of mitosis is called the G_2 phase. The G_2 phase provides a safety gap, allowing the cell to ensure that DNA replication is complete before going into mitosis. Mitosis, or M phase, is the next phase, during which the process of nuclear division occurs, leading up to the moment of cell division. The interval between the completion of mitosis and the beginning of DNA synthesis is called G_1 phase. During G_1 phase, the cell monitors its environment and its own size and, when the time is right, takes the step that commits it to DNA replication and completion of the division cycle. Phases S, G_2, M, and G_1 are the subdivisions of the standard cell cycle.

35. The answer is A. *(Biochemistry; fatty acid synthesis)*
Feedback inhibition of pathways is common throughout cellular metabolism. The ultimate product inhibits the committed step so that when sufficient product is available, the enzymatic sequence is completely stopped. This prevents energy from being lost by moving a substrate partly through the pathway. Enzyme phosphorylation, in response to elevation of cyclic adenosine monophosphate (cAMP), is also an important part of a variety of catabolic and anabolic pathways. Elevated levels of citrate indicate a high-energy status within the cell and, therefore, activate acetyl coenzyme A (CoA) carboxylase to increase fatty acid production. The enzymes that catalyze fatty acid synthesis exist as independent domains on one large polypeptide. This provides for the most efficient shuttling of substrate from one reaction to the next, and obviates the need for diffusion and random collision with the next enzyme. The acyl carrier protein (ACP) is a pantothenic acid derivative that is covalently bound to the growing chain. Biotin is the main carrier of carboxyl groups in nearly every reaction that requires transfer of activated bicarbonate anions. Niacin is important in the biosynthesis of nicotinamide–adenine dinucleotide (NADH), which is essential for reactions that oxidize hydroxyl groups into carbonyl groups.

36–37. The answers are: 36-C, 37-A. *(Pathology; peptic ulcer disease)*
Zollinger-Ellison syndrome was initially described in a person with refractory, erosive peptic ulcer disease. Most cases involve a pancreatic islet cell tumor that secretes gastrin, which is the most potent physiologic stimulator of parietal cell acid production. Aggressive medical treatment is sometimes not sufficient to block the copious production of acid in these patients, and usually the gastrin-secreting tumor must be extracted surgically or treated medically. Increased vagal tone results in increased acid production, but vagal hyperactivity is rarely sufficient to account for acid production of this magnitude. Increased release of histamine also leads to hyperactivity of the parietal cells. However, histamine is produced by mast cells located near the parietal cells, and mast cell tumors are not a common cause of Zollinger-Ellison syndrome. Pepsin is the proteolytic enzyme whose activation is pH dependent; hypersecretion of pepsin is uncommon and, in any case, would not lead to the refractory ulcers in this patient. Decreased mucosal production is probably involved in many cases of peptic ulcer disease, most notably those induced by stress or nonsteroidal anti-inflammatory drugs (NSAIDs). Locally produced prostaglandins are important in regulating the production of mucus by the cells lining the stomach, and stress as well as NSAIDs can inhibit prostaglandin production. However, peptic ulcer disease of this magnitude, particularly a condition that includes esophageal ulcers, could not be caused by insufficient mucous production.

The production of acid by parietal cells is regulated by the interplay of three main substances: histamine, gastrin, and acetylcholine, all of which can stimulate acid production. Parietal cells have receptors for all three signals, and each of the three signals can regulate release of the other signals independent of the parietal cell receptors. H_2-histamine receptor activation causes an elevation of cyclic adenosine monophosphate (cAMP) and the subsequent activation of cAMP-dependent protein kinases. Acetylcholine from the vagus nerve mediates its actions via muscarinic-type receptors. These muscarinic receptors, as well as their gastrin receptor analogues, mediate their signals through an elevation of free intracellular calcium. Acid production is a two-step process; in the first step, carbonic anhydrase splits the carbonic acid molecule into a bicarbonate anion and a hydrogen ion. In the second step, the movement of the bicarbonate anion into the blood causes the measurable and physiologically normal ''alkaline tide'' during meals (i.e., when the arterial pH increases slightly), and the hydrogen ion is pumped against a million-fold concentration gradient into the stomach by the hydrogen–potassium adenosine triphosphatase.

38–40. The answers are: 38-A, 39-E, 40-D. *(Pathology; metabolic acidosis and chronic renal failure)*
End-stage renal disease is the cause of death in up to 30% of patients with noninsulin-dependent diabetes mellitus. Chronic renal failure is characterized by increased glomerular filtration rate, proteinuria, and the systemic symptoms of urinary protein loss. Because the kidneys have a tremendous reserve for maintaining potassium balance, neither hypokalemia nor hyperkalemia is common in patients with renal failure. However, when potassium balance is lost, hyperkalemia is more common, generally resulting from acidosis, oliguria, or excess potassium ingestion. Proteinuria is one of the earliest findings in many types of kidney disease; the compromised glomeruli have leaky basement membranes, and albumin, as well as other small proteins, is lost from the serum. The liver increases production of all serum proteins in response to the loss. The mechanism causing triglyceride elevation is complex and poorly understood, but it is thought that the liver's production of lipoproteins is inappropriately increased in addition to the necessary increase in albumin production. Red blood cell production is dependent on the kidneys' synthesis of the growth factor erythropoietin. Although the reserve production of erythropoietin is substantial, most patients with end-stage disease have a clinically significant anemia. In the past, normochromic, normocytic anemia used to be a much more serious problem in patients with renal failure. With the development of recombinant erythropoietin, this problem is easily treatable. Patients with renal failure have a pungent odor in their sweat and on their breath called uremic fetor as a result of their elevated serum urea and creatinine.

Ammonia is one of the nontitratable acids in the urine and is a major route of acid excretion. Ammonia is synthesized in the cells of the kidney tubules and freely diffuses into the tubule fluid. Any free hydrogen ions are bound by the ammonia, making the charged ammonium ion, which does not diffuse back into the cells. Ammoniagenesis is tightly regulated by the kidney and is the major factor in the kidney's ability to handle large acid loads. The complete enzymatic pathway for urea synthesis is found only in hepatocytes. Urea synthesis plays no significant role in acid–base homeostasis; excretion of urea is the major route for disposal of nitrogenous wastes. Bicarbonate recycling by the tubule cells involves a complex set of transport processes. Carbonic anhydrase on the brush border of the proximal tubule cells synthesizes carbon dioxide and water from bicarbonate and hydrogen ion in the tubule fluid. The carbon dioxide diffuses into the cell, where another carbonic anhydrase synthesizes the bicarbonate anion from the incoming molecule and hydroxyl anion. The bicarbonate is transported with sodium into the bloodstream, whereas the hydrogen ion is secreted into the tubule fluid, resulting in a net reabsorption of bicarbonate. Pyruvate is a substrate for gluconeogenesis in the liver, and potassium is secreted in exchange for sodium reabsorption in the distal tubules.

In the initial phases of metabolic acidosis, the anion gap is small because the deficiency in serum bicarbonate is replaced by chloride anion. This phase is called hyperchloremic acidosis and reflects the initial stage in which some level of compensation is maintained. As the active transport of bicarbonate by the kidneys continues to drop, unmeasured anions like phosphate and sulfate begin to fill the gap. Because they are unmeasured, the apparent ''gap'' between the measured cations (i.e., sodium and potassium) and the measured anions (i.e., bicarbonate and chloride) starts to increase. The source of the phosphate that fills the anion gap is most likely the bone. Thus, hydrolysis of calcium salts in the bone provides the anions to compensate for the failure of the kidneys to synthesize ammonia and reabsorb bicarbonate. It is thought that metabolic acidosis plays a significant role in the pathophysiology, which leads to renal osteodystrophy. The synthesis of ammonia in the kidney tubules is important in acid secretion, and, as discussed above, it is seriously compromised in patients with renal failure.

41. The answer is E. *(Cell biology; cell cycle)*
There are two main classes of cyclins. One class includes the mitotic cyclins (e.g., cyclin B), which bind to cyclin-dependent kinases during G_2 of the cell cycle and are required for entry into mitosis. Another class is the G_1 cyclins (e.g., cyclin E, cyclin D_1, D_2, and D_3), which bind to cyclin-dependent kinases during G_1 of the cell cycle and are required for entry into the S phase of the cell cycle.

42–43. The answers are: 42-C, 43-D. *(Biostatistics; cross-sectional study of severity of disability in cerebrovascular accident and personality type)*
The patients participating in this study were simultaneously classified according to the severity of their disability and their personality type. Therefore, this is an example of a cross-sectional study.

When the data are in the form of counts (i.e., the number of people in each combination of categories), the chi-square test is used to test for the presence of a significant association between the two study variables. Both the paired and pooled *t* tests, as well as the analysis of variance, use continuous, not frequency, data to test for the equality of means. Correlation analysis estimates the magnitude of the association between two quantitative variables, whereas regression analysis is used to derive an equation for predicting the value of one variable based on values of the other.

44. The answer is C. *(Cell biology; cell cycle)*
Cyclin-dependent kinase inhibitors are proteins that bind to cyclin-dependent kinase complexes and inhibit their kinase function. Cyclin-dependent kinase inhibitors are classified as either the ink4 family of cyclin-dependent kinase inhibitors (e.g., p15, p16, p18, p19) or the p21 family of cyclin-dependent kinase inhibitors (e.g., p21, p27 kip1, p57 kip2). p53 is a tumor suppressor gene, also known as the ''guardian of the genome.'' It can bind DNA, act as a transcription factor, and induce the production of proteins (e.g., p21 cyclin-dependent kinase inhibitor), which is induced by DNA damage. However, p53 is not a cyclin-dependent kinase inhibitor itself.

45. The answer is D. *(Cell biology; cell cycle)*
The G_0 resting state of the cell cycle is a specialized, nongrowing state of the cell. The rate of protein synthesis is drastically reduced, often to as little as 20% of its value in proliferating cells. Slowly dividing cells can remain in G_0 state for weeks or years. In this state, the normal cells have lower levels of G_1 cyclins and cyclin-dependent kinases than cells in the G_1 phase of the cell cycle.

46–47. The answers are: 46-D, 47-B. *(Pharmacology; management of shock)*
Dobutamine is the agent of choice for a hypovolemic crisis. Other adrenergic-activating agents have two drawbacks. Many (e.g., epinephrine) are not β-receptor specific and, therefore, cause vasoconstriction, which is undesired because in these patients vasoconstriction is already severe and may be causing intestinal or renal damage. Other β-specific agents (e.g., isoproterenol) are chronotropic as well as inotropic. Because increased chronotropism carries a greater risk of ischemia, and because increased inotropism is a more efficient way to increase cardiac output, the selectively inotropic agent dobutamine is best suited. As an added benefit, dobutamine also activates an unusual class of dopaminergic receptors in the kidneys, causing vasodilation at a time when the kidneys may be suffering clinically significant ischemia. Albuterol is a

relatively selective agonist of the β_2 class of adrenergic receptors and is commonly prescribed to relieve the acute bronchoconstrictive symptoms during episodes of asthma and chronic obstructive pulmonary disease. Because the cardiac receptors are principally representatives of the β_1 subtype, albuterol would not offer any substantial cardiac effects. Propranolol is a nonselective β-adrenergic receptor antagonist used as a class II antiarrhythmic as well as an antianginal agent. It decreases cardiac output and is not indicated for the management of shock. Furosemide is a loop diuretic that can induce rapid and large increases in urine output and would be strictly contraindicated in this patient. Tubocurarine blocks neurotransmission at nicotinic cholinergic synapses and is used to provide muscular paralysis prior to intubation. It may be necessary to intubate patients during a hypovolemic crisis, but tubocurarine does not support the man's cardiovascular system.

In addition to the intestines, the kidneys are especially sensitive to hypovolemic shock that lasts 30 minutes to 1 hour. Acute tubular necrosis is the most common kidney lesion seen in patients recovering from hypovolemic shock, and hyperkalemia quickly ensues (primarily the result of oliguria). In the absence of a substantial external potassium load, most patients will only experience modest potassium accumulation, with rises in serum potassium of about 0.4 mM in a 24-hour period. As with all causes of kidney failure, serum blood urea nitrogen (BUN) and creatinine are markedly elevated (creatinine as high as 8–12; normal = 0.8–1.5). An antinuclear antibody screen is useful in diagnosing systemic lupus erythematosus. A positive antistreptolysin O (ASO) titer is generally adequate evidence to demonstrate a recent streptococcal infection and is especially useful in diagnosing acute rheumatic fever as well as post-streptococcal glomerulonephritis. A complete blood count provides information that may be important in diagnosing infection, anemia, or neoplasia. A digoxin level is important if digoxin toxicity is suspected. However, digoxin is most commonly prescribed to support patients with congestive heart failure, which is an unlikely condition in this 29-year-old man. Furthermore, digoxin toxicity is usually manifested in cardiac conduction disturbances and arrhythmias, not in renal failure.

48. The answer is D. *(Biostatistics; bias)*
Bias is a process at any stage of inference tending to produce results that systematically depart from the true values. It is not the result of random variation. Measurement bias occurs when the methods of measurement are consistently dissimilar among groups of patients. Confounding bias occurs when two factors or processes are associated or travel together, and the effect of one is confused or distorted by the effect of the other. Selection bias occurs when comparisons are made between groups of patients that differ with respect to determinants of the outcome other than those under study.

49. The answer is D. *(Biostatistics; confounding bias)*
Clinical manifestations of atherosclerosis are more likely to occur in patients with diabetes, whereas risk factors for cardiovascular diseases are higher in patients with diabetes. The clinical manifestation of atherosclerosis—myocardial infarction, sudden death, peripheral vascular disease, and stroke—are more likely to occur in patients with diabetes. Other risk factors for cardiovascular disease (e.g., blood pressure, excess weight, and high serum cholesterol) are increased in people with diabetes, too. This is an example of confounding bias: two factors are associated, and the effect of one is distorted by the effect of the other. Serum triglycerides as a risk factor for coronary heart disease but not independently of serum cholesterol is also an example of confounding bias. It is not an independent cause of coronary heart disease but is confounded with other factors (e.g., serum cholesterol), which is an independent cause of coronary heart disease. The fact that smoking cigarettes is a risk factor for coronary heart disease, and the exercise group smoked less is another example of confounding bias, because the group that exercised is confounded by the fact that they also smoked less. The association between oral contraceptives and thrombophlebitis, due to the way the history was reported, is an example of measurement bias, not confounding bias.

50. The answer is C. *(Pathology; post-streptococcal glomerulonephritis)*
Post-streptococcal glomerulonephritis is a relatively common complication of pharyngitis in children 6 to 10 years of age. Most cases are caused by group A β-hemolytic streptococci with specific types of M antigen. The child's puffiness is due to dramatically decreased glomerular filtration and the resultant oliguria with salt and water retention. As with all cases of nephritis, there is significant hematuria and proteinuria. The loss of protein combined with the salt and water retention produces the characteristic edema, and the increased blood volume is sufficient to explain her modest hypertension. Although systemic lupus erythematosus can be associated with glomerulonephritis, renal symptoms characteristic of the nephrotic syndrome are more common in the early stages; and, it would be unusual for an 8-year-old to present with lupus. Acute tubular necrosis can be associated with water retention, edema, and high blood pressure, but hematuria is not common in these patients. Furthermore, most cases of acute tubular necrosis are preceded by an identifiable ingestion of some acutely nephrotoxic agent or ischemic damage secondary to shock. Juvenile-onset diabetes frequently presents with renal symptoms, but these changes are usually nephrotic rather than nephritic in nature (i.e., lack of hematuria and more substantial proteinuria). The onset of diabetes is generally more gradual, and significant edema would probably evolve over a longer period of time. Finally, all cases of diabetes manifest with polyuria, and salt and fluid retention are rarely seen prior to the onset of chronic renal failure late in the disease. Isolated hyperaldosteronism is rare and would not be associated with hematuria.

51. The answer is E. *(Biostatistics; definitions of terms)*
Standard deviation is the absolute value of the average difference of individual values from the mean and is always more than the standard error of the mean, which is equal to the standard deviation divided by the square root of the population number. The mean is the sum of values divided by the number of values; mode is the most frequently occurring value. The median is the point where the number of observations above equals the number below. Range is the lowest and highest value in a distribution.

52. The answer is C. *(Biostatistics; cohort studies)*
In a cohort study, a group of people (cohort) is assembled, none of whom has experienced the outcome of interest. People in the cohort are classified according to those characteristics that might be related to the outcome. These people are observed over time to see which of them experience the outcome. A case series is a prevalence survey of a group of individuals with a particular disease performed at a single point in time. Case control studies compare the frequency of a purported risk factor in a group of cases and a group of controls. The case control design has the outcome of interest at the time that information on risk factors is sought.

53. The answer is D. *(Biostatistics; odds ratio)*
The odds ratio is one approach for comparing the frequency of exposure among cases and controls provides a measure of risk that is conceptually and mathematically similar to the relative risk. It is defined as the odds that a case is exposed divided by the odds that control is exposed with certain assumptions. This can be simplified to the product of the number of cases exposed multiplied by the number of noncases not exposed divided by the product of the number of noncases exposed multiplied by the number of cases not exposed (AD/BC). If the frequency of exposure is higher among cases, the odds ratio will exceed one, indicating risk. Thus, the stronger the association between exposure and disease, the higher the odds ratio. Conversely, if the frequency of exposures is lower among cases, the odds ratio will be less than one, indicating protection.

54–55. The answers are: 54-D, 55-B. *(Pancreatitis; alcoholism)*
The description of abdominal pain with guarding and hypoactive bowel sounds is classic for pancreatitis. Other causes of an acutely painful abdomen need to be considered, however. The absence of free air under

the diaphragm eliminates visceral perforation from the differential diagnosis in this patient with an acutely painful abdomen. Myocardial infarction is very unlikely in a 35-year-old woman with a negative family history for cardiac disease; furthermore, most patients do not describe the pain of infarction as stabbing but rather crushing. Similarly, an aortic aneurysm is generally a disease of older adults and is the result of chronic hypertension and atherosclerosis, which are unlikely in this woman of 35 years. The pain of renal colic is much different than what this patient described. Located primarily in the flank, it radiates to the groin in classic cases and is almost always described as a pain that comes severely in 10- to 20-minute waves. Renal colic is not usually worsened by lying supine.

Making a diagnosis of alcoholism is the responsibility of all physicians, since alcohol represents one of the most important causes of morbidity and mortality in the United States. Blackouts are frequently described by individuals who have drunk alcohol excessively on one or two occasions and are not sufficient reason to diagnose alcoholism in the absence of one of the other criteria listed. Each of the other problems (i.e., relationship problems, work problems, disease, arrests all related to alcohol) is a *Diagnostic and Statistical Manual IV (DSM-IV)* criterion for diagnosing alcoholism. The key unifying factor in all four of these problems is that a socially significant, undesirable repercussion of the drinking behavior had no effect in changing subsequent drinking.

56. The answer is B. (*Pharmacology; drug administration*)
There are two main routes of drug administration: enteral and parenteral. Parenteral administration is used for drugs that are poorly absorbed from the gastrointestinal tract and for agents that are unstable in the gastrointestinal tract. Intramuscular drug delivery is an example of parenteral drug administration. The intramuscular route is used for depot preparations, and when rapid onset of action is required (e.g., epinephrine in anaphylaxis). Sublingual is an enteral administration route in which the drug is placed under the tongue, allowing the drug to diffuse into the capillary network and enter the systemic circulation directly. The oral route (enteral) is when the drug is given by mouth. It is the most common route of administration, but it is the most complicated pathway to the tissues. Rectal administration (enteral) is when the drug is placed in the rectum for absorption. Fifty percent of the drainage of the rectal region bypasses the hepatic portal circulation; thus, the biotransformation of drugs that are metabolized by the liver is minimized.

57. The answer is B. (*Pharmacology; anesthetics*)
Ketamine is an intravenous general anesthetic. It is also a dissociative anesthetic in that patients appear awake but are unconscious and do not feel pain. Ketamine is not widely used because it increases cerebral blood flow and induces postoperative hallucinations. Halothane, ether, and nitrous oxide are inhaled general anesthetics. Inhaled general anesthetics are used primarily for the maintenance of anesthesia after administration of an intravenous agent. Procaine and lidocaine are local anesthetics. Local anesthetics are applied locally and block nerve conduction of sensory impulses from the periphery to the central nervous system. These drugs inhibit sodium channels of the nerve membrane.

58. The answer is F. (*Pharmacology; cholinergic agonists*)
Pralidoxime is a synthetic compound that can reactivate inhibited acetylcholinesterase. It binds to the inhibitor of acetylcholinesterase and pulls it off the inhibited enzyme. Isoflurophate covalently binds to acetylcholinesterase and irreversibly inhibits this enzyme. Edrophonium and neostigmine reversibly inhibit acetylcholinesterase. Acetylcholine is the neurotransmitter of parasympathetic and cholinergic nerves and is a cholinergic agonist. Pilocarpine is also a cholinergic agonist and is unaffected by acetylcholineesterase.

59. The answer is B. (*Pathology; α_1-antitrypsin deficiency*)
α_1-Antitrypsin deficiency may first present as acute hepatitis with impressive jaundice, elevated serum transaminases, and compromised blood clotting (especially in children). However, the phenotypic expression of

this genotype is variable, even in persons who are homozygous for the deficiency. Some patients with heterozygous genotypes, and even individuals with homozygous mutations, may experience emphysema and symptoms of chronic obstructive pulmonary disease before liver disease, especially if they smoked. All homozygous individuals who live into adulthood will have panacinar emphysema by their early forties. Although restriction fragment length polymorphisms (RFLPs) are useful in providing information for genetic counseling of the patient, the definitive diagnosis can be made by directly assaying the serum for protein activity. The pathophysiology seems to involve a deficiency of the protein's normal inhibitory effect on the serine proteases released by the neutrophils residing in the lung and liver. Because both tissues have antigen-presenting cells that are regularly active, there is a small population of neutrophils normally releasing proteases, nucleases, and elastases. In unaffected individuals, the antitrypsin protein irreversibly inhibits the destructive effects of elastases and proteases, thus checking the level of local tissue inflammation. In affected individuals, this small amount of inflammation grows unchecked, causing significant tissue destruction and the recruitment of more inflammatory effector cells. Since it is known that individuals who smoke have an increased number of neutrophils and macrophages in their lung tissue, smoking results in a significantly greater amount of damage than it would in an unaffected individual.

60. The answer is C. *(Pharmacology; alcohol withdrawal)*
Physical dependence on alcohol implies that withdrawal of the depressant results in clinically significant physical and behavioral changes. Benzodiazepines are appropriate as a substitute for the depressive effects of alcohol while the acute physical symptoms are still active (approximately 5–7 days). Chlordiazepoxide, a commonly prescribed benzodiazepine, is a good choice based upon its intermediate half-life and long history of use. The drug should be prescribed at a sedative dose and tapered over a 5-day period, so that the physician avoids exchanging one addiction for another. Phenytoin should not be routinely prescribed because seizures are an uncommon complication, and, in the few cases involving seizures, the episode had passed before adequate phenytoin levels were achieved. If the alcoholism coincides with clinically significant depression, nortriptyline may be appropriate in conjunction with appropriate counseling. However, nortriptyline is an antidepressant and is not directed at the delirium tremens. Haloperidol, a commonly prescribed antipsychotic, is not appropriate therapy for delirium tremens. Since morphine, a therapeutically useful narcotic analgesic, can be just as addictive as alcohol, it is certainly contraindicated.

61–63. The answers are: 61-B, 62-D, 63-D. *(Pharmacology; physiology; asthma diagnosis and treatment)*
Asthma is a potential underlying cause of episodic dyspnea associated with wheezing in an 11-year-old boy. Although it is often difficult to establish a diagnosis of asthma in the laboratory, a reduction in forced expiratory volumes (*curve 1*) that is reversible after the inhalation of a bronchodilator such as metaproterenol (*curve 2*) is consistent with a diagnosis of hyperreactive airway disease. Although variability in spirometric testing is common, a forced expiratory volume in 1 sec (FEV_1) of less than 1 L/min is of concern even in a patient of this age. Methacholine is a useful provocative agent that will reduce FEV_1 at a lower dose in an asthmatic patient than in normal subjects. Although cromolyn sodium and beclomethasone are useful agents in the therapy of asthma, neither agent is likely to produce acute reversal of airway obstruction.

Theophylline is one of a number of methylxanthines that is useful for the chronic therapy of asthma. Although it can increase intracellular levels of cyclic adenosine monophosphate (cAMP) via phosphodiesterase inhibition and relax bronchial smooth muscle, theophylline appears to affect symptoms of asthma via other mechanisms, including affecting adenosine receptors or intracellular calcium homeostasis. Propranolol is a β-adrenergic receptor antagonist that is contraindicated in patients with asthma because it may exacerbate their symptoms. Although local concentrations of histamine contribute to the pathogenesis of asthma, antihistamines do not have an accepted role in the therapy of asthma except to manage associated rhinitis. Bethanechol is a moderately long-acting parasympathomimetic and, as such, is contraindicated in asthmatics.

Ibuprofen and other nonsteroidal antiinflammatory agents (which inhibit cyclooxygenase) may also produce an airway narrowing effect (perhaps by shuttling arachidonic acid via the bronchoconstricting lipoxygenase pathway) and are often contraindicated in a subset (e.g., aspirin-hypersensitive) of asthmatics.

Stimulation of irritant receptors leads to reflex bronchoconstriction via a vagal reflex. Indeed, normal resting tone is set by the parasympathetic nervous system, and some aspects of hyperreactive airway disease are thought to involve a relatively high influence of vagal tone at the expense of sympathetic efferent bronchodilator activity. The intercostal and phrenic nerves are important nerves to the accessory respiratory muscle and the diaphragm, respectively.

64. The answer is D. *(Pharmacology; cholinergic antagonists)*
Scopolamine blocks muscarinic receptors causing inhibition of all parasympathetic functions. It also prevents motion sickness. Nicotine is a ganglionic blocker and acts at the nicotinic receptors in the autonomic ganglia. Nicotine depolarizes ganglia, resulting in stimulation of ganglia followed by paralysis of all ganglia. Tobucurarine, gallamine, and pancuronium are nondepolarizing (competitive) blockers of the cholinergic transmission between motor nerve endings and the nicotinic receptors on the neuromuscular end-plate of the skeletal muscle. Succinylcholine is a depolarizing neuromuscular blocking drug that attaches to the nicotinic receptor and acts like acetylcholine to depolarize the junction. However, unlike acetylcholine, succinylcholine persists at high concentrations at the synaptic cleft because it is resistant to acetylcholinesterase.

65. The answer is C. *(Pharmacology; cholinergic agonists)*
Isoflurophate covalently binds to acetylcholinesterase and irreversibly inhibits this enzyme. Edrophonium and neostigmine reversibly inhibit acetylcholinesterase. Carbachol, bethanechol, and pilocarpine are direct-acting cholinergic agonists that are resistant to metabolism by acetylcholinesterase.

66–67. The answers are: 66-C, 67-C. *(Microbiology; bacterial meningitis)*
The findings of fever, headache, nuchal rigidity, and lethargy with an acute onset and the lack of dramatic neurologic manifestations suggest acute bacterial meningitis. Viral meningitis causes much of the same symptomatology, but the onset typically is more insidious and the patient usually is less acutely ill. Patients with viral encephalitis display the same general symptomatology as those with viral meningitis, but encephalitis is differentiated by dramatic neurologic manifestations and a much poorer prognosis. Fungal meningitis is more chronic and frequently is seen with other systemic signs of mycotic disease. Brain abscess usually is seen with other foci of infection, and the patient typically has deficits that reflect the location of the lesion.

Streptococcus pneumoniae is the most common cause of bacterial meningitis among the elderly. *Haemophilus influenzae* type B is the most common cause of bacterial meningitis overall. Its incidence is highest in infants 6 to 12 months old and decreases with age; the incidence of meningitis caused by *H. influenzae* is low in adults. Meningococcal meningitis occurs primarily among young adults, and *Neisseria meningitidis* serogroups A, B, C, and Y cause most cases. *Staphylococcus aureus* occasionally causes meningitis but is a common cause of brain abscess.

68–70. The answers are: 68-E, 69-B, 70-E. *(Pathology; acute neurologic management; alcohol withdrawal)*
The most important action to take with the ataxic and confused homeless man is to determine what, if any, brain injuries he may have sustained. The scalp wound can be handled initially with a bandage before suturing. If a fracture is suspected, skull films can be obtained after an acute neurologic condition has been ruled out. A serum ethanol level is indicated, and though important, it is not a priority. Hygiene is relevant but not urgent.

Although all of the problems listed in the question must be considered in the differential diagnosis of this patient, the epidural hematoma is the most emergent potential problem listed. An epidural hematoma classically presents as an initial brief period of unconsciousness followed by a lucid period that is followed by unconsciousness. If a sufficient tear of the middle meningeal artery has occurred, death can ensue rapidly. The encephalopathies, including delirium, could progress to coma, but hepatic encephalopathy is not the most urgent choice listed.

Disulfiram (Antabuse) is used as a deterrent to further drinking; it is not a treatment for alcohol withdrawal. Hydration is important to prevent cardiovascular collapse. Benzodiazepines are cross-tolerant with barbiturates and ethanol and permit controlled withdrawal from ethanol. Changes in vital signs, including increased blood pressure, heart rate, and temperature, accompany ethanol withdrawal and should be monitored.

71–74. The answers are: 71-C, 72-B, 73-D, 74-D. *(Physiology; myocardial infarction)*
A fast rhythm with a wide complex is usually consistent with a ventricular tachycardia. It is highly likely that the 60-year-old man described in the question suffered a myocardial infarction associated with ventricular tachycardia. The treatment of choice for ventricular tachycardia associated with myocardial ischemia is lidocaine. Lidocaine is typical of a group of antiarrhythmic agents that block sodium ion channels that are the current-carrying processes responsible for depolarization in fast fibers of the heart (ventricular and atrial). It suppresses these channels in the infarct area in cells with abnormal resting membrane potential. Although the mechanism underlying this selectivity is poorly understood, it is thought that abnormal tissue ion channels tend to be in inactivated states, which would increase the binding and efficacy of use-dependent agents, or that damaged myocardial tissue tends to accumulate agents such as lidocaine to a greater extent. Agents such as diltiazem, propranolol, or digitalis affect electrical propagation and conduction in sinoatrial and atrioventricular nodal tissue, where parasympathetic input predominates, and calcium is the current carrying ion. Although propranolol has been shown to have some utility in reducing subsequent damage after myocardial infarction, it is contraindicated in patients with hypotension and potential poor left ventricular function. Epinephrine increases oxygen demands on the heart by directly stimulating beta receptors as well as increasing afterload, and, in this case, it appears to be contraindicated.

Creatine kinase (CK) is an enzyme that catalyzes the transfer of high energy phosphates and is found largely in tissues that use large amounts of energy. The two most common isoforms are CK-MM (muscle) and CK-BB (brain). There is an isoform that contains both M and B subunits (CK-MB), which is found only in the myocardium. In the heart, CK is approximately 85% CK-MB. An increase in both total CK and CK-MB (secondary to myocardial injury) has proven to be highly sensitive and specific for the diagnosis of myocardial infarction. Lactate dehydrogenase (LDH) is often elevated 48–72 hours after injury.

Significant injury to the anterior wall of the left ventricle may be due to occlusion (>70%) of the left anterior descending coronary artery. Alternatively, occlusion to a lesser degree of the left mainstem coronary artery may also produce the above condition. The left circumflex artery may affect the anterior wall but is more likely to involve inferior or posterior parts of the heart.

Low-dose aspirin has become an important component of pharmacotherapeutic approaches to reducing the risk of recurrent myocardial infarction. The desired effect is to irreversibly inhibit platelet cyclooxygenase (thereby reducing platelet-derived thromboxane A_2), while allowing for resynthesis of endothelial cell cyclooxygenase and maintaining a useful production of prostacyclin. Aspirin does not affect lipoxygenase activity and, therefore, it does not decrease circulating levels of any of the leukotrienes. Aspirin does not reduce normal body temperature.

75. The answer is B. *(Biochemistry; fatty acid metabolism)*
Because of a methyl group on the third carbon, phytanic acid cannot be metabolized through β-oxidation. Phytanic acid is converted to pristanic acid in peroxisomes by the decarboxylation of the hydroxylated intermediate. Pristanic acid can then be used as a substrate for β-oxidation, as can linoleic acid, arachidonic acid, palmitic acid, and decenoic acid. Phytanic acid is toxic if it is not metabolized.

76. The answer is D. *(Biochemistry; cholesterol biosynthesis)*
The rate-limiting and regulated step of cholesterol biosynthesis is the formation of mevalonate from 3-hydroxy-3-methylglutaryl coenzyme A (HMG CoA) catalyzed by HMG CoA reductase. This enzyme is inhibited by dietary cholesterol and endogenously synthesized cholesterol. A vegetarian diet, a diet low in cholesterol, and the administration of a bile acid–sequestering resin all result in a reduced intake of cholesterol, which will not inhibit HMG CoA reductase activity. Familial hypercholesterolemia is a result of a deficiency of low-density lipoprotein (LDL) receptors.

77–78. The answers are: 77-C, 78-C. *(Pathology; neurologic disease topography)*
Guillain-Barré syndrome presents with peripheral sensory defects as well as motor defects, which progress from distal areas of the body to involve more proximal regions. It usually follows a viral illness of unknown origin and affects mostly young people. Loss of deep tendon reflexes is also present. Guillain-Barré syndrome is thought to involve antimyelin autoantibodies against motor neurons that evolve after viral illness or influenza vaccine. There is a progressive mixed motor and sensory loss, even though motor neurons are the target of these antibodies, due to the inflammation of spinal nerves in which both motor and sensory fibers travel together.

Myasthenia gravis is a disease of the neuromuscular junction and most commonly presents with ocular symptoms, such as ptosis, diplopia, and dysarthria. It manifests as muscle fatigue without sensory symptoms. Deep tendon reflexes are diminished but not lost in this disease. Myasthenia gravis is an autoimmune disease, which involves acetylcholine (ACh) receptors in the postsynaptic neuromuscular junction.

Poliovirus is a picornavirus, which usually causes an intestinal disease that can progress to viremia and cause the destruction of anterior horn cells of the spinal cord, resulting in paralysis of the innervated muscles. It usually manifests as a purely muscular disorder, and deep tendon reflexes are absent only if the muscles involved in the reflex lose their motor innervation.

Raynaud's phenomenon is a peripheral vascular syndrome manifested by sensitivity to cold, livedo reticularis, and acrocyanosis. It occurs primarily in women in their late teens. The cause is unknown, but the condition is associated with vasospasms.

79–81. The answers are: 79-D, 80-E, 81-B. *(Physiology; chronic bronchitis; emphysema)*
Flow–volume curves from forced expiratory maneuvers provide useful information about the dynamic function of airways in health and disease. In the patient depicted in the figure, residual volume (and functional residual capacity) are elevated due to his underlying obstructive disease (bronchitis or emphysema). Loss of elastic recoil (due to underlying disease) and prolongation of expiration (in association with obstruction) usually lead to an increased functional residual capacity and total lung capacity and a decrease in vital capacity. A common pathophysiologic finding is a reduction in the flow rate at all lung volumes during expiration.

Although the clinical manifestations of obstructive disease are quite variable, many patients with bronchitis tend to retain CO_2 at some time during their disease. Patients of this type apparently have a diminished ventilatory drive secondary to peripheral or central chemoreceptors or altered afferent pathways. In spite of an increased work of breathing, these subjects attempt to conserve oxygen expenditure by not adequately increasing ventilation at the cost of an increased partial pressure of CO_2 (P_{CO_2}) [and decreased P_{O_2}]. In contrast to those patients that increase their minute volume (and thus maintain a normal P_{CO_2}), subjects such as this patient do not have very large physiologic dead spaces. However, patients with obstructive lung disease do perfuse poorly ventilated regions of lung. These high physiologic shunts generally have only modest effects on arterial P_{CO_2} (although they do contribute to the hypoxemia).

Chronic hypoxemia (often in conjunction with nocturnal desaturation during sleep apnea) leads to erythropoiesis and hypoxic pulmonary vasoconstriction. This desaturation and erythrocytosis produce cyanosis and can lead to right ventricular hypertrophy and right-sided heart failure. In such an event, functional tricuspid regurgitation may be detected by neck vein distention characterized by large v waves (and brisk y descents) as well as the heart sounds described above. Right-sided heart failure leads to an elevation in venous pressure. In spite of an increase in hematocrit, cyanosis and edema secondary to such failure produce the so-called "blue bloater" manifestation.

82. The answer is C. *(Pharmacology; adrenergic agonist)*
Ephedrine is a mixed-action adrenergic agent. It releases stored norepinephrine from nerve endings, and it directly stimulates both α- and β-adrenergic receptors. Clonidine, dopamine, and ritodrine are direct-acting adrenergic agents that directly bind α- or β-adrenergic receptors, producing effects similar to those that occur following stimulation of sympathetic nerves or release of the hormone epinephrine from the adrenal medulla. Amphetamine and tyramine are indirect-acting agonists that cause the release of norepinephrine from the cytoplasm or vesicles of adrenergic neurons. The norepinephrine release traverses the synapse and stimulates the α- and β-adrenergic receptors.

83. The answer is B. *(Pharmacology; adrenergic agonist)*
Dopamine is a catecholamine. Sympathomimetic amines that contain the 3,4-dihydroxybenezene group are catecholamines because 3,4-dihydroxybenezene is known as catechol. Catecholamines share the following properties: (1) they have a rapid onset of action, (2) they have a brief duration of action, (3) they are not administered orally, and (4) they do not penetrate the blood–brain barrier. Noncatecholamines (e.g., clonidine, ephedrine, albuterol, amphetamine, and metaproterenol), when compared to catecholamines, have a longer duration of action and can be administered orally.

84. The answer is D. *(Pathology; melanoma)*
The lesion described is that of a superficial, spreading melanoma. This form of melanoma often involves a rapidly expanding superficial lesion that contains shades of brown mixed with bluish-red or black. The border of the lesion is visible or palpably elevated. It is grossly distinguishable from other common pigmented lesions based on color, shape, and rate of growth. Although the back and extremities are common sites for detection of such a lesion, melanomas can arise in other areas of the body.

85. The answer is D. *(Pharmacology; adrenergic blockers)*
Prazosin produces a competitive block of α_1 receptors without blocking α_2 receptors. It is effective in the treatment of hypertension. Propranolol and atenolol are β-blockers and are competitive antagonists. Propranolol blocks both the β_1 and β_2 receptors, whereas atenolol is a cardioselective β-blocker that preferentially blocks β_1 receptors. Cocaine, guanethidine, and resperine affect neurotransmitter uptake or release. Cocaine blocks the Na^+–K^+-activated ATPase in the cellular membrane of the adrenergic neurons, which is required for cellular uptake of norepinephrine. Guanethidine inhibits the response of the adrenergic nerve to stimulation or to indirectly acting sympathomimetic amines by blocking the release of stored norepinephrine. Reserpine blocks the ability of adrenergic neurons to transport norepinephrine from the cytoplasm into storage vesicles. This causes depletion of norepinephrine in the adrenergic neuron, because monoamine oxidase in the neuron can degrade norepinephrine.

86. The answer is B. *(Pharmacology; barbiturates)*
Thiopental is a barbiturate with a rapid onset of action. Barbiturates are thought to interfere with sodium and potassium transport across cell membranes, leading to inhibition of the mesencephalic recticular activating system. Polysynaptic transmission is inhibited in all areas of the central nervous system (CNS). Barbiturates also potentiate gamma aminobutyric acid (GABA) action on chloride entry into the neuron. Diazepam and lorazepam are benzodiazepines. Benzodiazepines are anxiolytic drugs that inhibit the action of GABA a neurotransmitter. Ethanol is a CNS depressant, producing sedation and ultimately hypnosis with increasing

dosage. Buspirone actions are mediated by serotonin receptors, although it has some affinity for dopamine receptors. Hydroxyzine is an antihistamine with antiemetic activity.

87. The answer is B. *(Biochemistry; DNA replication)*
Topoisomerase enzymes are important for regulating the equilibrium between supercoiled and relaxed DNA. Okazaki fragments are annealed by the actions of a ligase, and the newly synthesized DNA is "proofread" by a subunit of DNA polymerase III. The RNA primer is required to initiate DNA synthesis and is thought to be synthesized by RNA polymerase.

88. The answer is F. *(Pharmacology; central nervous system stimulants)*
Tetrahydrocannabinol (THC) is a hallucinogen found in marijuana that produces euphoria followed by drowsiness and relaxation, depending on the social situation. Caffeine, amphetamine, theobromine, and nicotine are psychomotor stimulants. Psychomotor stimulants cause excitement and euphoria, decrease feelings of fatigue, and increase motor activity. Doxapram and nikethamide are convulsants and respiratory stimulants. Convulsants and respiratory stimulants have minimal effect on mental funtion, but produce exaggerated reflex responses, increased activity in the respiratory and vasomotor centers, and convulsions at high doses.

89–90. The answers are: 89-E, 90-A. *(Biochemistry; microbiology; cystic fibrosis)*
A deficiency in pancreatic lipases reduces the absorption of fat-soluble vitamins (A, D, and K). Vitamin K is critically important in the synthesis of clotting factors II, VII, IX, and a deficiency in vitamin K leads to bleeding diatheses manifested by a prolonged prothrombin time. Vitamins B_6 and C are water soluble and are less likely to be affected by pancreatic lipase deficiency.

Although clinical improvement from respiratory infections in cystic fibrosis occurs without eradication of bacteria from sputum during antibiotic therapy, it is standard procedure to treat the readily identifiable microorganisms. The gram-positive and particularly difficult to eradicate gram-negative bacteria (e.g., *Pseudomonas aeruginosa*) are often cultured from sputum, and a common regimen includes a β-lactam antibiotic, such as gentamicin, with a gram-negative antibiotic, such as the third-generation cephalosporin, ceftazidime. *P. aeruginosa* is often resistant to nitrofurantoin or nalidixic acid. Pentamidine is used for the treatment of protozoal infections, such as *Pneumocystis carinii*. Rifampin and isoniazid are used in the therapy of tuberculosis.

91. The answer is C. *(Pathology; neoplasia of the reproductive tract)*
Twenty-five percent of males in the United States have a tumor in the prostate gland. A prostatic tumor rarely occurs before age 40 years, but the incidence rises rapidly with advancing age. Seventy-five percent of prostatic tumors arise in the posterior lobe, are easily palpable, and, therefore, are detectable.

92–93. The answers are: 92-D, 93-D. *(Pathology; pheochromocytoma)*
The paroxysmal symptoms and detection of an abdominal mass within the adrenal gland are consistent with a diagnosis of pheochromocytoma, a relatively rare tumor of the chromaffin cells of the adrenal medulla. The cells of the adrenal cortex are generally not affected, although extra-adrenal chromaffin cells are often involved.

Pharmacotherapy to manage the clinical symptoms includes the use of an α-adrenergic receptor blocker (phenoxybenzamine) either alone or in combination with a β-blocker. β-blockers alone are contraindicated as they may leave the α-adrenoreceptor–mediated effects of the disorder unopposed. Clonidine is a useful test for the disorder; peripheral catecholamine levels will not be depressed after patients with pheochromocytoma take clonidine, whereas normal subjects will show a prompt decline. Methyldopa is likely to be converted in significant amounts to the weak vasoconstrictor alpha methyl norepinephrine, which may exacerbate the symptoms.

94. The answer is B. *(Pharmacology; organophosphate exposure)*
Organophosphates are highly toxic insecticides that occasionally affect agricultural workers. They are also frequently the primary agent in chemical weapons. They are highly lipid-soluble and are absorbed through virtually all body parts, including the skin. They produce a cholinergic crisis secondary to inhibition of acetylcholinesterase, which involves nicotinic and muscarinic receptors, both centrally and systemically. Atropine decreases some of the muscarine effects, including the bronchospasm and increased secretions of the airways. Mechanical ventilation may still be required if respiratory muscles are paralyzed. Pralidoxime, if given early enough, will help regenerate new cholinesterase and ultimately hasten reversal of the overdose.

95. The answer is C. *(Immunology; self-tolerance)*
The thymus is an antigenically privileged site, and thymocytes pass through only once; therefore, peripheral tolerance may be a necessary mechanism. There is no evidence that T cells leave and then come back to the thymus. Tolerance seems to be a negative-selection phenomenon, and it is believed that all selection initially takes place in the thymus.

96. The answer is A. *(Biochemistry; protein structure)*
Many polypeptides have a distinctive tertiary structure that provides insight into their function. Zinc fingers and leucine zippers are structural motifs that seem to be crucial in most proteins with DNA-binding functions. Current research indicates that the zinc fingers insert into the major groove of DNA between the bases. EF hands are structural motifs that are important in the calcium-binding properties of molecules like calmodulin, troponin C, and the ryanodine receptor. β-pleated sheets are frequently involved in the transport of hydrophobic molecules: α_1-microglobulin carries porphyrin rings, and apolipoproteins transfer cholesterol esters via β-pleated sheets. Gly-X-Y repeats are important in producing the tight triple helix of collagen. Glycine has only a hydrogen as its side chain and therefore allows the individual helices to be wound tightly without a bulky structure in the center. Immunoglobulin folds are important in the superfamily, which includes immunoglobulins, epidermal and nerve growth factors, and other proteins that have diverse functions.

97. The answer is D. *(Biochemistry; retroviruses)*
The retroviruses are unique in their diploid genetic structure, with two identical RNA molecules per virion. To initiate an effective infection, the virion-associated reverse transcriptase must produce a double-stranded DNA copy of the viral RNA, and that copy must be integrated into the host genome. Infectious virus then is produced from the integrated copy. The various viral antigens are made from messenger RNA (mRNA) produced from the DNA copy, and these antigens include both group-specific and host-specific reactive antigens. The viral RNA has plus polarity.

98. The answer is B. *(Hematology; chronic hemolytic anemia and iron overload)*
Patients with a long-standing history of chronic hemolytic anemia (e.g., sickle cell disease or β-thalassemia major) generally have a substantially enlarged spleen, which exacerbates their condition by destroying abnormal but functional erythrocytes. Splenectomy, however, greatly increases the patient's susceptibility to infection by encapsulated organisms because the spleen is a major site of antigen presentation. Congestive heart failure can result from many factors, including iron overload, chronic high-output demand, and mild hypoxia. The heart rate is typically fast and has an enlarged stroke volume in an effort to increase tissue oxygenation. These increased demands are made in the presence of blood, which is poor at delivering oxygen to the overworked myocardium. Increased absorption, as well as regular transfusions, combine to cause fairly severe iron overload. Cardiac myocytes, particularly in the conducting system, suffer damage principally related to iron toxicity. The liver and pancreas are also susceptible to the effects of systemic iron excess. Emphysema is not related to iron toxicity, high-output cardiac failure, or chronic hypoxia.

99. The answer is D. *(Immunology; immunoglobulin properties)*
The biological significance of immunoglobulin D (IgD) remains obscure. It has no properties that set it apart from any other immunoglobulin, and it has not yet been implicated in any specific disease states. Immunoglobulin M (IgM) antibodies against immunoglobulin G (IgG) are known as rheumatoid factors and are frequently seen in a variety of autoimmune related diseases. IgG is the main serum antibody, and it remains elevated long after the antigen has disappeared. IgM is the "first responder" in the body's production of humoral immunity and is found in the highest titers during the first 10 days following antigen presentation. IgA is especially important in defending against enteric pathogens, and IgE-mediated hypersensitivity results in allergic rhinitis.

100. The answer is D. *(Hematology; α-thalassemias)*
None of the common hemoglobinopathies are sex-linked because none of the subunits are encoded on the X chromosome. Two copies of the α-globin subunit gene are located on chromosome 16, and there are two chromosomes from each parent. On each chromosome, the proximity of the two identical α-subunit genes results in a high frequency of recombination, which, in turn, leads to an increased frequency of nonhomologous recombination and deletion. Thus deletions are the most common cause of α-thalassemia. Because restriction fragment length polymorphisms are very sensitive to deletions, they are useful in identifying the genotypes for genetic counseling. The α-thalassemias are most common in Asians and blacks, with the most severe cases occurring in Asians. The severity is governed by the number of normal genes remaining; when one of the genes is missing, it is a completely silent carrier state. Deletion of two genes results in a mild hypochromic anemia, which is clinically silent and is detected only by a routine complete blood count. The more severe forms of the disease [i.e., hemoglobin H disease (Hb H), and hydrops fetalis] result from a loss of three or four of the genes, respectively. Hb H is the abnormal hemoglobin composed of four β subunits instead of two β and two α. Hb H disease causes a hemolytic anemia that is generally well compensated. Hydrops fetalis is incompatible with life, and these infants usually die in utero. The severe forms are more common in Asians because they more often carry the homozygous deletion haplotype (αα/—); therefore, they can pass on a chromosome that has no functional α genes. Black people with the carrier state are more frequently heterozygous in both alleles (α-/α-).

101. The answer is E. *(Pathology; multiple endocrine neoplasia)*
Zollinger-Ellison syndrome is a gastrin-secreting, pancreatic islet-cell tumor often associated with multiple endocrine neoplasia (MEN) type I. The primary components of MEN IIa are pheochromocytoma and medullary carcinoma of the thyroid, whereas MEN IIb is characterized by pheochromocytoma and medullary carcinoma as well as the unusual neural tumors of the facial mucosal surfaces. MEN I is characterized by parathyroid tumors, pituitary adenomas, and pancreatic islet-cell tumors. All three types of MEN are hereditary, and the genes have been tentatively assigned to chromosome 10 for type II and chromosome 11 for type I. The patterns of inheritance are variable, as is the expression of disease phenotypes. Some patients have all of the characteristic tumors, whereas others have only one or two of the classically described neoplastic growths. The medullary cells (e.g., adrenal and thyroid), as well as the glia involved in the neuromas, arise embryologically from the neural crest. Thus, it is thought that a neoplastic clone may give rise to all three types of tumors.

102. The answer is B. *(Pathology; nephrotic syndrome)*
Nephrotic syndrome is the name given to the set of clinical symptoms that includes proteinuria, generalized edema, hypoalbuminemia, and hyperlipidemia. Several different pathologic lesions of the kidney can be seen when a renal biopsy is performed on a patient with nephrotic syndrome, but the most common is focal segmental glomerulosclerosis. People with systemic diseases (e.g., diabetes and systemic lupus erythematosus) can also have nephrotic syndrome. Nephrotic syndrome specifically excludes hematuria, whether micro-

scopic or gross, which indicates a more serious lesion of the glomerular filtration apparatus and is indicative of nephritis, not nephrosis.

103. The answer is E. *(Pathology; effects of chronic alcohol abuse)*
Alcoholism is a major source of morbidity and mortality in the United States. Cerebellar degeneration and ataxia, often seen in association with profound anterograde amnesia, is known as the Wernicke-Korsakoff syndrome. Demyelination seems to be critical to the cerebellar component of the disease, but the lesion causing the memory loss is still ill-defined. Esophagitis associated with vomiting and chronic reflux is a common complaint of alcoholics, but the more serious Mallory-Weiss tears (usually secondary to fierce retching) involve the rupture of a submucosal vein resulting in acute, voluminous blood loss. Testicular atrophy and amenorrhea are often the result of liver degeneration and the concomitant reduction in steroid metabolism. High estrogen levels result in feedback inhibition of hypothalamic gonadotropin releasing hormone (GnRH) secretion. Chronic alcohol abuse also results in mild hypertension for reasons that are still unclear. Protein malnutrition and the synthesis of fatty acids from ethanol combine to produce the commonly seen elevation in serum triglycerides. Bronchogenic carcinoma is one of the few serious pathologic entities not associated with alcoholism.

104. The answer is D. *(Pathology; acute pancreatitis)*
α_1-Antitrypsin deficiency is commonly associated with damage to the liver and lungs, but not the pancreas. Clearly, alcohol ingestion can cause acute pancreatitis, and several bouts of alcohol-induced subacute pancreatitis may allow chronic pancreatic failure to emerge without a clinically symptomatic episode of acute pancreatitis. Elevated serum triglycerides are found more often in people with pancreatitis than in the general population, but the reason for this phenomenon is not understood. The backup of bile into the pancreatic duct may be the reason for pancreatitis associated with biliary tract disease, but the complete sequence of events is poorly understood. Cholestasis is probably part of the reason for the increased incidence of pancreatitis following abdominal surgery, but again, the exact mechanism is not clear. Trauma or surgery, which lead to damaged pancreatic tissue, almost invariably cause some level of pancreatitis because the pancreas is full of digestive enzymes that are extraordinarily destructive if inappropriately released.

105. The answer is C. *(Immunology; immunoglobulins)*
Immunoglobulin E (IgE) has a serum half-life of 2 days, making it the shortest lived immunoglobulin. The low serum levels of this class of immunoglobulin are due to both a high affinity for mast cells and basophils and a low rate of synthesis. It is elevated in certain parasitic infections, such as *Ascaris* infections, and is not an agglutinating or complement-fixing antibody.

106. The answer is E. *(Microbiology; antimicrobials and pseudomembranous colitis)*
The patient is likely suffering from antibiotic-associated pseudomembranous colitis (note the patient's diarrhea and deterioration following antibiotic therapy). Sigmoidoscopic examination, Gram stain of feces for white blood cells, a *Clostridium difficile* toxin test, and isolating the patient are appropriate procedures to follow for this patient. However, changing the antibiotic from a cephalosporin to clindamycin is inappropriate because *C. difficile* is not sensitive to clindamycin.

107. The answer is D. *(Pathology; agnogenic myeloid metaplasia)*
Bone marrow hypocellularity and teardrop-shaped erythrocytes are pathognomonic for agnogenic myeloid metaplasia with myelofibrosis. Leukocyte alkaline phosphatase levels are normal or elevated until the final stages of the disease. The liver does not usually undergo any significant change in size, whereas the spleen is almost always markedly enlarged as it becomes the principal site of extramedullary hematopoiesis.

108. The answer is A. *(Pharmacology; characteristics of warfarin)*
Warfarin affects normal synthesis of clotting factors in the liver, and its coagulant effects can be reversed by vitamin K. It is well-absorbed orally but will cross the placenta and may affect the fetus. It is used on a chronic basis for deep venous thrombosis and long-term care postmyocardial infarction because its onset of action is slow. Another useful anticoagulant is heparin, which is a large water-soluble polymer that must be given parenterally and does not cross the placenta. It is primarily used for acute anticoagulant therapy because its onset of action is rapid. It can be reversed by the administration of protamine. The main action of heparin is thought to involve catalyzing the activation of antithrombin III in blood, thereby inhibiting thrombin and factor Xa.

109. The answer is D. *(Biochemistry; antioxidants)*
Transketolase is a part of the nonoxidative phase of the hexose monophosphate shunt and has no known role in protecting red blood cells from oxygen insult. A number of enzymes are involved in the protection of red blood cells from oxygen insult by hydrogen peroxide. Glutathione peroxidase catalyzes the reduction of hydrogen peroxide to water. The reduced nicotinamide-adenine dinucleotide phosphate (NADPH) utilized by glutathione reductase to regenerate reduced glutathione is produced in the 6-phosphogluconate dehydrogenase reaction. Catalase results in the decomposition of hydrogen peroxide to water and molecular oxygen.

110. The answer is D. *(Immunology; Arthus reaction)*
The Arthus reaction requires relatively large amounts of antibody and antigen, which then form insoluble complexes and begin to accumulate endogenously. When the aggregates are large enough, the complement cascade is activated. The formation of complement fragments C3a and C5a causes an increase in vascular permeability with resulting edema. Neutrophils and platelets accumulate at the site of the reaction. The activated neutrophils release a host of proteases and collagenases, resulting in rupture of the vessel wall, hemorrhage, and local necrosis. Serum sickness is the most common type III reaction, and the Arthus reaction is the least common.

111. The answer is D. *(Pharmacology; zidovudine and treatment of AIDS)*
Zidovudine (ZDV) is currently the most important agent available for the palliation of AIDS. ZDV is phosphorylated to a deoxynucleoside derivative, which inhibits viral RNA-dependent DNA polymerase. Its selectivity is a function of its specificity for reverse transcriptase compared to human DNA polymerase. Granulocytopenia and anemia occur in up to 45% of treated patients, and resistance does occur to the drug after prolonged therapy. ZDV delays the development of signs and symptoms of AIDS in patients who are asymptomatic and improves the clinical symptoms of patients with AIDS at most stages in their disease. Thus, the incidence of opportunistic infections decreases, and there are some improvements in neurologic deficits, AIDS-associated thrombocytopenia, psoriasis, and lymphocytic interstitial pneumonia.

112. The answer is B. *(Physiology; vascular permeability; inflammation)*
Eosinophil chemotactic factor (ECF) is a set of tetrapeptides that produces a chemotactic gradient to attract eosinophils but has no effect on vascular permeability. Histamine and serotonin increase vascular permeability by causing post-capillary venular contraction. Slow-reacting substance of anaphylaxis (leukotrienes C_4 and D_4) are the only eicosanoids that directly increase vascular permeability. Both serotonin and slow-reacting substance of anaphylaxis increase vascular permeability.

113. The answer is E. *(Pathology; chronic obstructive pulmonary disease)*
Risk for chronic obstructive pulmonary disease (COPD) with various degrees of emphysema or chronic bronchitis is strongly associated with cigarette smoking and exposure to irritating substances in the environment (e.g., sulfur dioxide) or workplace (e.g., silica, cotton or grain dust, toluene diisocyanate). Usually, it

is associated with older age-groups, especially individuals with preexisting lung disease. A genetically linked deficiency in α_1-antitrypsin is strongly linked to premature obstructive pulmonary disease. Although intravenous drug abuse is associated with pulmonary complications, including acute respiratory failure and opportunistic infections accompanying immunodeficiency-like syndromes in certain individuals, it is not usually considered a risk factor for COPD.

114. The answer is C. *(Genetics; Duchenne muscular dystrophy)*
In Duchenne muscular dystrophy (DMD) the amount of dystrophin (a 400-kilodalton protein of unknown function but thought to be involved in Ca^{2+} regulation) is reduced from its normal 0.002% of total protein. Derangement of Ca^{2+} homeostasis is thought to be the cause of the excessive shortening of the sarcomeres. The affected muscle groups hypertrophy due to replacement of muscle mass by fibrofatty tissue. DMD is most often transmitted from a female carrier to the affected male (about 1 per 3500 liveborn males) by X-linked recessive inheritance (myotonic dystrophy is associated with mutations on chromosome 19), although approximately one-third of the cases appear to be due to spontaneously arising mutations.

115. The answer is D. *(Immunology; virulence factors; group A streptococci)*
The symptoms and clinical microbiology results indicate that the child has scarlet fever caused by a group A streptococcus (*Streptococcus pyogenes*) infection. This organism causes hemolysis by producing extracellular hemolysins such as streptolysin O. Other important virulence factors of this organism include membrane-bound protein (M protein) [which is antiphagocytic and also helps mediate adhesion], lipoteichoic acid (which also mediates adhesion), and a hyaluronic acid capsule. The erythrogenic toxins responsible for scarlet fever rash are not hemolytic.

116. The answer is E. *(Pathology; Cushing's syndrome)*
Cushing's syndrome may be caused by hypothalamic or pituitary pathology or both, adrenal adenoma (or carcinoma), and exogenous glucocorticoid administration. In pediatric cases, severe growth retardation may occur before closure of the epiphysis during puberty. Hypersecretion of adrenocorticotropic hormone (ACTH) from the pituitary gland, due to either an underlying tumor or overstimulation from corticotropin releasing factor (CRF) of hypothalamic origin, stimulates the adrenal cortex to release excessive amounts of glucocorticoids (and mineralocorticoids). Other sites of excessive ACTH secretion, including tumors of nonendocrine origin, may be important. A useful initial screen to detect the presence of the syndrome is to inject dexamethasone and then to monitor the expected suppression of cortisol (due to pituitary inhibition) in plasma the following day. Patients with various forms of Cushing's syndrome and a responsive adrenal cortex will not undergo the predicted suppression until considerably higher amounts of dexamethasone are administered. Subsequent tests [including urinary secretion and administration of metyrapone (cortisol synthesis inhibitor)] and diagnostic procedures will help to identify the source of the excessive cortisol production.

117. The answer is E. *(Biochemistry; protein synthesis)*
Protein synthesis occurs in both the cytoplasm and the mitochondria of cells and requires large amounts of energy. In addition to requiring adenosine triphosphate (ATP) for the formation of aminoacyl transfer RNA (tRNA), guanosine triphosphate (GTP) is required for initiation, formation, translocation, and termination of the peptide bond. Protein synthesis requires messenger RNA (mRNA), tRNA, and ribosomal RNA (rRNA). Peptide-bond formation involves the transfer of the nascent polypeptide chain from one tRNA to the amino group of another aminoacyl tRNA. This reaction is accomplished by the enzyme complex known as peptidyl-transferase, which is an integral part of the 50S ribosomal subunits.

118. The answer is C. *(Histology; osteoclasts; bone metabolism)*
Osteoclasts are stimulated by parathyroid hormone and inhibited by calcitonin. Osteoclasts are multinucleated

cells found on the surface of bone, often in Howship's lacuna. They are bone-resorbing cells involved in remodeling bone and in calcium homeostasis, and probably are derived from the macrophage–monocyte system.

119. The answer is C. *(Pharmacology; antibacterial drug use during pregnancy)*
High levels of amoxicillin in the urine can be achieved because penicillins are eliminated mainly unmetabolized via the kidney. There is minimal risk for the fetus using this or other penicillins, although these agents do cross the placental barrier. Sulfonamides should be avoided due to displacement of bilirubin from serum albumin and resultant deposition of bilirubin in the central nervous system (CNS) [kernicterus] of the fetus and newborn, who do not yet have an intact blood–brain barrier. Minocycline should be avoided since tetracyclines are possibly teratogenic and can cause altered bone growth due to high calcium binding. Gentamicin can damage the eighth nerve in the fetus, leading to hearing impairment.

120. The answer is D. *(Immunology; immunologic disorders)*
Graves' disease is a thyroid disorder, but it is not known to be associated with thymomas. Thymomas, 90% of which are benign, are associated with myasthenia gravis, systemic lupus erythematosus, hypogammaglobulinemia, neutrophil agranulocytosis, and polymyositis. The significance of the association with these diseases, in particular myasthenia gravis, remains obscure, although removal of the thymus sometimes leads to regression of this disease.

121. The answer is C. *(Immunology; HIV)*
The human immunodeficiency virus (HIV) has a demonstrated ability to infect any cell with a CD4 receptor, which includes T-helper cells, macrophages, and a subset of brain cells. The virus particle attaches to the cell via the CD4 receptor and gains entry through membrane fusion; it does not require endocytosis. During the replication process, a large amount of viral glycoprotein is produced, which becomes integrated into the host cell membrane. This can either lead to a budding of new virus or fusion with another uninfected CD4$^+$ cell. One infected cell can fuse in this fashion with a large number of uninfected cells, rendering them immunologically inactive.

122–126. The answers are: 122-E, 123-B, 124-C, 125-A, 126-D. *(Neuroanatomy; brain function evaluation)*
Short-term memory is dependent on an ability to concentrate. Information for short-term memory is stored in the hippocampus and temporal lobe. Digit repetition measures attention and requires an intact RAS in the pons and midbrain. (Rare deep medial frontal lobe lesions can cause indifference and inattention.) Interpretation of proverbs requires the use of brain areas where the highest cortical function appears to be located. The analytic and conceptual skills are largely based in the prefrontal cortex.

The copying of a design requires many areas of the brain—namely, the visual or occipital cortex, the parietal association areas, and the prefrontal and frontal cortices. Damage to the right parietal lobe results in greater impairment in this task than a similar lesion on the left side. A good performance indicates integrity of many neural structures; therefore, this test is a good screening method. Poor performance requires appraisal of each area involved (e.g., is the problem related to poor motor control of writing? is there a problem with the analysis of the design?).

Although serial 7s subtraction is used by some as a test of concentration (i.e., a test of brain stem RAS integrity), this utilization is an underestimate of the complexity of the task. The ability to calculate is highly dependent on intelligence and education; therefore, the task is calling on brain areas other than the RAS—namely, calculating abilities in the left parietal lobe and recall of mathematical facts in memory storage areas.

127. The answer is E. *(Microbiology; Chlamydia trachomatis)*
Chlamydia trachomatis cannot synthesize adenosine triphosphate (ATP) or oxidize the reduced form of nicotinamide–adenosine dinucleotide (NADH) and is an obligate intracellular parasite. *C. trachomatis* organisms are internalized by host cells but evade destruction by preventing lysosomal fusion with the phagosome. *C. trachomatis* infections can be treated with tetracyclines, erythromycin, sulfonamides, sulfamethoxazole–trimethoprim, or rifampin.

128. The answer is B. *(Cell biology; viruses)*
A virus is a cellular parasite and, therefore, cannot reproduce itself. A virus must infect a host cell and utilize the host cell's transcription machinery to replicate itself. The infectious viral particle, known as a virion, consists of either RNA or DNA (not both) and is surrounded by a protein shell known as a capsid. A virus interacts with a host cell by binding to a specific cellular receptor and transferring its genetic material into the host. The virus can then manipulate the host's transcription machinery to allow synthesis and replication of its own viral proteins.

129. The answer is D. *(Cell biology; prokaryotes and eukaryotes)*
Both prokaryotic and eukaryotic cells are surrounded by a phospholipid bilayer to form a plasma membrane. The internal membranes in prokaryotic cells are all connected to the outer plasma membrane, whereas eukaryotic cells contain extensive internal membranes that are unconnected. These internal membranes of eukaryotes enclose subcellular structures known as organelles. The outer plasma membrane acts as a barrier to the cell, which allows only certain substances to enter (e.g., oxygen, carbon dioxide, water). To obtain the essential macromolecules, a cell must use membrane transporters that allow substances (e.g., inorganic ions, sugars, and amino acids) to permeate the cell. Prokaryotic cellular DNA is in the form of a single circular molecule within a single chromosome. In contrast, eukaryotic DNA is a single, linear, double-stranded molecule divided between two or more chromosomes contained in a membrane-bound nucleus.

130. The answer is C. *(Cell biology; β_1-adrenergic receptors)*
β-adrenergic receptors bind catecholamines (e.g., epinephrine and isoproterenol) to activate adenylate cyclase and elevate levels of cyclic adenosine monophosphate (cAMP) within a cell. There are two types of β-adrenergic receptors: typically β_1 and β_2 receptors. β_1 receptors bind catecholamines and the order of affinities is isoproterenol > norepinephrine > epinephrine, whereas the affinities for the β_2 receptors are isoproterenol > epinephrine > norepinephrine. β_1 receptors are located on cardiac muscle cells, whereas β_2 receptors are typically found on smooth muscle cells in bronchial airways. Upon agonist binding, β_1 receptors induce increased heart rate and contractility. This effect can be blocked by antagonists (e.g., practolol, a known β-blocker) to slow heart contractions in patients with cardiac arrhythmias and angina. β_2 agonists (e.g., terbutaline) open air passages in patients with asthma by relaxing bronchial smooth muscle.

131. The answer is A. *(Cell biology; transcription)*
Many protein transcription factors are required to form a pre-initiation complex at the TATA box to initiate RNA polymerase II transcription. However, only TFIID binds directly to the TATA box region of the DNA. This transcription factor must bind to the TATA box first, forming a stable complex between TFIID and the DNA. A second transcription factor, TFIIB, then binds to RNA polymerase II and associates with the DNA at the TFIID-TATA box site. TFIIB acts as an ATPase, which induces melting of the DNA to form an open complex. Transcription then begins in the presence of TFIIE and is assisted in elongation by the transcription factor TFIIS.

132–136. The answers are: 132-C, 133-B, 134-A, 135-B, 136-C. *(Behavioral science; family therapies)*
The family therapies can be roughly divided into three schools. The behavioral–psychoeducational approaches

are grounded in social learning theory and frequently will instruct patients in the principles of this theory during treatment. The structural–strategic therapies view family problems as misguided and dysfunctional attempts to adapt to current life circumstances. Clarification of current relationship patterns, such as alliances and coalitions, and cognitive reframing are techniques associated with these therapies. The intergenerational–experiential therapies view family problems as rooted in the family's fixation at a particular stage of development; therapy attempts to discover the cause of this fixation by examining transgenerational patterns and elaborating the family's identity.

137. The answer is D. (*Cell biology; mitosis*)
Cellular genetic material is equally distributed during cell division by a process known as mitosis. Mitosis is divided into several stages: prophase, metaphase, anaphase, and telophase. During early prophase, centrioles begin moving toward opposite poles of the cell as the nuclear membrane begins to disaggregate. As the cell reaches middle and late prophase, chromosomes are condensed and can be visualized as two chromatids joined at the centromeres. Microtublar spindles also begin to form. In metaphase, the chromosomes move toward the equator of the cell. The two sister chromatids separate into independent chromosomes at anaphase not telephase. Each chromatid contains a centromere bound by a spindle fiber that links the chromatid to the pole of the cell to which it will migrate. As the cell elongates, cytokinesis begins, and a cleavage furrow forms. At telophase, two new daughter cells are formed, each containing one copy of each chromosome.

138. The answer is E. (*Cell biology; protein synthesis*)
Protein synthesis in eukaryotic cells occurs by translation of messenger RNA (mRNA) in three stages: initiation, elongation, and termination. In the termination stage, a single transcription factor recognizes the stop codon UAG in the mRNA sequence and signals the release of the peptidyl-transfer RNA used to add each additional amino acid. This subsequently releases the newly synthesized polypeptide chain. Once the ribosome detaches from the mRNA, guanosine triphosphate (GTP) is hydrolyzed, which provides enough energy to divide the ribosome into two subunits.

139. The answer is B. (*Cell biology; structure of polypeptides*)
Polypeptides can be arranged in four different structure types. Primary structure refers to the linear arrangement of a polypeptide chain along with the available corresponding cysteine side chains. Secondary structure consists of two different forms: α-helix and β-pleated sheet. Tertiary structure combines these secondary structures into complex and compact domains. The combination of several polypeptide chains into one molecule is an example of a quaternary structure.

140–144. The answers are: 140-D, 141-A, 142-B, 143-B, 144-C. (*Genetics; insulin-dependent diabetes mellitus*)
Approximately 95% of patients with insulin-dependent diabetes mellitus (IDDM) have human leukocyte antigen (HLA) DR4. HLA DR3/DR4 heterozygotes are particularly susceptible to IDDM, and the DR3/DR4 antigens account for more than half the genetic contribution underlying IDDM.

If a proband with IDDM and his sibling share no haplotype, the risk to the sibling of developing IDDM is approximately 2% . The risk is 5% to a sibling who does share one HLA haplotype with a proband affected with IDDM. Approximately half of the normal population has HLA DR3 or HLA DR4; the empiric risk for developing IDDM is approximately 5% to a sibling for whom no HLA typing is available.

If the proband and sibling both share DR3 and DR4, the risk to the sibling of developing IDDM is approximately 20%. Clearly, the HLA haplotype alone does not underlie the genetics of IDDM, and there must be other genes that also contribute to the development of the disease.

145–149. The answers are: 145-E, 146-A, 147-B, 148-E, 149-A. *(Toxicology; heavy metal poisoning)*
Elemental mercury is volatile at room temperature and is efficiently absorbed through the lungs. Other inorganic and organic forms of mercury are found in industrial processes, foodstuffs, medicines, paints, and cosmetics. These forms usually cause toxicity after gastrointestinal exposure. Metallothionein synthesis is increased after exposure to mercury, and this results in a protective effect against tissue damage. Exposure to the vapor results in airway inflammation and pneumonitis; chronic exposure to the vapor produces toxicity principally in the central nervous system (CNS). [The neuropsychiatric signs commonly observed in felt hat workers, who were exposed to mercury vapor, led to the expression, "mad as a hatter."] The other forms of mercury can cause corrosive damage to the skin and gastrointestinal tract as well as the CNS manifestations. Gastric lavage and chelation therapy (with N-acetylpenicillamine or dimercaprol) should be considered in the treatment protocol.

The toxic metal arsenic is commonly encountered in a variety of forms (i.e., inorganic, organic, vapor); it produces toxicity in nearly every organ system by tightly binding to sulfhydryl groups as well as by interfering with oxidative phosphorylation. Exposure to arsenic vapor can lead to the rapid onset of severe hemolysis and hematuria. Exposure to the organic and inorganic forms (i.e., through skin or gastrointestinal absorption) can produce acute or chronic symptoms depending on the dose and duration of exposure. Gastric lavage, penicillamine, dimercaprol, and hemodialysis all should be considered for the effective management of arsenic toxicity.

The largest epidemic of lead poisoning in history followed the introduction of lead into paints as a color stabilizer. More than 2 million preschool children are annually affected in the United States. Lead toxicity in all tissues is related to its disruption of sulfhydryl groups in proteins. In adults, chronic exposure leads to abdominal pain, anemia, renal disease, ataxia, and memory loss. Childhood poisoning frequently presents with abdominal pain and anemia, but the CNS effects are most important. Unfortunately, subclinical toxicity is most common; the lead poisoning retards CNS development without causing any symptoms that might bring an affected patient to medical attention. Mental retardation, language deficits, cognitive dysfunction, and abnormal behavior are all common manifestations of long-term exposure to lead during the critical preschool years.

Exposure to cadmium is generally related to occupation or pollution from local refining or mining operations. Toxicity can follow ingestion or inhalation; acute symptoms can quickly follow relatively large doses, whereas chronic symptoms are often associated with cumulative exposure.

Tin is not a common cause of heavy metal toxicity.

150–154. The answers are: 150-D, 151-F, 152-A, 153-B, 154-C. *(Biochemistry; hormonal regulation of the menstrual cycle)*
The outer, stratified squamous epithelia are characteristic of thecal cells (*D*), and the inner, columnar epithelia are characteristic of granulosa cells (*E*). Luteinizing hormone (LH; *B*) exerts its primary effects on thecal cells, whereas follicle-stimulating hormone (FSH; *C*) exerts its primary effects on granulosa cells.

Thecal cells play a key role in estrogen synthesis because granulosa cells cannot produce estradiol from cholesterol: They need the androgen precursors from the thecal cells. During the follicular phase, estradiol participates in both a positive and negative feedback loop with the hypothalamic-pituitary-ovarian axis. Follicular estradiol (*F*) increases the pituitary gland's LH response to hypothalamic gonadotropin-releasing hormone (GnRH) while decreasing its FSH response. The same GnRH (*A*) pulsatile secretions during this period result in progressively larger LH (*B*) secretions until the LH surge occurs, which induces ovulation. FSH also has a surge, which corresponds with the LH surge and ovulation, but the LH surge alone is sufficient to induce ovulation.

FSH (*C*) is responsible for recruiting follicles at the beginning of the menstrual cycle. According to the current model, the follicle with the greatest sensitivity to FSH quickly develops the capacity to increase its estradiol production despite the negative feedback effect of estradiol on pituitary FSH secretion. Thus, as other follicles stop the maturation process due to decreased availability of FSH, one follicle produces increasing amounts of estradiol independent of FSH stimulation.

155. The answer is E. *(Cell biology; cell membranes)*
Biomembranes are made up of an enclosed phospholipid bilayer. The hydrocarbon side chains of the phospholipids pack together to minimize exposure to water. This allows the hydrophilic side chains to associate with the aqueous surroundings. The large hydrophobic side chains of cholesterol insert themselves within the membrane, orienting the hydrophilic head toward the water to make the membranes more fluid in nature. Carbohydrate chains that are covalently bonded to lipids form glycolipids in cell membranes, which can serve as antigens for recognition of specific antibodies. Proteins that contain stretches of hydrophobic amino acids associate with membranes as integral membrane proteins to form cellular components (e.g., channels and transporters). DNA is confined to the nucleus of cells because of the nuclear membrane; it is not associated with cell membranes.

156. The answer is D. *(Cell biology; cell membranes)*
The inner and outer leaflets of biologic membranes have different lipid compositions, inducing lipid asymmetry. A phospholipid cannot move spontaneously from the cytoplasmic leaflet to the exoplasmic leaflet in the endoplasmic reticulum (ER) because the hydrophilic head group cannot pass through the hydrophobic bilayer. This does not occur through membrane budding because this is a process by which phospholipids are transferred from one organelle to another by vesicles. It also does not occur through phospholipid exchange proteins because these proteins also remove phospholipids from one membrane and release them to another membrane or organelle. The movement of a phospholipid in the ER into the exoplasmic leaflet is catalyzed by the flippase protein so that movement occurs within a few minutes.

157. The answer is C. *(Pathology; hypercalcemia of malignancy)*
Certain malignancies cause hypercalcemia. Frequently, the hypercalcemia is induced by elevated levels of parathyroid hormone (PTH)-related protein that is produced by the tumor. This protein has an amino-terminal end that has many of the same actions as PTH. Thus, its effects, particularly on the bone and kidneys, cause an increase in serum calcium. PTH is rarely produced by tumors outside the parathyroid glands. In fact, PTH levels are reduced in hypercalcemia of malignancy due to the inhibition of the parathyroid glands by the high concentration of calcium. Calcitriol is frequently reduced because PTH is a major stimulus for the formation of calcitriol. However, in some lymphomas, the production of excess calcitriol is the cause of the hypercalcemia. Serum phosphorus concentrations may be low in hypercalcemia of malignancy due to the increased renal excretion. The level of hypercalcemia, when caused by malignancy, may be higher than that normally caused by primary hyperparathyroidism, because multiple factors are often produced by the tumor that act synergistically to cause greater increases (e.g., interleukin-1, interleukin-6, and tumor necrosis factor-α).

158. The answer is G. *(Biochemistry; vitamin D metabolism)*
Vitamin D is a fat-soluble vitamin that comes from diet. It is made from cholesterol with the help of sunlight. It is converted to the 25-hydroxyvitamin D form in the liver, a process that is regulated by substrate availability. Then it is converted to its most active form—1,25-dihydroxyvitamin D (calcitriol)—in the proximal tubules of the kidneys and, to a lesser extent, in macrophages and mononuclear cells. This step is stimulated by parathyroid hormone (PTH) and phosphate depletion. Feedback inhibition also occurs with 1,25-dihydroxyvitamin D inhibiting both its own production and the synthesis of PTH. The actions of vitamin D are mediated by a cytosolic receptor that translocates to the nucleus on binding with vitamin D. Its functions are to increase calcium and phosphorus absorption in the intestine, to synergistically act with PTH in the bone to increase

calcium and phosphate release, and to suppress helper T cells when produced locally by activated macrophages and mononuclear cells.

159. The answer is D. *(Pathology; pheochromocytoma)*
The patient has a pheochromocytoma. Heart palpitations, abdominal pain, and weight loss are other symptoms associated with these tumors. Although about 10% of pheochromocytomas are associated with a familial syndrome, they are not seen in multiple endocrine neoplasia (MEN) syndrome type I. They may be seen in MEN type II A or B, as is medullary carcinoma of the thyroid. Pheochromocytomas are usually located in the adrenal medulla, but may be found elsewhere in the body. They excrete epinephrine and norepinephrine, not cortisol. The 24-hour urinary excretion is a better measure of catecholamine production than are the plasma levels because the latter is more easily affected by the current emotional status of the patient and the venipuncture. Although a computed tomography scan is often helpful in forming the diagnosis and treatment plan for a patient with pheochromocytoma, intravenous contrast material may precipitate a hypertensive crisis; therefore, the contrast material should be avoided if possible. Because a pheochromocytoma is a life-threatening disease for which there is a treatment, patients showing several of the signs and symptoms should be evaluated promptly.

160. The answer is F. *(Endocrinology; adrenal steroid hormone production)*
A 17-α-hydroxylase deficiency causes decreased cortisol production and increased deoxycorticosterone and corticosterone production. The excess of the latter two hormones is due to the lack of feedback inhibition of cortisol on the pituitary and hypothalamus. A 3-β-dehydrogenase deficiency does not allow the production of either cortisol or aldosterone; only androgens are produced. A 21-hydroxylase deficiency does not allow cortisol or aldosterone production, whereas dehydroepiandrosterone (DHEA) and androstenedione are produced in excess. A 17,20-desmolase deficiency blocks androgen synthesis, not that of aldosterone or cortisol. Aromatase deficiency does not block cortisol production or lead to an increase in androgen production. An 18-hydroxylase deficiency blocks the synthesis of aldosterone, not cortisol.

161. The answer is F. *(Endocrinology; diabetic ketoacidosis)*
Diabetic ketoacidosis (DKA) is a complication of type I diabetes mellitus, that is preventable in a patient who is following the proper therapeutic regimen. DKA may also be a part of the initial presentation of diabetes mellitus. The condition is usually brought on by a precipitating event (e.g., infection, failure to take enough insulin, and possibly emotional stress). Hypokalemia is a concern in patients with DKA. The potassium level should be monitored closely, even if initially normal, because the serum concentration may drop with rehydration. The administration of bicarbonate to a patient with DKA is controversial except in severe acidosis. However, it should not be given as a bolus, as that would shift the Bohr curve strongly to the left in this setting of low BPG and decrease oxygen delivery to the brain. Instead, it should be given slowly, and the increase should be monitored closely. Rehydration therapy may be started before insulin is given, as this allows assessment of the effects that rehydration has on glucose levels.

162. The answer is B. *(Behavioral medicine; modifying consequences to change behavior)*
The most effective use of positive reinforcement is to give it frequently and easily and then gradually become stringent. This method is called shaping. It is more effective than giving continual praise regardless of the result or only giving praise when the final goal is reached. Using negative reinforcement makes a person's undesired behavior more likely to occur (i.e., the desired behavior becomes difficult). Punishment reduces the undesired behavior, but is ineffective if it is not directly related to the behavior.

163. The answer is D. *(Behavioral medicine; obesity)*
Recent data indicate that obese individuals eat a higher proportion of calories from fat, although their overall calorie intake may not be increased. The obese person may have larger fat cells, more of them, or both,

when compared to a person of average weight. There is no evidence that the number of gut cells differs. The number of calories burned during exercise depends on the distance traveled and the weight that was moved. Thus, a heavier individual burns more calories walking 1 mile than a lighter individual. Assuming that the same distance is traveled, the speed of the exercise is irrelevant to the number of calories that are burned.

164–168. The answers are: 164-B, 165-D, 166-E, 167-C, 168-A. *(Hematology; blood typing)*
The couple in family 164 can only be the parents of infant B. Infant A, C, D, or E cannot be their child because those children are Rh$^+$, and both the mother and father are Rh$^-$.

The couple in family 165 can only be the parents of infant D. The child of family 165 must have just the N antigen in the MN group. Infant D is the one who has only the N antigen.

The couple in family 166 could be the parents of infant B, C, or E. However, infant B must belong to family 164, and infant C must belong to family 167, since infants A, B, D, and E all have the N blood group antigen, which neither the mother nor the father in family 167 has. Therefore, infant E must belong to family 166. The couple in family 166 cannot be the parents of infant A, who has blood type O, because the child must inherit the gene for either the A or the B antigen from his mother. The couple in family 166 cannot be the parents of infant D, because he must have inherited the gene for either the A or the B blood group antigen from his father, and the father has the O antigen.

The couple in family 168 could be the parents of infant A or B, but infant B must belong to family 164, therefore infant A must be family 168's child. The couple in family 168 cannot be the parents of infant C because he did not inherit the gene for the N blood group antigen, which the father must have transmitted to his son. The couple in family 168 cannot be the parents of infant D or E because both infants have a gene for the B blood group, which neither the mother nor the father in family 168 has.

169–172. The answers are: 169-E, 170-A, 171-C, 172-B. *(Behavioral science; psychological stages of neoplastic disease)*
It is important for the physician to recognize the psychosocial stages that patients with neoplastic disease may experience, because the goals and difficulties of each phase differ. The diagnostic phase requires the physician's attention to possible patient denial of the disease and to ultimate acceptance of the need for treatment. The actual treatments of neoplastic disease often involve serious side effects (malaise, nausea, vomiting) that may promote noncompliance. The period of remission may involve anxious waiting for signs of the disease, which can lead to hypochondriacal complaints and lack of return to full functioning. Patients in the terminal phase of cancer need to be in a supportive setting with adequate palliation of pain and discomfort.

173–177. The answers are: 173-D, 174-C, 175-A, 176-F, 177-B. *(Biochemistry; protein synthesis, post-translational modification, and targeting)*
Protein synthesis begins in the nucleus, where the gene in question is first transcribed into messenger RNA (mRNA). The nascent transcript generally contains introns, which are pieces of the transcript that do not code for amino acid sequences. The introns are removed in a process known as exon splicing. The correctly spliced mRNA transcript leaves the nucleus and is bound to a free ribosome.

After the correct addition of the first eight to twenty amino acids, a special signal is encountered in most of the proteins that are destined for lysosomes, secretion, or the plasma membrane. This signal peptide causes the ribosome to stop translating the transcript and move to the endoplasmic reticulum (ER). ER with aggregations of ribosomes is frequently called "rough ER" because of its dense, speckled appearance. Proteins that are ultimately destined for the cytoplasm (e.g., hexokinase) do not have a special signal, and their translation is finished on free ribosomes void of any ER interaction.

Following synthesis on the rough ER, proteins destined for one of the three special targets frequently have sugar moieties added to asparagine on the nitrogen side chain. This N-linked glycosylation occurs in the lumen of the rough ER; then the protein is sent to the Golgi complex. Although its function is still being studied, it is clear that the Golgi complex is the key site for sorting proteins that are emerging from the rough ER. The N-linked sugars are modified, and additional sugars are frequently added to the oxygen-based side chains of serine or threonine (O-linked glycosylation). Fatty acids and other lipid moieties are often added in the lumen of the Golgi complex, too (i.e., acylation). These various modifications may contribute to the protein's function or structural stability. Sometimes, they serve as signals for targeting mechanisms.

Mannose 6-phosphate was the first targeting signal to be well established. Mannose 6-phosphate moieties are essential for an enzyme to be transferred into the lysosomal lumen. Patients with lysosomal storage diseases frequently have a defect in this targeting mechanism. Usually, the enzyme has a defective signal so that it is synthesized but not concentrated in the site where it serves its degradative function.

Proteins destined for the mitochondria and nucleus are nearly all synthesized in the cytosol on free ribosomes. Therefore, they are generally not glycosylated or acylated. The signal for transporting these proteins to their respective compartments is usually found in the amino acid sequence. A very short nuclear localization sequence causes proteins to be sequestered in the nucleus; one of several signals targets a mitochondrial protein to its appropriate destination (e.g., the inner membrane, matrix, outer membrane, intermembranous space).

178–180. The answers are: 178-B, 179-E, 180-A. *(Neuropathology)*
Neurofibrillary tangles are not unique to Alzheimer's disease as they are also seen in Down syndrome, normal aging, and pugilistic dementia; however, they uniquely occur in high concentrations in the hippocampus of Alzheimer's patients. Multinucleated giant cells occur in patients with AIDS who have encephalitis. Lewy bodies and eosinophilic cytoplasmic inclusions in the substantia nigra are characteristic of Parkinson's disease. Prions, proteins devoid of nucleic acid that are infectious, are associated with Creutzfeldt-Jakob dementia. Pick's bodies stain silver and are inclusions within neurons.

Test IV

QUESTIONS

DIRECTIONS: *One best answer questions* consist of numbered items or incomplete statements followed by answers or by completions of the statement. Select the ONE lettered answer or completion that is BEST in each case.

Matching questions consist of a list of four to twenty-six lettered options (some of which may be in figures) followed by several numbered items. For each numbered item, select the ONE lettered option that is most closely associated with it. Each lettered option may be selected once, more than once, or not at all.

Questions 1–3

A child presents to the pediatrician for evaluation of "difficulty walking." Examination reveals a waddling gait, proximal muscle weakness, pseudohypertrophy of the calf muscles, and a Gower maneuver upon standing from a sitting position. A tentative diagnosis of Duchenne muscular dystrophy (DMD) is made, pending the results of serum enzyme studies, electromyography, and muscle biopsy. A family pedigree is illustrated below.

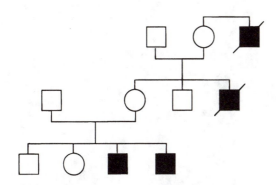

1. According to the pedigree, the mode of inheritance of DMD is

(A) autosomal recessive
(B) autosomal dominant
(C) X-linked
(D) nonpenetrant
(E) none of the above

2. What is the chance that the mother is a carrier for DMD?

(A) 25%
(B) 50%
(C) 75%
(D) 100%
(E) None of the above

3. What is the chance that the next male child will carry the gene that causes the disease?

(A) None
(B) 50%
(C) 75%
(D) 100%
(E) None of the above

4. All of the following are true statements about the cyclin B–cdc2 kinase complex EXCEPT

(A) destruction of the cyclin B inactivates the cyclin B–cdc2 kinase activity
(B) freshly synthesized cyclin B allows the reactivation of the cyclin B–cdc2 kinase complex
(C) the cyclin B–cdc2 kinase complex is important in the cell entering mitosis
(D) activated cyclin B–cdc2 kinase complex causes a G_1 arrest in the cell cycle
(E) cyclin B–cdc2 kinase can be inhibited by tyrosine phosphorylation

5. A 53-year-old man complains of shortness of breath when climbing stairs and a productive cough. He has had respiratory infections each of the past 2 years, has smoked two packs of cigarettes per day for the past 35 years, is obese, and looks somewhat cyanotic. Which one of the following statements is most likely correct?

(A) The patient has a low forced expiratory volume in 1 second (FEV_1), but a normal FEV_1/forced vital capacity (FVC) ratio
(B) The patient has restrictive rather than obstructive pulmonary disease
(C) The patient is likely to have emphysematous disease rather than bronchitic disease
(D) The patient has elevated hemoglobin and hematocrit levels
(E) The patient has α_1-antitrypsin deficiency
(F) The patient's history of smoking has no relationship to his current disease

6. The violaceous skin nodule apparent in the photomicrograph below, which was taken from a young individual, is most likely

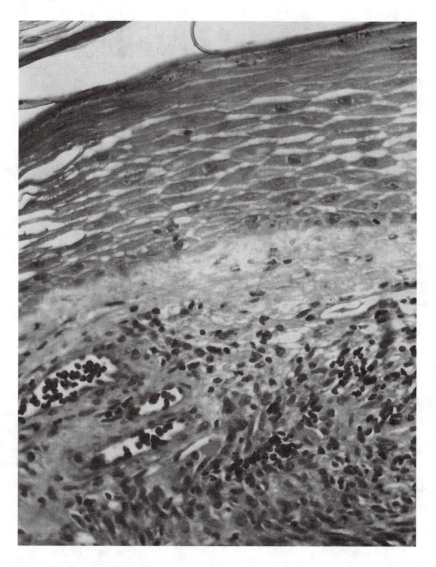

(A) seen on the back of infants' necks

(B) a highly malignant pigmented melanoma

(C) seen in men infected with human immunodeficiency virus (HIV)

(D) due to radiation therapy that was administered over 10 years ago

7. Which one of the following statements concerning referred pain is true?

(A) Pain from the transverse colon is usually referred to a midline area below the umbilicus
(B) Somatic pain is usually referred in a diffuse, poorly localized pattern
(C) Diaphragmatic pain is usually referred to the inguinal area
(D) The mechanism of referred pain is well understood

Questions 8–10

An 18-year-old college freshman has been ''acting strangely'' for several months, according to his roommates. His grades are deteriorating, and he avoids social interactions. He talks about being the devil's accomplice. He is unshaven, and his clothes are messy.

8. The first diagnosis to consider with this patient is

(A) schizophrenia
(B) mania
(C) schizoaffective disorder
(D) major depression
(E) phencyclidine psychosis

9. Further history reveals periods of staring spells and olfactory hallucinations. Based on these symptoms, the physician should order which of the following tests?

(A) Bender Gestalt test
(B) Thematic apperception test
(C) Electroencephalogram
(D) Halstead-Reitan battery
(E) Brain stem evoked potentials

10. A reasonable medication trial for complex partial seizures is

(A) haloperidol
(B) carbamazepine
(C) imipramine
(D) alprazolam
(E) clonidine

11. The term that describes the adherence of neutrophils and monocytes to the vascular endothelium before movement into the extravascular space is

(A) margination
(B) diapedesis
(C) pavementing
(D) migration
(E) clotting

12. A fluorescent probe that binds to glucocorticoid receptors is applied to cells. The probe is freely diffusible throughout the cell and has no effect on the glucocorticoid receptor. If the cell has not been previously stimulated by glucocorticoids, where is the most intense fluorescence?

(A) Cell membrane
(B) Cytosol
(C) Nuclear membrane
(D) Nucleus
(E) Nucleus and cytosol

13. A middle-aged woman presented with a throbbing headache and bilateral tenderness over her forehead. Knobby cords were palpated at the sides and were biopsied. The tissue is pictured in the micrograph below. The correct diagnosis is

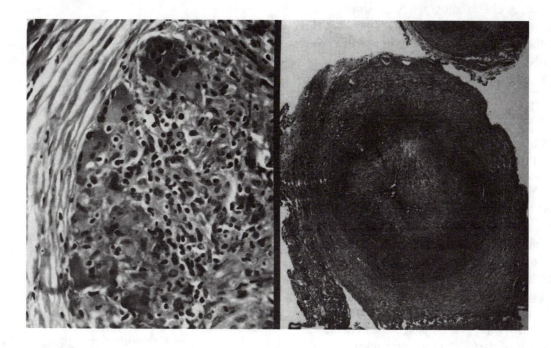

(A) temporal arteritis
(B) foreign body giant cell reaction to an inject-ed substance
(C) Mönckeberg's arteriosclerosis
(D) Takayasu's arteritis

14. Cromolyn sodium is now the first-line agent for the treatment of mild to moderate asthma, especially asthma in children associated with allergenic causes. Although its mechanism of action is unclear, cromolyn sodium's widespread use is due to its

(A) bioavailability after oral administration
(B) direct bronchodilating effect, making it useful in acute emergencies
(C) prophylactic potential secondary to inhibition of the release of inflammatory mediators
(D) immediate effect to reduce bronchospasm
(E) antimuscarinic effects

15. A patient's symptoms are pleuritic chest pain, nonproductive cough, diminished breath sounds at the base bilaterally, and a dullness to percussion. A chest radiograph is consistent with a pleural effusion. A thoracentesis is performed. All of the following results are interpreted correctly EXCEPT

(A) the pleural fluid has high levels of protein and lactate dehydrogenase (LDH); therefore, it is an exudate
(B) the pleural fluid has a high level of LDH, but the protein level is within the normal range; therefore, the fluid is a transudate
(C) the pleural fluid has a low level of glucose (30 mg/dl) and a low pH (6.5); therefore, a chest tube should be inserted because of the likelihood of empyema
(D) the pleural fluid contains blood, so the hematocrit should be checked
(E) the pleural fluid has an amylase level that is higher than serum levels; therefore, pancreatic disease and esophageal varices are at the top of the differential diagnoses
(F) the pleural fluid has moderately increased triglycerides; therefore, lipoprotein electrophoresis should be performed

Questions 16–18

A patient presents with epigastric and right upper quadrant pain. The pain is most intense 2–4 hours after eating and is reduced by the ingestion of antacids. The patient states that he has passed black tarry stools (melena) within the last week.

16. Fiberoptic endoscopy reveals a yellowish crater surrounded by a rim of erythema that is 3 cm distal to the pylorus. Accordingly, an ulcer has been identified in the patient's

(A) fundus
(B) antrum
(C) duodenum
(D) jejunum
(E) ileum

17. Hypertrophy of which of the following submucosal structures often accompanies denudation of the epithelium in peptic ulcer?

(A) Brunner's glands
(B) Meissner's plexus
(C) Auerbach's plexus
(D) Peyer's patches
(E) Paneth's cells

18. Possible pharmacotherapy for this patient may include

(A) bethanechol
(B) diphenhydramine
(C) indomethacin
(D) ranitidine
(E) dexamethasone

19. The most important prognostic factor for human cancer is

(A) the patient's age
(B) tumor stage
(C) lymphocytic infiltration
(D) vascular invasion
(E) the mitotic index

20. Growth hormone (GH; somatotropic hormone; somatotropin) is synthesized and stored in large amounts in the anterior pituitary gland (adenohypophysis). Which of the following statements accurately describes GH?

(A) It is secreted continuously
(B) Synthesis is stimulated by the action of somatostatin
(C) Receptors have a limited distribution outside the central nervous system (CNS)
(D) It stimulates cartilage and bone growth via somatomedin
(E) It has a proinsulin-like effect in addition to its other actions

21. A 29-year-old intravenous drug abuser presented with bilateral fluffy lung infiltrates. A transbronchial biopsy was performed. A Grocott-Gomori methenamine–silver nitrate stain was performed on the lung tissue (pictured below). The diagnosis is

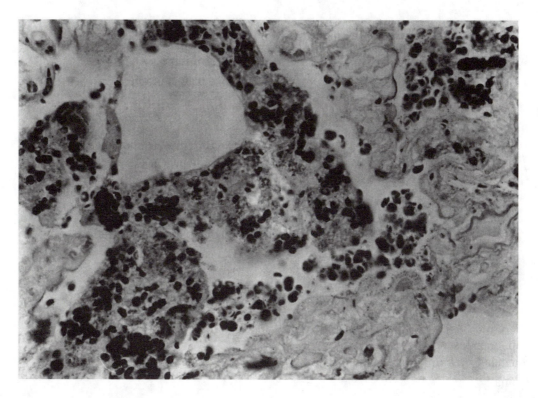

(A) atypical mycobacterial infection

(B) cytomegalovirus (CMV) pneumonitis

(C) nocardial abscess

(D) pneumocystis pneumonia

(E) legionnaires' disease

22. A 24-year-old black woman presented with chest pain; her chest radiograph revealed mediastinal lymphadenopathy. A lymph node biopsy from the anterior mediastinum was obtained by mediastinoscopy, and the tissue sample is portrayed in the photomicrograph below. The correct diagnosis is

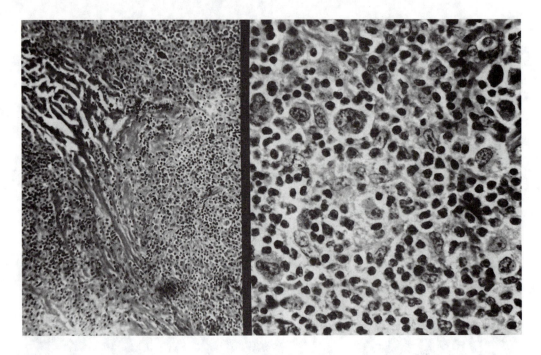

(A) sarcoidosis

(B) thymoma

(C) sclerosing mediastinitis

(D) Hodgkin's disease

23. Which of the following statements regarding the proximal tubular epithelium illustrated below is most likely to be correct?

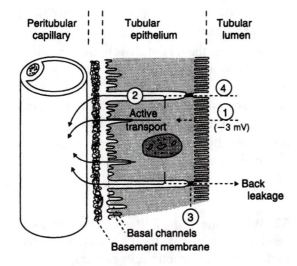

(A) The ion whose movement is depicted in (*1*) is Na$^+$

(B) The process depicted at site (*2*) is aldosterone-sensitive

(C) The cell is impermeable to water because of the tight junctions shown in (*3*)

(D) The process depicted at site (*4*) is affected by antidiuretic hormone (ADH)

(E) The intracellular potential is similar to the tubular lumen potential (-3 mV)

24. Of the following statements regarding thoracic outlet syndrome, which one is true?

(A) It results from an irregularly shaped first thoracic rib

(B) Compression of the left phrenic nerve may occur

(C) Numbness and tingling occur along a median nerve distribution

(D) Compression of the subclavian artery may occur

25. Glucose stimulation of beta cells in the endocrine pancreas subsequently causes

(A) enhancement of gluconeogenesis in the liver

(B) increased glycogenolysis by the liver

(C) stimulation of the release of glucagon

(D) decreased oxidation of amino acids in the liver

Questions 26–27

A 55-year-old patient presents with weakness, weight loss, and bone pain of 3 months' duration. Head x-rays show many well-demarcated osteolytic lesions.

26. All of the following symptoms would help to confirm the diagnosis of this disease EXCEPT

(A) the presence of monoclonal proteins weighing 55,000 daltons in the serum and urine

(B) a history of recurrent bacterial infections

(C) a spike in a particular isotype region in the electrophoretic pattern of serum proteins

(D) the presence of Bence Jones protein in the serum or urine

27. In approximately 55% of patients presenting with multiple myeloma, the major membrane-bound carrier protein, or monoclonal protein, would be

(A) immunoglobulin M (IgM)

(B) IgD

(C) IgE

(D) IgA

(E) IgG

28. Monitoring aminoglycoside serum levels is requisite for the systemic use of the drugs because

(A) they are extensively metabolized by hepatic enzymes

(B) they are rapidly eliminated

(C) they can cause severe hypersensitivity reactions

(D) their therapeutic index is low, and toxicity is easily manifest

(E) they rapidly cross the blood–brain barrier

29. Tamoxifen can control the growth of some forms of female breast cancer by

(A) inhibiting estrogen synthesis

(B) inhibiting androgen-induced DNA transcription

(C) competing for estrogen receptors

(D) inhibiting the secretion of luteinizing hormone (LH)

(E) stimulating nuclear transcription

30. Propranolol (a β-blocker) may be used with nitroglycerin (glyceryl trinitrate; GTN) in concurrent therapy for typical (exertional) angina because propranolol

(A) is a potent vasodilator of coronary arteries

(B) increases conduction in the atria and atrioventricular node

(C) blocks the reflex tachycardia that occurs with the use of GTN

(D) dilates constricted airways

(E) is positively inotropic

31. Phenytoin (Dilantin) is effective in most forms of epilepsy (with the exception of absence seizures) because it

(A) directly binds to chloride channels in the central nervous system (CNS)

(B) enhances the inhibitory actions of γ-aminobutyric acid (GABA) at its receptor in the CNS

(C) affects Na^+ conductance in neurons via voltage-sensitive Na^+-channel inhibition

(D) is usually started concurrently with phenobarbital therapy

32. Which one of the following statements concerning the synthesis of different types of RNA molecules in eukaryotic cells is true?

(A) RNA polymerase I produces mainly messenger RNA (mRNA)

(B) RNA polymerase III produces ribosomal RNA (rRNA)

(C) RNA polymerase II produces transfer RNA (tRNA)

(D) None of the above

33. Which one of the following drugs or chemicals has been associated with the induction of aplastic anemia?

(A) Acetaminophen

(B) Methyldopa

(C) Benzene

(D) Penicillin

(E) Thiouracil

34. A monoclonal antibody (immunoglobulin G; IgG) that neutralizes endotoxin has been produced. This antibody has tremendous therapeutic potential for patients suffering septic shock from endotoxemia, and it might be useful in treating patients who have which one of the following diseases?

(A) Pulmonary anthrax
(B) Whooping cough
(C) Cholera
(D) Leprosy
(E) Bubonic plague

35. Which of the following proteins bind to penicillin?

(A) Alanine racemase
(B) 30S Ribosomes
(C) Peptidoglycan
(D) Porin
(E) Transpeptidase

36. A medical student received a deep laceration in an altercation at a party. He reports having had a DTP (diphtheria-tetanus-pertussis) series in childhood. The most appropriate treatment would be

(A) injection of human tetanus immunoglobulin G (IgG)
(B) injection of equine tetanus IgG
(C) intravenous administration of an aminoglycoside
(D) injection of tetanus toxoid

37. Which of the following statements concerning acetylsalicylic acid (aspirin), the prototype of a group of nonsteroidal anti-inflammatory agents that are also analgesic and antipyretic, is correct?

(A) Aspirin is a potent lipoxygenase inhibitor
(B) The major adverse effect of aspirin is gastrointestinal bleeding
(C) Aspirin can reduce normal body temperature
(D) Aspirin is a competitive inhibitor of platelet cyclooxygenase

38. Which one of the following statements concerning messenger RNA (mRNA) splicing is true?

(A) Alternate splicing, producing two different mRNA molecules from the same gene, is a common occurrence in most mammalian genes
(B) Spliceosomes are collections of small nuclear ribonucleoproteins (snRNPs) located near ribosomes on the rough endoplasmic reticulum
(C) U1 snRNP binds to a nucleotide segment on the 5' end of the intron to be spliced
(D) Spliceosomes recognize splicing sites by the large 50–80 base-pair sequences on the 5' and 3' regions of introns

39. The most common tumor of the appendix, which is pictured below, is

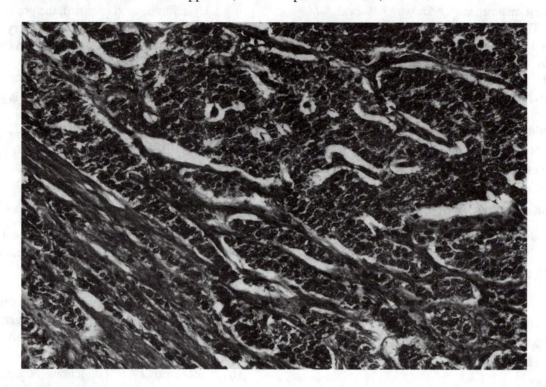

(A) a carcinoid tumor

(B) an adenocarcinoma

(C) a mucocele

(D) an inflammatory pseudotumor

40. Which one of the following conditions would result in a negative nitrogen balance?

(A) Consumption of dietary proteins that are deficient in glycine

(B) Normal intake of dietary protein accompanied by defective cholecystokinin–pancreozymin (CCK–PZ) production

(C) Nitrogen consumption that exceeds nitrogen excretion

(D) A tyrosine supplement in the diet of a child with phenylketonuria (PKU)

(E) A 50% reduction in the hydrochloric acid (HCl) content of gastric juice

41. Translation of a synthetic polyribonucleotide containing the repeating sequence CAA in a cell-free protein synthesizing system produced three homopolypeptides: polyglutamine, polyasparagine, and polythreonine. If the codons for glutamine and asparagine are CAA and AAC, respectively, which of the following triplets is a codon for threonine?

(A) AAC

(B) CAA

(C) CAC

(D) CCA

(E) ACA

Questions 42–43

It is hypothesized that nocturnal body temperatures are linearly related to body weight in 60- to 70-year-old women. Nursing records are reviewed for weights in kilograms and 4 a.m. temperatures in degrees Celsius.

42. These variables are considered to be

(A) continuous
(B) nonparametric
(C) constants
(D) reciprocal
(E) outliers

43. The null hypothesis for the study question described would state that there is

(A) an expected correlation between body weight and temperature
(B) an effect of aging on temperatures in obese elderly women
(C) no relation between temperature and body weight
(D) an inverse relation between body weight and nocturnal temperature
(E) a probability ($P < 0.05$) that body weight is related to nocturnal temperature

44. *Pseudomonas aeruginosa*, *Staphylococcus aureus*, and *Serratia marcescens* all produce which one of the following substances?

(A) Endotoxins
(B) Enterotoxins
(C) Lipoteichoic acids
(D) Mycolic acids
(E) Pigments

45. Resistance to phagocytosis is among the most important properties for virulence of many bacteria. *Mycobacterium tuberculosis* is very resistant to phagocytic killing and actually grows in macrophages. The successful antiphagocytic strategy employed by *M. tuberculosis* clearly involves which one of the following mechanisms?

(A) Production of protein exotoxins to kill or impair the phagocyte
(B) Prevention of phagosome–lysosome fusion
(C) Elaboration of immunoglobulin A (IgA) protease
(D) Production of the antiphagocytic polysaccharide capsule
(E) Escape from the phagolysosome into the cytoplasm

46. Injection of a pharmacologically effective amount of an antimuscarinic agent, like atropine, may

(A) increase bronchial glandular secretions
(B) increase heart rate
(C) cause paralysis in some skeletal muscles
(D) constrict the pupil
(E) promote sweating

47. G proteins are involved with various cellular signaling pathways and are known to hydrolyze

(A) adenosine triphosphate (ATP)
(B) guanosine triphosphate (GTP)
(C) adenosine diphosphate (ADP)
(D) guanosine diphosphate (GDP)
(E) adenosine monophosphate (AMP)

48. A peripheral lung nodule was resected from a 50-year-old man. The tumor, pictured below, is best classified as

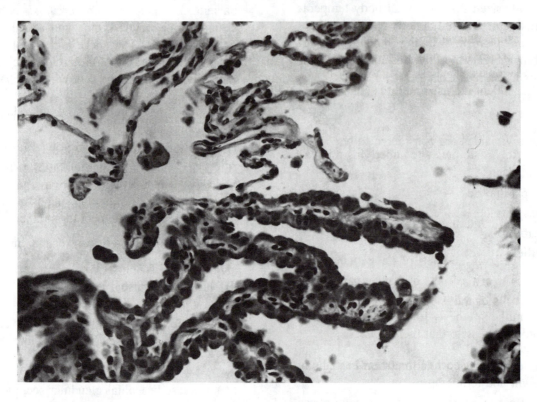

(A) small cell carcinoma

(B) undifferentiated large cell carcinoma

(C) adenoid cystic carcinoma

(D) bronchioloalveolar carcinoma

(E) diffuse large cell lymphoma

49. A lymph node removed from a 32-year-old man shows diffuse large cell lymphoma. Which of the following clinical scenarios most likely characterizes this patient?

(A) Disseminated disease at presentation; prolonged survival and eventual death owing to lymphoma or its complications

(B) Rapid development of circulating immature blasts, requiring aggressive cytotoxic therapy

(C) Greater than 90% chance of being alive 10 years after diagnosis

(D) Rapid death if therapy is unsuccessful; approximately 50% chance for long-term survival if therapy achieves complete response

(E) Spontaneous remission in 20% of patients

Questions 50–53

A young adult visits his physician with complaints of polyuria and unexplained weight loss. Fasting plasma glucose is greater than 140 mg/dl (on two occasions), and an oral glucose tolerance test is consistent with a diagnosis of type I insulin-dependent diabetes mellitus (IDDM).

50. The likely histologic site underlying this patient's disorder is

(A) pancreatic acini
(B) zymogen-containing cells of the pancreatic acinus
(C) alpha cells of the islets of Langerhans
(D) beta cells of the islets of Langerhans
(E) delta cells of the islets of Langerhans

51. An important aspect of treatment in this patient is

(A) a single daily injection of an insulin zinc suspension (Lente insulin)
(B) glipizide
(C) abstinence from dietary carbohydrates
(D) increased intake of saturated fats
(E) avoidance of exercise

52. An endogenous hormone that tends to decrease circulating blood glucose is

(A) glucagon
(B) growth hormone (GH)
(C) somatostatin
(D) epinephrine
(E) thyroid hormone

53. Despite vigorous therapy, all of the following are potential chronic complications of IDDM EXCEPT

(A) intercapillary glomerulosclerosis
(B) proliferative retinopathy
(C) atherosclerosis
(D) peripheral polyneuropathy
(E) pulmonary hypertension

54. Surfactant is a substance that is critical for normal lung function. All of the following statements about surfactant are true EXCEPT

(A) surfactant is made up of mostly lipids and a smaller percentage of protein, the most abundant lipid being dipalmitoyl phosphatidylcholine
(B) surfactant is synthesized by the alveolar type II epithelial cells; damage to these cells in patients with adult respiratory distress syndrome (ARDS) can lead to increased alveolar collapse
(C) surfactant increases pulmonary compliance by decreasing alveolar surface tension
(D) surfactant forms a lipid bilayer with interspersed protein molecules that lines the alveolar surface, thereby preventing atelectasis and facilitating gas exchange
(E) the hydrophobic tails of the dipalmitoyl phosphatidylcholine are pointed toward the air, whereas the hydrophilic heads are pointed toward the cell and aqueous hypophase
(F) surfactant replacement is an available therapy for neonatal respiratory distress syndrome (RDS)

55. Halothane has blood:gas and oil:gas partition coefficients of 2.4 and 220, respectively. Methoxyflurane has blood:gas and oil:gas coefficients of 13 and 950, respectively. Which of the following statements regarding these volatile anesthetics is correct?

(A) Both result in faster induction than does nitrous oxide (blood:gas partition coefficient of 0.47)
(B) The minimal alveolar concentration of halothane is less than that of methoxyflurane
(C) Both agents are useful because they do not have any cardiodepressant effects
(D) Recovery from methoxyflurane is faster than that from halothane
(E) An increase in ventilatory rate makes the onset of anesthesia more rapid for either agent

56. Restriction enzymes have which one of the following characteristics? They

(A) can cleave only circular DNA
(B) generate either staggered (sticky) or blunt ends upon cleaving DNA
(C) cleave different DNAs randomly
(D) can cleave different DNAs only once
(E) can cleave both DNA and RNA

57. A chronically ill 43-year-old patient with a relapse of multiple sclerosis has been in the hospital for 4 weeks. He has angered the nurses by being very demanding, including calling them "every 5 minutes" for minor reasons and complaining that they do not respond promptly. To remedy this situation, the physician must

(A) instruct the patient to behave better
(B) order a sedating medication
(C) arrange for the nurses to visit the patient for 3 minutes every hour
(D) warn the patient that he will be transferred to another hospital if he does not straighten out

58. A 74-year-old man presents with hypertension, diabetes mellitus with retinopathy, and chronic obstructive pulmonary disease (COPD). He admits to drinking four bottles of beer a day. He has been living alone for the past year since his wife died. His primary care physician should be especially and immediately concerned about the risk of

(A) renal insufficiency
(B) silent myocardial infarction
(C) suicide
(D) peripheral neuropathy
(E) pneumonia

59. The graph below measures the number of viable bacterial cells in a control culture and cultures of exponentially growing cells to which antibiotics were added at the point indicated by the *arrow*. The antibiotic added to the culture to produce *curve A* was which one of the following?

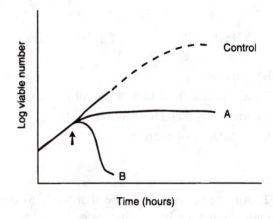

(A) Polymyxin B
(B) Cephalothin
(C) Chloramphenicol
(D) Methicillin
(E) Vancomycin

60. According to the Henderson-Hasselbalch equation:

$$pH = 6.1 + \log [HCO_3^-]/0.03 \times P_{CO_2}$$

The apparent dissociation constant, pK′, in blood is 6.1; and the solubility constant for CO_2 in plasma at 38°C is 0.03 mmol/L/mm Hg. If a patient has a plasma $[HCO_3^-]$ of 37 mmol/L and arterial P_{CO_2} of 60 mm Hg, then the patient is most likely to have (recall log 10 = 1; log 20 = 1.3; log 30 = 1.5; normal values of $[HCO_3^-]$ = 25 mmol/L; P_{CO_2} = 40 mm Hg)

(A) respiratory alkalosis

(B) respiratory acidosis

(C) fully compensated respiratory acidosis

(D) metabolic alkalosis

(E) metabolic acidosis

61. The ability of erythrocytes to pump Na^+ from the cytoplasm into the plasma compartment would be compromised most directly by a total deficiency of

(A) stearoyl coenzyme A (CoA) desaturase

(B) diphosphoglycerate kinase

(C) pyruvate carboxylase

(D) glucose 6-phosphatase

(E) malate dehydrogenase

62. A total of 25 hypertensive patients are followed over a 2-week period for the effects of a diuretic drug on K^+ concentrations. The statistical test used to compare the K^+ serum levels before and after medication is most likely to be

(A) discriminant analysis

(B) paired t-test

(C) regression analysis

(D) chi-squared test

(E) Pearson correlation

Questions 63–64

A 22-year-old male college student visits the student health service complaining of extreme fatigue, sore throat, difficulty concentrating, and fever to 39°C over the last week. Physical examination is unremarkable except for mild lymph node enlargement in the axillary, cervical, and inguinal regions and a palpable spleen tip. A blood count shows hemoglobin of 10 g/dl, platelets of 105,000/µl, and white cell count of 22,000/µl with 60% lymphoid cells. The laboratory blood profile also shows an absolute red cell count of 2.3×10^6/µl, mean red cell volume of 125 femtoliters (fl), and mean cell hemoglobin concentration of 43 g/dl.

63. What is the most likely diagnosis for this patient?

(A) Infectious lymphocytosis

(B) *Bordetella pertussis* infection

(C) Cytomegalovirus (CMV) mononucleosis syndrome

(D) Mononucleosis secondary to Epstein-Barr virus (EBV) infection (infectious mononucleosis)

(E) Mononucleosis secondary to *Toxoplasma gondii* infection

64. Which of the following is the most likely cause of this patient's anemia (Hb 10 g/dl)?

(A) Immune-mediated

(B) Compromise of erythroid production secondary to EBV infection of bone marrow precursors

(C) Virus-associated hemophagocytic syndrome

(D) Slow gastrointestinal blood loss since the start of illness owing to thrombocytopenia

(E) Disseminated intravascular coagulation (DIC)

65. The eclipse phase of the virus replication cycle has which one of the following characteristics? It

(A) is defined as that time period after which the first virus particles are assembled

(B) denotes the time between virus entry into the cell and the time virus particles appear extracellularly

(C) is that part of the replication cycle during which virus particles cannot be recovered from the infected cells

(D) is comparable to the metaphase portion of mitosis

66. Light microscopy requires the use of special techniques, such as stains, to visualize cells and cell components. Which of the following cellular components can be visualized after staining for catalase?

(A) Golgi complex

(B) Lysosomes

(C) Rough endoplasmic reticulum

(D) Smooth endoplasmic reticulum

(E) Peroxisomes

67. Dinitrochlorobenzene was applied to a patient's skin over a 1-cm^2 area on the right forearm. Approximately 2 weeks later, a pruritic rash occurred at the site. It can be concluded that

(A) the patient lacks all T-cell–mediated immune function

(B) the patient suffers from DiGeorge syndrome

(C) the reaction would require an additional 2 weeks to develop on subsequent exposure to dinitrochlorobenzene

(D) the reaction observed was most likely caused by CD4+ T cells

Questions 68–69

An ophthalmologic examination of a 60-year-old man complaining of vision problems reveals increased intraocular pressure (25 mm Hg) with optic disk changes and visual field defects. These findings strongly suggest primary open-angle glaucoma for which pharmacotherapy is considered.

68. The underlying cause of the patient's condition is a decreased outflow facility of the aqueous humor. A primary anatomic structure involved with the histopathologic changes that account for this problem is the

(A) conjunctiva

(B) cornea

(C) canal of Schlemm

(D) ciliary process

(E) choroidal vessel

69. Pharmacotherapy for the patient is initially designed to open trabecular meshwork by contracting the ciliary muscle. A useful agent for this purpose is

(A) atropine

(B) succinylcholine

(C) pilocarpine

(D) dexamethasone

(E) tubocurarine

70. Which one of the following statements about mechanical ventilation is true?

(A) Hypoxemic respiratory failure is an indication for mechanical ventilation, but hypercarbic respiratory failure is not

(B) A backup respiratory rate is set for the assist-control, but not the synchronized intermittent mandatory ventilation mode

(C) When using the assist-control mode, every breath that the patient takes will be of a set volume

(D) Pressure support ventilation is the mode that is most commonly used when initiating mechanical ventilation in acutely ill individuals

(E) A potential disadvantage of using positive end-expiratory pressure is that it may increase cardiac output, but decrease oxygen delivery to the tissues

(F) With mechanical ventilation, it is not possible to accurately control the oxygen concentration of the air that is inhaled by the patient

71. The peripheral nerve tumor pictured below is best classified as a

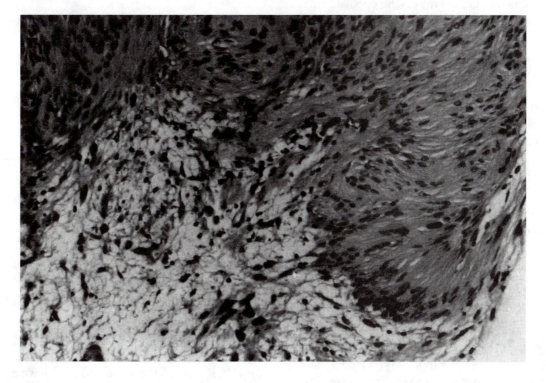

(A) neurofibroma
(B) traumatic neuroma
(C) neurilemoma
(D) triton tumor

72. Triglycerides are neutral fats of animals and food plants; they make up approximately 90% of the dietary intake of fats. An important step in their digestion in the gastrointestinal tract is

(A) significant hydrolysis by gastric lipases
(B) breakdown by biliary enzymes
(C) formation of fatty acids and monoglyceride by pancreatic lipase
(D) active transport of fatty acid products in the intestinal brush border

73. Which of the tracts listed below, whose fibers traverse the spinal cord, brain stem, and higher structures, is thought to cross to the opposite side of the central nervous system (CNS) twice?

(A) The anterior spinocerebellar tract, which conveys unconscious sensory information from joints, tendons, and muscles
(B) The spinal thalamic tract, which conveys conscious sensory information of pain and temperature
(C) The cuneocerebellar tract, which conveys conscious muscle and joint sensory information
(D) The vestibulospinal tract, which conveys efferent fibers

74. A 29-year-old white woman comes to the physician's office stating that she recently discovered a gap in her memory of 2 hours. She tells the physician that her friends informed her that she has been acting inappropriately. Suddenly the patient becomes confused but remains docile. She asks the physician from where the overwhelming smell of rotten food is emanating. The patient most likely suffers from

(A) Klüver-Bucy syndrome of the temporal lobes
(B) temporal lobe epilepsy
(C) jacksonian epileptic seizures
(D) petit mal seizures

75. A 5-year-old child in Bangladesh drinks untreated river water and develops cholera. Which of the following scenarios is most likely to occur?

(A) Recovery following treatment is slow because *Vibrio cholerae* causes chronic intracellular infections
(B) Microscopic examination of stools reveals leukocytes
(C) Disease symptoms arise due to cholera toxin-mediated elevation in cyclic adenosine monophosphate (cAMP) levels in intestinal cells
(D) *V. cholerae* attaches to the dental flora

76. Centrioles are replicated in which phase of the cell cycle?

(A) G_0 phase
(B) G_1 phase
(C) S phase
(D) G_2 phase
(E) M phase

77. Which one of the following statements about energy storage and transfer is true?

(A) Adenosine triphosphate (ATP) can be synthesized from adenosine diphosphate (ADP) by phosphate transfer from 3-phosphoglycerate
(B) Phosphocreatine is an important energy source for muscle tissues
(C) Reactions that have a $K_{eq} > 1$ have a positive $\Delta G°$
(D) When ATP is hydrolyzed to adenosine monophosphate (AMP) and inorganic pyrophosphate (PP_i), the reaction is endergonic and will proceed spontaneously
(E) The energy of hydrolysis for phosphoenolpyruvate is less than that for pyrophosphate

78. The extraction of β-hydroxybutyrate from blood and its oxidation to carbon dioxide and water requires the participation of

(A) β-hydroxybutyrate dehydrogenase and 3-hydroxy-3-methylglutaryl coenzyme A (HMG CoA) lyase
(B) acetoacetate thiokinase and β-hydroxybutyrate dehydrogenase
(C) HMG CoA synthase and thiolase
(D) short-chain fatty acetyl CoA dehydrogenase and thiolase
(E) succinyl CoA: acetoacetate acyltransferase and HMG CoA lyase

Questions 79–81

A 43-year-old man who is being treated with hydrochlorothiazide for control of mild edema presents to the physician complaining of malaise, fatigue, muscular weakness, and muscle cramps. Blood tests reveal elevated creatinine with an even greater elevation in blood urea nitrogen, high blood urate, and altered blood electrolytes.

79. What is the primary anatomic site of action of hydrochlorothiazide?

(A) Proximal tubules
(B) Early distal tubules
(C) Late distal tubules
(D) Thick ascending limb of the loop of Henle
(E) Collecting ducts

80. The patient's complaints most likely reflect the most serious adverse effect of diuretic therapy, which is

(A) hyperglycemia
(B) hyperuricemia
(C) drug hypersensitivity
(D) hyperkalemia
(E) hypokalemia

81. To correct this patient's problem, the physician must consider all of the following therapeutic choices EXCEPT

(A) K^+ supplementation
(B) digitalis
(C) spironolactone
(D) reduced dosage of hydrochlorothiazide
(E) amiloride

82. An investigator has isolated a bacterium that, in the absence of glucose, constitutively produces the proteins coded for by the lac operon. Which of the following statements explains this observation?

(A) The promoter has a mutation that prevents RNA polymerase from binding
(B) There is a missense mutation in the gene for β-galactosidase
(C) The gene for the catabolite activator protein is mutated and inactive
(D) There is a mutation in the attenuator sequence
(E) The gene for the repressor protein is mutated and inactive

83. An adolescent patient attends weekly individual, psychodynamic psychotherapy sessions. When he begins to feel too close to and dependent on the psychiatrist, he often misses a scheduled appointment. This behavior is an example of

(A) acting out
(B) antisocial personality
(C) repression
(D) suppression
(E) identification with the aggressor

84. Which of the statements concerning the disaccharide pictured below is most accurate? It

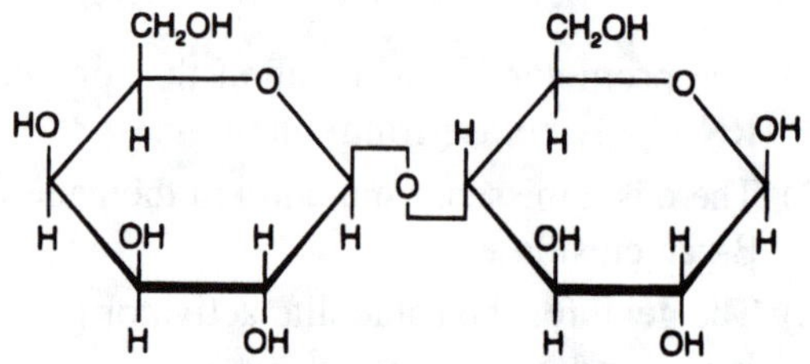

(A) yields a negative result in the Fehling-Benedict reducing sugar test
(B) is cleaved by isomaltose
(C) is a β-galactoside
(D) is digested and absorbed by a lactase-deficient child
(E) is a good source of calories for a 2-week-old child with galactosemia

85. A 42-year-old woman with breast cancer was treated with radiation and currently is receiving chemotherapy. She complained of some left-sided chest pain, which was determined not to be of cardiac origin. On the fourth day, several vesicles appeared on her left thorax, following a rib in distribution; she also had several smaller vesicles at other sites (scalp, leg, forearm). Her physician diagnosed varicella-zoster virus (VZV) infection and started treatment with acyclovir. Which one of the following statements best describes the VZV in this case?

(A) Thymidine kinase–negative VZV mutants are likely to render the treatment ineffective
(B) The initial exposure to VZV in childhood could not have led to viral latency in the dorsal ganglia
(C) The lesions outside the dermatomal distribution are likely explained by depressed cell-mediated immunity
(D) The VZV was the most likely causal factor in the patient's breast cancer
(E) The acyclovir will alkylate the VZV DNA

86. A 62-year-old woman died of congestive heart failure due to severe mitral stenosis. At autopsy, sections of the heart revealed the lesions shown in the photomicrograph below. This suggests a previous history of which one of the following conditions?

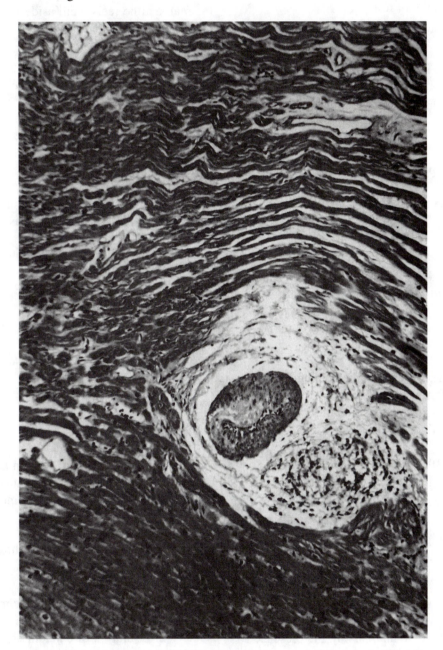

(A) Amyloidosis

(B) Rheumatic fever

(C) Polyarteritis nodosa

(D) Myocardial infarction

87. Which of the following tests is the major projective instrument of personality assessment?

(A) Rorschach inkblot test
(B) Minnesota Multiphasic Personality Inventory
(C) Thematic apperception test
(D) Sentence completion test
(E) Projective drawings

88. Proof of the presence of active disease caused by *Mycobacterium tuberculosis* is provided by which one of the following diagnostic measures?

(A) The tuberculin test
(B) Clinical findings (e.g., weight loss, night sweats, cough, low-grade fever)
(C) Finding acid-fast organisms in sputum
(D) Isolation of *M. tuberculosis*

89. Several workers at a chemical manufacturing facility were referred to a physician for evaluation of connective tissue neoplasms. This physician could expect to find

(A) antigenic cross-reactivity between tumors
(B) distinct antigenic specificity for each tumor
(C) antigenic cross-reactivity between these tumors and those induced by ultraviolet light
(D) distinct antigenic specificity for different cells from the same tumor

90. Hodgkin's lymphoma can be distinguished from other forms of lymphoma by the presence of

(A) Reed-Sternberg cells
(B) the Philadelphia chromosome
(C) Auer rods
(D) decreased quantities of leukocyte alkaline phosphatase

91. An 86-year-old man has diminished vibratory sensation at the knees and toes, although his reflexes are intact, temperature sensation is normal, and he feels well, aside from having headaches. What is the most likely explanation?

(A) Peripheral neuropathy
(B) Normal age-related change
(C) Spinal cord lesion
(D) Small strokes
(E) Brain or brain stem tumor

92. The pressor response to an indirect-acting sympathomimetic agent, such as amphetamine, is

(A) associated with marked tolerance (tachyphylaxis)
(B) decreased in the presence of a monoamine oxidase (MAO) inhibitor
(C) potentiated by an uptake 1 inhibitor, such as imipramine
(D) potentiated by pretreatment with reserpine
(E) related to its direct effects on postsynaptic receptors

93. The introduction of foreign DNA into bacteria is an important tool in molecular biology. Which of the following statements concerning nucleic acid transfer is true?

(A) Transformation is the technique whereby a bacteriophage is used to introduce DNA into a bacteria
(B) Transduction is the technique whereby "competent" bacterial cells are suspended in a solution of calcium chloride and DNA
(C) The most common DNA used in transformation is plasmid DNA
(D) Conjugation is the technique whereby a bacteriophage is used to introduce DNA into a bacteria

Questions 94–100

A 27-year-old man who has torn his anterior cruciate ligament (ACL) while skiing is sent to the operating room for ACL replacement and reconstruction. The anesthesiologist selects halothane.

94. Important adverse effects of halothane include all of the following EXCEPT

(A) depression of respiratory drive
(B) lowering of ventilatory response to carbon dioxide
(C) malignant hyperthermia in genetically sensitive individuals
(D) lowering of the seizure threshold
(E) depressed myocardial contractility

95. Induction of anesthesia is smooth, and the operation begins. Before any incision is made, the surgical resident informs the surgeon that this surgery is to be performed on the

(A) ankle
(B) knee
(C) hip
(D) elbow
(E) shoulder

96. The ACL stabilizes this joint by attaching the

(A) medial malleolus of the tibia to the talus
(B) lateral malleolus of the fibula to the talus
(C) head of the femur to the innominate (hip) bone
(D) femur to the fibula
(E) femur to the tibia

97. The head of the femur is attached to the innominate bone at the cup-shaped region known as the

(A) ilioischial fossa
(B) iliofemoral fossa
(C) ischial depression
(D) acetabulum
(E) sella turcica

98. The primary site of long bone growth occurs at the

(A) epiphysis
(B) diaphysis
(C) epiphyseal plate
(D) medullary cavity
(E) primary ossification center

99. All of the following bones are carpal bones EXCEPT

(A) capitate
(B) cuboid
(C) trapezium
(D) trapezoid

100. All of the following statements are true for compact bone EXCEPT that it

(A) is made up of parallel bony columns
(B) contains neurovascular channels
(C) is composed of a network of trabeculae
(D) contains haversian canals
(E) contains osteocytes that communicate via gap junctions

101. Which of the following tests is contraindicated in patients with intracranial neoplasms?

(A) Computed tomography (CT) of the head because of the use of contrast dye
(B) Nuclear magnetic resonance (NMR) because of the length of time a patient must remain supine during testing
(C) Lumbar puncture to examine cerebrospinal proteins and relieve hydrocephalus
(D) X-ray imaging of the skull because the radiation may shrink the tumor and cause hemorrhaging

102. A 3-year-old boy is febrile, breathing slowly, has a bark-like cough and inspiratory stridor. These symptoms have developed during the past 36 hours. He has been vaccinated against *Haemophilus influenzae* type b. Which one of the following statements is correct?

(A) The boy has epiglottitis and should be intubated immediately
(B) Cold air and quick temperature changes will make this boy appear much worse
(C) The organism causing this illness is respiratory syncytial virus
(D) The boy should be placed in a humidified room, and supplemental oxygen and racemic epinephrine should be considered if his condition continues to worsen
(E) The etiology of this disease is most commonly bacterial
(F) Croup can be eliminated from the differential diagnosis due to the inspiratory stridor because abnormal lung sounds are heard only during expiration in patients with croup

103. The figure below is a stylized diagram of the juxtaglomerular apparatus of the kidney. A decrease in the flow of glomerular filtrate into the tubules might cause which one of the following actions?

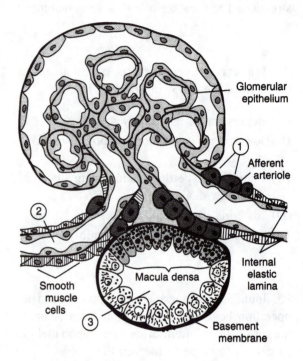

(A) Renin released from *1*
(B) Vasodilation of *2*
(C) An increase in Na^+ concentration at *3*
(D) A reflexive vasoconstriction of the afferent arteriole

104. A quantitative Gram stain revealed many fewer cells than expected from the turbidity of a bacterial culture. The decrease in cells was most likely due to

(A) inactivation of the cytochromes
(B) digestion of the bacterial cell wall by autolytic processes
(C) presence of gram-negative organisms in the culture
(D) presence of bacterial spores in the culture

105. According to Fick's law, oxygen consumption is equal to the product of blood flow and arteriovenous oxygen difference. If the lungs absorb 300 ml/min of oxygen, arterial oxygen content is 20 ml/100 ml blood, pulmonary arterial oxygen content is 15 ml/100 ml blood, and heart rate is 60/min, then stroke volume is

(A) 50 ml
(B) 60 ml
(C) 100 ml
(D) 5 L/min
(E) 6 L/min

106. Capsule production is essential for the virulence of many pathogenic bacteria. Which of the following statements best describes bacterial capsules?

(A) The most important function of the *Streptococcus pneumoniae* capsule is adhesion
(B) The capsule of *Haemophilus influenzae* type B stimulates a T-cell–dependent immune response
(C) Opsonizing antibodies are often directed against *S. pneumoniae* capsules
(D) The capsule of group B *Neisseria meningitidis* is protein
(E) The DTP (diphtheria-tetanus-pertussis) vaccine currently licensed contains purified *Bordetella pertussis* capsules

107. True statements about the side chains of amino acids that are found in proteins include which one of the following?

(A) Serine provides strong buffering capacity at pH 7.0
(B) Alanine absorbs ultraviolet light
(C) Glutamic acid and aspartic acid differ significantly in their isoelectric pH (pI)
(D) Proline often produces a bend in the protein chain
(E) Only D-amino acids are incorporated into protein

108. A 56-year-old woman with a history of ovarian cancer treated by chemotherapy several years ago presents to a clinic with complaints of fatigue and the recent development of small hemorrhages on her arms. She has the following lab values: hemoglobin, 9.6 g/dl; white blood cells, 2900/μl; platelets, 56,000/μl. A bone marrow aspirate is hypercellular and contains approximately 10% blasts (normal < 5%) with megaloblastic morphologic changes in the red cell precursors and megakaryocytes with abnormal nuclei. Cytogenetic analysis reveals a clone with a deletion of the long arm of chromosome 7. What diagnosis best fits this woman's condition?

(A) Preleukemia (myelodysplastic syndrome)
(B) Megaloblastic anemia
(C) Acute lymphocytic leukemia
(D) Acute nonlymphocytic (myeloid) leukemia
(E) Chronic myelogenous leukemia

109. Of the drugs listed below, which one is thought to function through a receptor?

(A) Mannitol
(B) Dimercaprol
(C) Cimetidine
(D) Ethylenediaminetetraacetic acid (EDTA)

110. According to the figure below, which one of the following conditions would result in a shift of the oxygen saturation curve from *a* to *b*?

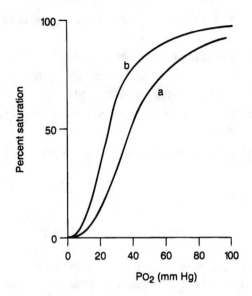

(A) A change in pH from 7.6 to 7.4

(B) A change in P_{CO_2} from 30 to 40 torr

(C) An increase in the concentration of 2,3-diphosphoglycerate (DPG)

(D) The presence of fetal hemoglobin ($\alpha_2\gamma_2$)

(E) The oxidation of the heme iron from Fe^{2+} to Fe^{3+}

111. Which one of the following muscles raises the soft palate during swallowing?

(A) Levator veli palatini

(B) Palatoglossus

(C) Palatopharyngeus

(D) Superior constrictor

112. A 32-year-old man is unemployed and lives in a personal care boarding home. He has a 10-year history of undifferentiated schizophrenia, and has been observed pacing around the house and fidgeting whenever seated. Recently, he received his monthly injection of fluphenazine. The most likely cause of his agitation is

(A) anxiety

(B) restless legs syndrome

(C) akathisia

(D) undiagnosed hyperthyroidism

(E) worsening psychosis

113. Which one of the following statements best describes chondroblasts?

(A) They are endosteal cells capable of secreting proteoglycan

(B) They are perichondrial cells capable of secreting type II collagen

(C) They are periosteal cells capable of secreting type I collagen

(D) They show little mitotic activity

(E) They are filled with rough endoplasmic reticulum but lack a Golgi apparatus

114. A previously healthy 27-year-old woman is seen because of a petechial rash. She denies recent bleeding and has had no recent illnesses. Hemoglobin, hematocrit, and white blood cell counts are normal. Examination of the peripheral blood smear reveals normal red and white blood cells and is remarkable only for a paucity of platelets. The most likely diagnosis in this patient is

(A) aleukemic leukemia

(B) idiopathic thrombocytopenic purpura (ITP)

(C) Glanzmann's thrombasthenia

(D) amegakaryocytic thrombocytopenia

(E) drug-induced thrombocytopenia

Questions 115–120

A 50-year-old man presents to the emergency room with severe epigastric pain, low-grade fever, tachycardia, and mild hypotension. The patient relates a history of moderate to heavy social drinking. The chief resident suspects acute pancreatitis.

115. The single most important laboratory finding to confirm the diagnosis of pancreatitis would be

(A) hyperlipidemia
(B) hyperbilirubinemia
(C) elevated serum amylase
(D) elevated serum phospholipase A
(E) elevated serum alkaline phosphatase

116. Which of the following polypeptide hormones is stimulated by increased acid from the stomach and subsequently stimulates the release of pancreatic juice rich in electrolytes and water?

(A) Gastrin
(B) Secretin
(C) Cholecystokinin
(D) Pancreozymin
(E) Vasoactive intestinal polypeptide (VIP)

117. Which of the following hormones is produced by the duodenal and upper jejunal mucosa and stimulates the release of pancreatic juice rich in digestive enzymes?

(A) Cholecystokinin
(B) Secretin
(C) Glucagon
(D) Pancreatic polypeptide
(E) VIP

118. Neuronal control of pancreatic exocrine function is mediated by

(A) VIP
(B) dopamine
(C) serotonin
(D) substance P
(E) acetylcholine (ACh)

119. Of the following statements about secretin, a polypeptide that has a significant effect on pancreatic secretion, which one is correct?

(A) It is synthesized in the pancreatic acinar cells
(B) It causes the pancreas to secrete large amounts of enzyme
(C) Its release is caused by the presence of fats and amino acids in the upper small intestine
(D) It causes the pancreas to secrete large amounts of bicarbonate ion (HCO_3^-)
(E) It is stored in an active form within S cells of the duodenum

120. The principal reason that the pancreas does not autodigest is that

(A) proteolytic enzymes are secreted as proenzymes
(B) pancreatic acini and ducts secrete a protective mucopolysaccharide, which lines their walls
(C) the pancreas maintains a slightly alkaline pH, rendering the digestive enzymes inactive
(D) pancreatic parenchyma is high in hydroxyproline, which is resistant to proteolysis
(E) proper enzyme substrates are not present

121. A complement fixation test is performed on a patient's serum by first adding influenza type A virus antigen and then adding complement, followed by antibody-coated sheep red blood cells (SRBC), which are then lysed. A possible explanation for this would be

(A) the patient has no immunoglobulin E (IgE) or IgA anti-influenza type A antibodies

(B) the patient's serum contains an antibody that cross-reacts with SRBC

(C) the patient has no complement fixable anti-influenza type A antibodies

(D) the patient's serum contains high levels of IgM, which cause SRBC lysis

122. Volume and pressure (alveolar; pleural) for a normal respiratory cycle are shown in the figure below. Which one of the following statements about respiration is correct?

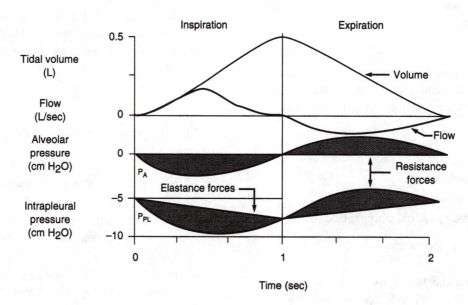

(A) Inspiration is the result of a passive process

(B) Gas flow is greatest at the end of inspiration

(C) Elastic recoil of the lung is identical at the beginning and end of inspiration

(D) During expiration, alveolar pressure becomes greater than atmospheric pressure

123. Which one of the following areas in a eukaryotic cell is a site of RNA processing?

(A) Mitochondria
(B) Golgi complex
(C) Rough endoplasmic reticulum
(D) Endosome

124. In humans, the major route of nitrogen metabolism from amino acids to urea involves which one of the following sets of enzymes?

(A) Amino acid oxidases and arginase
(B) Glutaminase and amino acid oxidases
(C) Glutamate dehydrogenase and transaminases
(D) Transaminase and glutaminase
(E) Glutamine synthetase and urease

125. Multiple mechanisms in the body maintain oxygen and carbon dioxide levels within a normal range. All of the following statements about those mechanisms are correct EXCEPT

(A) the aortic bodies are the primary sensors of decreases in arterial oxygen tension
(B) the Hering-Breuer reflex functions to terminate respiration and involves pulmonary stretch receptors and vagal afferents; however, this system is not important under normal resting conditions
(C) central chemoreceptors located on the ventral medullary surface are the major mediators of the response to hypercapnia
(D) during metabolic acidosis, peripheral chemoreceptors cause hyperventilation to compensate with a respiratory alkalosis
(E) a person who has an increased elastic load will attempt to compensate by taking small breaths at a high rate
(F) the responsiveness to ventilatory stimuli is reduced during sleep

126. The micrograph below is a portion of the liver biopsied from a 42-year-old man. The microscopic features seen are most likely due to

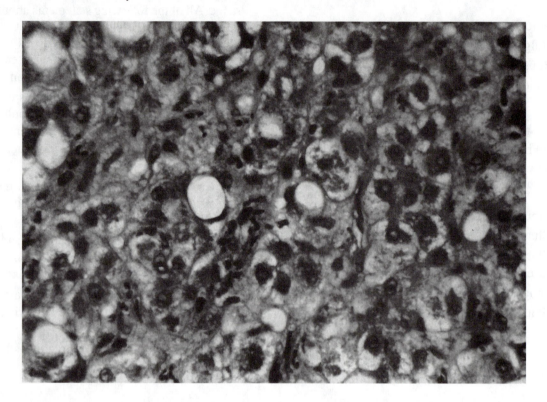

(A) exposure to carbon tetrachloride

(B) acetaminophen toxicity

(C) ethanol use

(D) acute rejection of a liver allograft

127. All of the following statements concerning the response of immunoglobulins to viruses in vivo are true EXCEPT that they

(A) displace attached viruses from the host cell

(B) inhibit the action of viral enzymes

(C) induce complement-mediated lysis of infected host cells

(D) retard the infectivity of viruses for host cells

128. Cholesterol biosynthesis occurs in the cytosol of many cells of the body, primarily in the liver, and entails all of the following steps EXCEPT that it

(A) forms lanosterol from squalene and then converts it to cholesterol
(B) requires reduced nicotinamide-adenine dinucleotide phosphate (NADPH) as a source of reducing equivalents
(C) forms 3-hydroxy-3-methylglutaryl coenzyme A (HMG CoA) from acetoacetyl CoA
(D) forms squalene from isoprenoid units
(E) uses HMG CoA reductase for catalysis of HMG CoA to mevinolin

129. Angiotensin-converting enzyme (ACE) hydrolyzes angiotensin I to angiotensin II. Possible explanations why inhibition of this enzyme with specific peptide inhibitors (i.e., captopril) reduces blood pressure in some subjects include all of the following EXCEPT

(A) decreased production of a vasoconstrictor (angiotensin II)
(B) increased synthesis and release of aldosterone
(C) centrally mediated decrease in water uptake
(D) inhibition of synaptic transmission in peripheral sympathetic nervous system

130. All of the following substances readily diffuse through cell membranes EXCEPT

(A) oxygen
(B) carbon dioxide
(C) glucose
(D) water
(E) nitrogen

131. A 43-year-old man complains of snoring, excessive daytime sleepiness, although he gets 8 hours of sleep per night and does not do any extreme physical activity. Polysomnography shows that he has an apnea index of 40 with a persistent effort to breathe. All of the following statements are true EXCEPT

(A) the patient meets the diagnostic criteria for obstructive sleep apnea syndrome
(B) the patient has an increased risk of myocardial infarction and stroke if he does not receive treatment for his sleep disorder
(C) a thyroid-stimulating hormone test to check for hypothyroidism could have been performed before the polysomnography
(D) weight loss and reduction of alcohol consumption may reduce the patient's symptoms
(E) the patient should sleep supine to reduce his symptoms
(F) surgical intervention (e.g., uvulopalatopharyngoplasty) should be considered if the patient is refractory to other treatment

132. A fecal specimen is cultured from a person with diarrhea, and *Shigella dysenteriae* and *Giardia lamblia* are isolated. All of the following statements about *Shigella* and *Giardia* are true EXCEPT

(A) *Shigella* has a peptidoglycan-containing cell wall but *G. lamblia* does not
(B) *Shigella* and *Giardia* both have DNA and RNA
(C) *Shigella* and *Giardia* both have sterol-containing plasma membranes
(D) *Shigella* has a lipopolysaccharide but *Giardia* does not
(E) *Shigella* has 70S ribosomes but *Giardia* has 80S ribosomes

133. All of the following statements about enzymes are true EXCEPT that

(A) V_{max} is a measure of catalytic efficiency
(B) K_m is a measure of the enzyme's affinity for the substrate
(C) formation of the substrate complex results in rearrangement of specific functional groups of the enzyme
(D) the reaction rate is accelerated by increasing the activation energy
(E) ionizable amino acid side chains are frequently used as general acids and bases in catalysis

134. Adult respiratory distress syndrome (ARDS) shows all of the following morphologic signs EXCEPT

(A) pulmonary edema
(B) hyaline membrane formation
(C) proliferation of type II pneumocytes
(D) alveolar wall damage
(E) decreased permeability of the pulmonary capillary endothelium

135. Type II pneumocytes have all of the following characteristics EXCEPT

(A) they elaborate pulmonary surfactant
(B) they exhibit surface microvilli
(C) they make up most of the alveolar surface area
(D) they contain osmiophilic lamellar bodies
(E) defects in these cells contribute to infant and adult respiratory distress

136. All of the following intracellular substances are second messengers in mammalian cells EXCEPT

(A) inositol 1,4,5-triphosphate (IP_3)
(B) cyclic adenosine monophosphate (cAMP)
(C) Ca^{2+}
(D) diacylglycerol (DAG)
(E) *c-fos*

137. Embolism of a cerebral artery most commonly occurs from all of the following situations EXCEPT

(A) atheromatous plaques of the vertebral artery
(B) atheromatous plaques of the internal carotid artery
(C) endocarditis of the mitral valve
(D) atheromatous plaques of the abdominal aorta

138. Which one of the following statements regarding pulmonary emboli is true?

(A) Pulmonary emboli can usually be diagnosed by the clinical presentation
(B) The most common source of pulmonary emboli is the internal jugular vein
(C) Risk factors for pulmonary emboli include indwelling catheters, sickle cell disease, and hypocoagulable states
(D) Pulmonary angiography is considered the "gold standard" test for the diagnosis of pulmonary emboli
(E) Pulmonary emboli lead to a decrease in pulmonary vascular resistance
(F) All pulmonary emboli share a characteristic abnormality on chest radiograph

139. All of the following statements about RNA are correct EXCEPT

(A) a messenger RNA (mRNA) molecule is translated once and is then degraded
(B) ribosomal RNA (rRNA) is formed by transcription of a family of repeated nuclear genes
(C) the ribosome, which is a complex of RNA and protein, is the site of protein synthesis
(D) three different RNA polymerase enzymes are required for sustained protein synthesis in human cells
(E) transfer RNA (tRNA) molecules contain an anticodon loop that pairs with the triplet codon of mRNA

140. All of the following statements about hormone receptors are true EXCEPT that they

(A) may elicit their biologic response without being fully saturated with hormone
(B) may be desensitized by phosphorylation
(C) determine the specificity of cellular responses to hormones
(D) are deficient in Addison's disease
(E) are frequently transmembrane proteins

141. All of the following statements concerning the subthalamus are true EXCEPT

(A) it contains the cranial ends of the nerve cells of the red nucleus
(B) it has important connections with the corpus striatum and, thus, is involved with voluntary muscle control
(C) it contains the cranial ends of the nerve cells of the substantia nigra
(D) it has important connections with the cerebellum and, thus, is involved with voluntary muscle control

Questions 142–146

(A) Ectoderm
(B) Mesoderm
(C) Endoderm
(D) Neuroectoderm

Match each of the following structures with its germ layer of origin.

142. Melanocytes

143. Adrenal cortex

144. Liver

145. Thyroid gland

146. Gonads

Questions 147–149

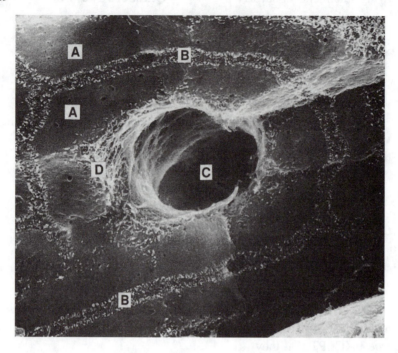

Match each description below with the appropriate lettered structure in the scanning electron micrograph of liver parenchymal tissue.

147. Receives blood from the portal vein and hepatic artery and drains blood into the central vein

148. A liver parenchymal cell

149. A bile canaliculus surrounded by tight junctions that form the blood–bile barrier

Questions 150–154

(A) Combined hyperlipidemia
(B) Hypertriglyceridemia
(C) Type III hyperlipoproteinemia
(D) Hypercholesterolemia
(E) Lipoprotein lipase deficiency

For each lipoprotein type listed below, select the genetic disorder that is most likely to be associated with it.

150. Chylomicrons

151. Low-density lipoproteins (LDL)

152. Chylomicron remnants and intermediate-density lipoproteins (IDL)

153. Very low-density lipoproteins (VLDL)

154. VLDL and chylomicrons

Questions 155–159

(A) Serotonin and catecholamines in the cerebral cortex
(B) γ-Aminobutyric acid (GABA) and glycine in the spinal cord
(C) Substance P in the dorsal horns
(D) Dopamine in the basal ganglia
(E) Serotonin in the spinal cord

Match each procedure or operation with the neurotransmitter that it would deplete.

155. Destruction of spinal interneurons (by controlled hypoxia)

156. Section of dorsal roots

157. Section of the medial forebrain bundle

158. Destruction of the substantia nigra

159. Destruction of the medullary raphe

Questions 160–163
(A) *ros*
(B) *erbB*
(C) *trk*
(D) *sis*
(E) *kit*
(F) *jun*

Oncogenesis, the production of tumors, occurs because of the loss of cellular signaling, which is frequently caused by a protein that functions as an uncontrolled growth factor receptor. Match the normal physiologic receptor with the oncogene that it most closely resembles functionally and structurally.

160. Insulin receptor

161. Nerve growth factor (NGF) receptor

162. Epidermal growth factor (EGF) receptor

163. Platelet-derived growth factor (PDGF) receptor

Questions 164–169

(A) *Treponema pallidum*
(B) *Treponema pertenue*
(C) *Treponema carateum*
(D) *Leptospira interrogans*
(E) *Borrelia recurrentis*

Match each disease below with its etiologic agent

164. Relapsing fever

165. Bejel

166. Pinta

167. Syphilis

168. Fort Bragg fever

169. Yaws

Questions 170–175

(A) S_1 louder than S_2
(B) S_2 louder than S_1
(C) Aortic valvular ejection sound
(D) Pulmonic valvular ejection sound

The first heart sound (S_1) is composed of sounds from tricuspid and mitral valve closure. The second heart sound (S_2) is the sound of the aortic and pulmonic valves closing. For each cardiovascular abnormality listed below, select the heart sounds with which it is most likely to be associated.

170. Mitral valve stenosis

171. Aortic stenosis

172. Acute aortic regurgitation

173. Severe hypertension

174. Anemia

175. Hyperthyroidism

Questions 176–179

(A) Onion-skin thickening of the arterioles
(B) Tophus
(C) Human leukocyte antigen DR4 (HLA-DR4)
(D) Heberden's nodes

Match the forms of joint disease listed below with the characteristic typically associated with it.

176. Rheumatoid arthritis

177. Osteoarthritis

178. Lyme arthritis

179. Gouty arthritis

180. All of the following statements about local potentials are true EXCEPT

(A) voltage-gated sodium- and potassium-ion channels are involved
(B) the duration is variable (5 seconds to several minutes)
(C) its form is a graded response
(D) its propagation is passive with local decay
(E) the amplitude is small (0.1–10 mv)

ANSWER KEY

1-C	31-C	61-B	91-B	121-C
2-D	32-D	62-B	92-A	122-D
3-B	33-C	63-D	93-C	123-A
4-D	34-E	64-A	94-D	124-C
5-D	35-E	65-C	95-B	125-A
6-C	36-D	66-E	96-E	126-C
7-A	37-B	67-D	97-D	127-A
8-D	38-C	68-C	98-C	128-E
9-C	39-A	69-C	99-B	129-B
10-B	40-B	70-C	100-C	130-C
11-C	41-E	71-C	101-C	131-E
12-B	42-A	72-C	102-D	132-C
13-A	43-C	73-A	103-A	133-D
14-C	44-E	74-B	104-D	134-E
15-B	45-B	75-C	105-C	135-C
16-C	46-B	76-C	106-C	136-E
17-A	47-B	77-B	107-D	137-D
18-D	48-D	78-B	108-A	138-D
19-B	49-D	79-B	109-C	139-A
20-D	50-D	80-E	110-D	140-D
21-D	51-A	81-B	111-A	141-D
22-D	52-C	82-E	112-C	142-D
23-A	53-E	83-A	113-B	143-B
24-D	54-D	84-C	114-B	144-C
25-D	55-E	85-C	115-C	145-C
26-A	56-B	86-B	116-B	146-B
27-E	57-C	87-A	117-A	147-C
28-D	58-C	88-D	118-E	148-A
29-C	59-C	89-B	119-D	149-B
30-C	60-C	90-A	120-A	150-E

151-D	157-A	163-E	169-B	175-A
152-C	158-D	164-E	170-A	176-C
153-B	159-E	165-A	171-C	177-D
154-A	160-A	166-C	172-B	178-A
155-B	161-C	167-A	173-B	179-B
156-C	162-B	168-D	174-A	180-A

ANSWERS AND EXPLANATIONS

1–3. The answers are: 1-C, 2-D, 3-B. *(Genetics; Duchenne muscular dystrophy)*
Duchenne muscular dystrophy (DMD), or childhood muscular dystrophy, classically occurs only in boys with a pattern of X-linked inheritance. This pattern can be deduced from the pedigree that accompanies the question because all of the affected individuals are males, the mothers and fathers are not affected, and the affected males are on the maternal side of the family.

In X-linked diseases, mothers are always carriers because the mutant gene is on the X chromosome. The male child either receives the X chromosome with the mutant gene and gets the disease or receives a normal X chromosome and does not get the disease. Males cannot be carriers of X-linked disorders. A female carrier has a 50% chance of giving her chromosome that bears the mutant gene to each of her children.

4. The answer is D. *(Cell biology; cell cycle)*
The cyclin B–cdc2 complex controls entry into mitosis. During the S phase, cyclin B is synthesized, reaching its maximal levels at G_2 phase of the cell cycle when the majority of cyclin B binds cdc2. The cyclin B–cdc2 complex is then phosphorylated and dephosphorylated in a complex series of events to reach activation and drive the cell into mitosis. The threonine 161 residue must be phosphorylated, and the tyrosine 14 and threonine 15 residue must be dephosphorylated for cyclin B–cdc2 activation. The cyclin B–cdc2 complex is deactivated at the end of mitosis by the destruction of the cyclin B of the complex. The cyclin B–cdc2 complex has no role in the G_1 phase of the cell cycle.

5. The answer is D. *(Physiology; chronic bronchitis)*
The symptoms presented in this case are typical of chronic bronchitis. The age and smoking history make α_1-antitrypsin deficiency unlikely, as this person would have presented these symptoms sooner. His obesity, productive cough, and cyanosis are more typical of chronic bronchitis than emphysema. Both of these diseases are obstructive rather than restrictive; therefore, one would expect a low forced expiratory volume in 1 second (FEV_1) and a low FEV_1/forced vital capacity (FVC) ratio. In addition, the hemoglobin and hematocrit levels in patients with chronic bronchitis are often elevated in an attempt to compensate for the chronic hypoxia due to hypoventilation. Smoking is by far the most important risk factor for this condition.

6. The answer is C. *(Histopathology; Kaposi's sarcoma)*
Kaposi's sarcoma was initially described as a cutaneous hemorrhagic nodule usually occurring on the lower extremities of elderly men. Kaposi's sarcoma is now recognized as being associated with human immunodeficiency virus (HIV) infection and afflicting primarily men with the virus. It is recognized histologically by irregular fascicles of spindle cells in the dermis, which are accompanied by extravasated erythrocytes that impart a purple color. Kaposi's sarcoma is believed to be derived from endothelial cells, perhaps lymphatic endothelium. Unlike angiosarcomas, it does not form anastomosing vascular channels.

7. The answer is A. *(Neurobiology; referred pain)*
Referred pain is not well understood. Somatic referred pain is very well localized and intense. Visceral referred pain is the opposite and is thought to be conveyed by autonomic fibers. Diaphragmatic pain is usually referred to the shoulder.

8–10. The answers are: 8-D, 9-C, 10-B. *(Behavioral science, pharmacology; epilepsy)*
Major depression is the first diagnosis to consider because, in the case presented in the question, the subacute time course, self-neglect, social withdrawal, and psychotic symptoms indicate a possible depression. Major depression, even depression associated with psychotic symptoms, is treatable and has a good prognosis. There is no mention of drug abuse to suggest phencyclidine psychosis and no euphoria or increased sociability to suggest mania. The time during which symptoms have occurred has not been long enough to suggest schizophrenia or schizoaffective disorder.

The symptoms listed in the questions suggest complex partial seizures of the temporal lobe. Considering the psychotic symptoms and social withdrawal, epilepsy with schizophreniform interictal disorder might also be considered. The evoked potentials and the projective or cognitive tests would not be helpful.

Carbamazepine is the preferred treatment for complex partial seizures. The antipsychotic drug haloperidol should be added only if the psychotic symptoms do not respond to the antiepileptic agent. Haloperidol and the antidepressant imipramine lower the seizure threshold. The antipanic drug alprazolam is not indicated, although some other types of benzodiazepines are used as antiepileptics.

11. The answer is C. *(Immunology; inflammation and cellular margination)*
As the vascular phase of the inflammatory response progresses, neutrophils and monocytes move toward the periphery of the microcirculatory vessels (a process referred to as margination) and adhere to, or pavement, the vascular endothelium in preparation for migration into the extravascular space. To migrate, leukocytes develop pseudopods and move, without accompanying loss of fluid, through gaps between the endothelial cells—a process termed diapedesis. In the latter part of the vascular phase, increased vascular permeability causes loss of plasma with resultant venous stasis and, eventually, clotting in the small capillaries local to the inflamed area.

12. The answer is B. *(Cell biology; hormone receptors)*
The cytosol would contain the most fluorescence. Glucocorticoid receptors are soluble receptors and are not associated with the plasma membrane. Glucocorticoids diffuse into cells, bind to receptors in the cytosol, and then translocate to the nucleus. Inside the nucleus this hormone-receptor complex regulates transcription via binding to specific sequences of DNA.

13. The answer is A. *(Histopathology; temporal arteritis)*
Temporal (giant cell) arteritis may be one component of the syndrome of polymyalgia rheumatica. Patients present with headache, tenderness over the temporal artery, visual loss (if retinal vessels are affected), and facial pain. Histologically, a granulomatous reaction is seen within the vessel wall associated with a mixed neutrophilic and lymphocytic infiltrate. Giant cells appear to phagocytize portions of elastica, and the vessel may be thrombosed in its late stage (*right*). Clinical response to steroids is excellent. Mönckeberg's arteriosclerosis shows medial calcification of arteries and is not an arteritis, whereas Takayasu's arteritis ("pulseless disease") involves the aortic arch and its major branches.

14. The answer is C. *(Pharmacology; asthma)*
Cromolyn sodium inhibits degranulation of mast cells and, in other poorly understood ways, interferes with the inflammatory process now assumed to be critical to moderate asthma caused by a variety of allergens and other conditions. Cromolyn is not absorbed from the gut and must be administered topically to the lung where it acts prophylactically to inhibit bronchospasm caused by inhaled allergens, exercise, or altered environmental conditions. It does not directly relax bronchial smooth muscle in vivo or in vitro and, thus, is of little use in acute emergencies of bronchial hyperreactivity. However, prophylactically, it will reduce the bronchial response to a number of spasmogens.

15. The answer is B. *(Physiology; transudates and exudates)*
When performing a thoracentesis, differentiation between transudates and exudates should always be an initial part of the analysis. To do this task, the protein and lactate dehydrogenase (LDH) levels of the pleural fluid and serum must be determined. If either the protein or LDH levels of the pleural fluid or either of their ratios to the serum levels are elevated, then the fluid should be classified as an exudate. All of these values should be normal in the setting of a transudate. Low glucose levels and low pH are typical of parapneumonic effusions and may indicate empyema or a grossly purulent effusion. This type of effusion with an infectious

cause requires drainage with a chest tube because it may progress rapidly to become loculated. The appearance of blood in pleural fluid is an indication for checking the hematocrit of the fluid to determine if there is a hemothorax. Elevated amylase in pleural effusion is frequently caused by either pancreatic disease or esophageal varices, so the patient should be evaluated for these complications. Elevated triglycerides are suggestive of chylothorax if they are moderately elevated (50–110 mg/dl) and diagnostic if they are greater than 110 mg/dl. Lipoprotein electrophoresis is useful in the setting of a moderate elevation of triglycerides to determine the contribution of chylomicrons.

16–18. The answers are: 16-C, 17-A, 18-D. *(Pathology; pharmacology; peptic ulcer disease)*
A number of physiologic, genetic, and other factors increase the risk of gastric (and duodenal) peptic ulcers. The evidence that *H. pylori* plays a principle role is compelling. Smoking and caffeine are known to adversely affect the morbidity, mortality, and healing rates of peptic ulcers. In general, first-degree relatives of peptic ulcer patients as well as males have a threefold to fourfold increased risk of developing this disorder. Paradoxically, in gastric ulcer disease, acid secretion is not elevated. It is possible that excess secreted hydrogen ion is reabsorbed across the injured gastric mucosa. In general, a defect in gastric mucosal defense is the more important local physiologic factor promoting ulceration at this site.

In the patient described in the question, direct visualization identified a duodenal ulcer, a very common cause of right upper quadrant pain and melena. Denudation of the mucosal epithelium is the hallmark of histologic changes in peptic ulcer disease and, in duodenal ulcer, is often accompanied by hypertrophy of submucosal Brunner's glands (mucus-secreting glands).

The agents of choice for duodenal ulcer include antimicrobial agents, such as amoxicillin, tetracycline, and clarithromycin and histamine (H_2) antagonists, including ranitidine and cimetidine. Other useful agents, alone or in combination with anti–*H. pylori* agents and H_2 antagonists, include anticholinergic drugs, "proton pump" inhibitors (benzimidazoles), antacids, and cytoprotective analogues of prostaglandins E_1, E_2, and prostacyclin.

19. The answer is B. *(Pathology; tumor)*
In most human cancers, the stage of the disease, not the age of the patient, is the most important prognostic factor. Stage refers to the extent, or degree of spread, of the disease in the patient (i.e., localized, regional, or distant). Tumor grade (i.e., differentiation), mitotic count, and extent of invasion correlate with the stage of the tumor, in that high-grade (i.e., less differentiated) tumors and highly invasive tumors tend to be high-stage lesions.

20. The answer is D. *(Physiology; growth hormone)*
Growth hormone stimulates cartilage and bone growth via somatomedin, an intermediary peptide. It is secreted periodically, like many other pituitary hormones, and is affected in a negative fashion by somatostatin, a hypothalamic peptide. Unlike other anterior pituitary hormones, cellular targets for growth hormone are relatively ubiquitous. Somatomedin, synthesized in the liver and possibly other sites (e.g., muscle), is an important mediator of the growth effects of the hormone on cartilage and bone. Indeed, growth hormone has no direct effects on these cells by itself. Growth hormone has a large array of effects on amino acid, fat, and carbohydrate activities and, in general, displays anti–insulin-like actions.

21. The answer is D. *(Microbiology; pneumocystis pneumonia)*
Pneumocystis pneumonia is caused by *Pneumocystis carinii*, a microorganism of uncertain classification that belongs to either the protozoa or fungi. It forms four to seven microcysts within a frothy honeycomb-like alveolar exudate in the air spaces. These cysts contain numerous sporozoites, which are released from the cysts at maturation. Pneumocystis pneumonia is commonly seen in individuals infected with human immunodeficiency virus (HIV), a condition that would be suspected in an individual with a history of intravenous drug abuse.

22. The answer is D. *(Histopathology; Hodgkin's disease)*
The photomicrograph of the woman's biopsy shows classic features of nodular-sclerosing Hodgkin's disease. The node is divided into irregular nodules by broad bands of dense collagen (*left*). In the panel on the *right*, the nodal infiltrate is composed of lymphocytes, plasma cells, eosinophils, and multilobated cells with prominent red nucleoli, called Reed-Sternberg cells. Although Reed-Sternberg cells are not pathognomonic of this disease, they are diagnostic when seen in this appropriate inflammatory milieu. The nodular sclerosis type of Hodgkin's disease usually presents with a large mediastinal mass and involvement of adjacent lymph node groups (e.g., supraclavicular nodes).

23. The answer is A. *(Physiology; Na$^+$ transport and renal epithelial physiology)*
Na$^+$ is transported from the tubular lumen to the peritubular capillary by an electrochemical gradient that is largely generated by the action of the Na$^+$, K$^+$-ATPase activity at the basolateral surface. The cell is freely permeable to water and chloride, thereby reabsorbing a virtually isosmotic fraction of tubular luminal fluid. The attraction of Na$^+$ creates a very large intracellular negative potential (approximately -70 mV). There is no significant hormone dependence of ion transport in these cells on either aldosterone or antidiuretic hormone (ADH).

24. The answer is D. *(Anatomy; thoracic outlet syndrome)*
Thoracic outlet syndrome describes compression of the lower trunk of the brachial plexus and the subclavian artery by an anomalous thirteenth (cervical) rib. Sensory changes occur over the distribution of the ulnar nerve; the phrenic nerves are not involved.

25. The answer is D. *(Biochemistry; gluconeogenesis and glycolysis)*
Stimulation of beta cells by glucose results in the release of insulin. Insulin has numerous effects on virtually every tissue, and its overall effect is the conservation of body fuel supplies. It does this by promoting the uptake and storage of glucose, amino acids, and fats. In the liver, it decreases gluconeogenesis and glycogenolysis and promotes glycolysis. In addition, it promotes lipogenesis in the liver and fat cells and is antilipolytic. It is also an important anabolic protein hormone while simultaneously inhibiting the breakdown of amino acids. It inhibits the release of glucagon from neighboring alpha cells.

26–27. The answers are: 26-A, 27-E. *(Immunology; multiple myeloma; immunoglobulin abnormalities)*
Well-demarcated or "punched out" osteolytic lesions are almost pathognomonic for multiple myeloma. In 99% of the patients with multiple myeloma, electrophoretic analysis of the serum proteins shows an increase in one of the immunoglobulin classes or light chains, approximately 23,000 daltons (Bence Jones protein), in the urine. The presence of 55,000-dalton monoclonal proteins is indicative of heavy-chain disease, a different type of monoclonal gammopathy that is not associated with osteolytic lesions. Although not specific for this disease, patients with multiple myeloma do suffer from a suppression of synthesis of normal antibodies and are, thus, susceptible to recurrent bacterial and viral infections.

In approximately 55% of people diagnosed with multiple myeloma, the membrane-bound protein (M protein) is immunoglobulin G (IgG), and in 25%, the M protein is IgA and rarely IgM, IgD, or IgE. In the remaining 20%, Bence Jones proteinuria without the serum M protein is seen.

28. The answer is D. *(Pharmacology; aminoglycosides; therapeutic index)*
Aminoglycosides can cause severe nephrotoxicity and ototoxicity. Their therapeutic index is low; peak and trough levels are commonly monitored to allow for dose adjustments or a change in timing of administration. Aminoglycosides are eliminated rapidly with a serum half-life of 1–5 hours. However, rapid clearance is not the major determinant for therapeutic monitoring. Aminoglycosides are not extensively metabolized. Because they are polar molecules, they are lipid insoluble and do not cross the blood–brain barrier. The incidence of hypersensitivity reactions is extremely low.

29. The answer is C. *(Pharmacology; neoplasia and hormone action)*
Tamoxifen has become the drug of choice for the initial endocrine management of breast cancer as well as a useful adjuvant therapy for the palliative management of advanced breast cancer. It is relatively nontoxic, and patients with breast tumors containing estrogen receptors are most likely to respond to the drug. The drug binds to the estrogen receptor in the nucleus but does not stimulate transcription. The tamoxifen–estrogen receptor complex does not readily dissociate, thereby affecting estrogen receptor recycling. In premenopausal women, competition with estrogen receptors in the anterior pituitary and hypothalamus disrupts normal feedback inhibition of gonadotropin-releasing hormone, thereby enhancing gonadotropin release.

30. The answer is C. *(Pharmacology; angina therapy)*
Nitroglycerin (glyceryl trinitrate; GTN) is most effective by decreasing preload in angina. At high concentrations, some benefit in angina is obtained from GTN by reducing afterload. However, this latter effect is often accompanied by reflex tachycardia that may disrupt the improvement in myocardial oxygen consumption and supply achieved by GTN. Propranolol is useful in blocking this reflex effect because it is negatively inotropic and negatively chronotropic. Propranolol may be accompanied by coronary artery vasospasm after removing β-receptor–mediated dilation and leaving unopposed a coronary artery α-receptor–mediated vasoconstriction.

31. The answer is C. *(Pharmacology; antiepileptics)*
Phenytoin decreases resting Na^+ flux as well as the flow of Na^+ currents during chemical depolarization or action potential. In the central nervous system (CNS), this results in depression of the generation and transmission of repetitive action potentials in epileptic foci. It is usually the drug of choice for all seizures except absence seizures and, in general, is started alone to assess its efficacy. Phenytoin is associated with potential teratogenic effects (fetal hydantoin syndrome). Other agents like diazepam or phenobarbital affect chloride channels by interacting with γ-aminobutyric acid (GABA) at its receptor site.

32. The answer is D. *(Biochemistry; RNA synthesis)*
RNA polymerase I produces ribosomal RNA (rRNA). RNA polymerase II produces mostly messenger RNA (mRNA). RNA polymerase III makes transfer RNA (tRNA) and other small RNAs. The reason that mammalian cells use three different types of RNA polymerases is not known.

33. The answer is C. *(Pharmacology; toxicology and aplastic anemia)*
Benzene is associated with the induction of aplastic anemia by damaging myeloid stem cells. Thiouracil is associated with agranulocytosis, primarily because of its ability to decrease production or increase destruction of neutrophils. Penicillin acts as a hapten, which produces erythrocyte destruction via warm antibody autoimmune hemolysis. In contrast, methyldopa stimulates the production of antibodies against intrinsic red blood cell antigens. Ingestion of an excessive quantity of acetaminophen is followed by the production of toxic metabolites, which first decrease hepatic glutathione levels and then cause a centrilobular necrosis due to biomolecular adduct formation.

34. The answer is E. *(Immunology; monoclonal antibodies and gram-negative bacteria)*
A monoclonal antibody, such as immunoglobulin G (IgG), would be useful only against organisms producing lipopolysaccharide, namely gram-negative bacteria. The organism would have to produce a disease state through bacteremia since IgG would only be present in the circulatory system. Organisms such as *Bordetella pertussis*, the causative agent of whooping cough, and *Vibrio cholerae*, the agent of cholera, are gram-negative but do not invade the bloodstream. Pulmonary anthrax is caused by *Bacillus anthracis*, which is a gram-positive organism. Leprosy is caused by *Mycobacterium leprae*, which is acid-fast, not gram-negative. Bubonic plague, however, is caused by *Yersinia pestis*, a gram-negative organism that multiplies in the bloodstream, spreading through to the lymphatics. *Y. pestis* has many virulence factors, including lipopolysaccharide.

35. The answer is E. *(Pharmacology; mechanism of action of penicillin)*
The principles of antibiotic action are perhaps best exemplified by penicillin. Antibiotics act by specifically binding to macromolecules only found in the parasite. Transpeptidase is the only penicillin-binding protein listed; it is inactivated when binding occurs.

36. The answer is D. *(Immunology; passive immunity; vaccination)*
The most appropriate treatment for the medical student described in the question would be an injection of tetanus toxoid, which would trigger an anamnestic response because of the DTP (diphtheria-tetanus-pertussis) administration in childhood. If there is no history of DTP immunization, passive immunity can be induced by the administration of heterologous (e.g., equine) or homologous (i.e., human) antibodies. Type I and type III reactions can result from heterologous administration. Aminoglycosides are given for infections caused by gram-negative bacteria. The tetanus toxoid is produced by *Clostridium tetani*, a gram-positive rod.

37. The answer is B. *(Pharmacology; adverse effects of aspirin)*
The major adverse effect of aspirin is gastrointestinal bleeding. Inhibition of local cytoprotective arachidonic acid metabolites (prostaglandin E_2 and prostacyclin) in the gastric mucosa contributes to this adverse effect and can be offset by simultaneously using exogenous synthetic prostanoids. In addition, aspirin has a direct irritating effect on the mucosa. Nonsteroidal anti-inflammatory agents in general have little effect on lipoxygenase activity but do affect cyclooxygenase. In particular, aspirin is an irreversible inhibitor of this enzyme in platelets (and other cell types) by acetylating the α-amino group of the terminal serine. This irreversible inhibition has significant implications in that platelet function will not be restored to normal until a new enzyme has been synthesized. Aspirin has little effect on normal body temperature but reduces abnormally elevated body temperatures secondary to alterations in central thermoregulation.

38. The answer is C. *(Biochemistry; RNA splicing)*
The splicing reaction takes place in the nucleus of the cell before capping and polyadenylation as part of the post-transcriptional modification of eukaryotic RNA. U1 small nuclear ribonucleoprotein (snRNP) recognizes a 9 base-pair region of the introns involved and is thought to precipitate the organized formation of the large particle termed the spliceosome on the RNA. The splicing reaction then cuts the intron at the 5' end and forms a "lariat" structure by covalently binding the cut 5' end of the intron to a sequence on the 3' end. The intron is then cut again at the 3' end and thus is cut out of the RNA.

39. The answer is A. *(Pathology; carcinoid of the appendix)*
The most common tumor of the appendix is a carcinoid tumor. The neoplastic cells show neuroendocrine differentiation. The cells grow in nests and are associated with a delicate, branching vascular network. The nuclei of the cells have a "salt and pepper" chromatin distribution. Typically, the cytoplasm of the cells contains granules, which are visible by special stains. Silver salts turn the granules black; thus, they are argyrophilic. The behavior of these tumors is related to their depth of invasion into the muscular wall and serosal adipose tissue.

40. The answer is B. *(Biochemistry; nitrogen metabolism)*
Negative nitrogen balance would result from defective cholecystokinin–pancreozymin (CCK–PZ) production when the consumption of dietary protein is normal. Negative nitrogen balance occurs when the excretion of nitrogen exceeds the intake of nitrogen. A number of conditions can cause a negative nitrogen balance, including a deficiency in any one of the essential amino acids or a defect in the intestinal phase of protein digestion and absorption. CCK–PZ is essential for stimulating the secretion of inactive pancreatic zymogens, which become active proteases in the small intestine. The intestinal phase of digestion is essential to maintain-

ing nitrogen balance; the gastric phase appears to have little, if any, impact. For example, gastric resection can be performed without affecting nitrogen balance. In phenylketonuria (PKU), tyrosine becomes an essential amino acid and must be supplied in the diet.

41. The answer is E. *(Biochemistry; protein synthesis)*
The synthetic polynucleotide sequence of CAACAACAACAA ... could be read by the in vitro protein synthesizing system starting at the first C, the first A, or the second A. In the first case, the first triplet codon would be CAA, which codes for glutamine. In the second case, the first triplet codon would be AAC, which codes for asparagine; and in the last case, the first triplet codon would be ACA, which codes for threonine.

42–43. The answers are: 42-A, 43-C. *(Biostatistics; continuous variables; null hypothesis)*
The variables described in the question are continuous in that their values are along a continuum as are age and IQ, as opposed to being categorical. Categorical variables, such as sex, race, and marital status, require the use of nonparametric statistical tests, such as the chi-squared test.

A null hypothesis is the hypothesis that an observed difference is due to chance alone and not to a systematic cause. In the study question, the null hypothesis is that there is no relationship between temperature and body weight. The study is designed to disprove the null hypothesis. The null hypothesis does not involve a P value, although a cutoff is generally chosen to show the likelihood that an association between variables is not due to chance alone (i.e., $P = 0.05$ means that there is a 5% probability that the two events or measurements are similar due to chance alone).

44. The answer is E. *(Microbiology; bacterial pigment production)*
Pseudomonas aeruginosa, *Staphylococcus aureus*, and *Serratia marcescens* are all pigment producers. Pigment production by bacteria is associated with both gram-positive and gram-negative organisms. *P. aeruginosa* and *S. marcescens* produce endotoxins, and only *S. aureus* produces enterotoxin and lipoteichoic acids. None of the organisms listed produce mycolic acids.

45. The answer is B. *(Microbiology; mycobacteria)*
Mycobacterium tuberculosis produces factors such as sulfatides, which inhibit the fusion of phagosomes with lysosomes. In addition to inhibiting phagosome–lysosome fusion, *M. tuberculosis* escapes engulfment by lysosomes. The organisms are also resistant to phagocytic killing because of their tough cell surface.

46. The answer is B. *(Pharmacology; antimuscarinic agents)*
Atropine may abolish the parasympathetic input that normally maintains a relatively slow heart rate. Indeed, atropine is often used intraoperatively (and in emergencies) to increase heart rate. Atropine inhibits secretions from salivary, lacrimal, bronchial, and sweat glands. It causes mydriasis and cycloplegia. It has no effect on skeletal muscle in which neuromuscular transmission involves acetylcholine (ACh) and nicotinic, not muscarinic, receptors.

47. The answer is B. *(Cell biology; G proteins and signal transduction)*
Guanosine triphosphate (GTP)–binding proteins (G proteins) are involved with the process of signal transduction and are the target of toxins, such as pertussis and cholera toxins. G proteins are activated when bound to GTP and deactivate via the hydrolysis of GTP to form guanosine diphosphate (GDP).

48. The answer is D. *(Pathology; bronchioloalveolar carcinoma)*
Bronchioloalveolar carcinomas are well-differentiated adenocarcinomas, which grow in a nondestructive fashion over the matrix of the alveolar septa, replacing normal pneumocytes. This pattern has been called lepidic growth. Bronchioloalveolar carcinomas also have a propensity for aerogenous and lymphatic spread, and widespread intrapulmonary metastases may occur.

49. The answer is D. *(Pathology; therapeutic effects in neoplasia)*
Paradoxically, patients with histologically "unfavorable" high-grade lymphomas show long-term survival if a complete clinical remission can be attained. However, it is rare to attain cure in histologically low-grade "favorable" non-Hodgkin's lymphomas: Patients die gradually from bone marrow compromise or lymphoma over many years. Long-term survival after 5 years for diffuse large cell lymphomas is roughly 50%. Those who do not attain complete remission usually die within several years. Spontaneous remissions are rarely seen in aggressive lymphomas.

50–53. The answers are: 50-D, 51-A, 52-C, 53-E. *(Pathology, pharmacology, pathophysiology; diabetes mellitus)*
The beta cells of the islets of Langerhans are the major site of insulin production in the pancreas. In insulin-dependent diabetes mellitus (IDDM), these cells are affected by genetic, autoimmune, viral, or other environmental factors so that they produce inadequate or no insulin.

Patients with type I IDDM are often started on daily injections of an intermediate-acting insulin preparation. Oral hypoglycemic agents such as glipizide are contraindicated in this group. Although abstinence from carbohydrates was initially thought appropriate, dietary manipulations now generally involve maintaining a complex carbohydrate diet with an emphasis on minimizing the intake of fats, especially saturated fats. Exercise normalizes peripheral tissue sensitivity to exogenous insulin.

Alpha cells of the endocrine pancreas secrete glucagon, which increases blood glucose by increasing glycogenolysis and gluconeogenesis in the liver. Growth hormone (GH) opposes the action of insulin by interfering with the body's ability to use glucose. Somatostatin suppresses glucagon secretion and, therefore, tends to decrease blood glucose.

Despite control of blood glucose levels with exogenous insulin, diet, and exercise in patients with IDDM, chronic changes in the microcirculation (especially in the kidney and eye) and macrocirculation (e.g., atherosclerosis) frequently occur. In addition, peripheral polyneuropathy is the most common diabetic neuropathy noted and appears to be associated with accumulation of sorbitol within Schwann cells. Currently, there is no association of IDDM and pulmonary hypertension.

54. The answer is D. *(Physiology; surfactant)*
Surfactant is a mixture of approximately 90% lipids (about half being dipalmitoyl phosphatidylcholine) and approximately 10% proteins. It increases pulmonary compliance by decreasing alveolar surface tension. Surfactant is synthesized by the alveolar type II epithelial cells. Reduced or excessive production by these cells can lead to conditions such as respiratory distress syndrome (RDS) of the newborn and pulmonary alveolar proteinosis, respectively. Decreases in surfactant production are involved in the pathogenesis of adult respiratory distress syndrome (ARDS). Surfactant is secreted in a multilamellar form, and then it transforms into a lattice-like tubular myelin on top of which forms a lipid monolayer. The dipalmitoyl phosphatidylcholine within this monolayer is oriented so that the hydrophobic tails point toward the air-filled alveoli. Surfactant replacement therapy is available and currently recommended in both neonatal RDS and prophylactically in premature infants that are at high risk of having RDS.

55. The answer is E. *(Pharmacology; characteristics of volatile anesthetics)*
Halothane and methoxyflurane are typical inhalational drugs, which tend to depress both the cardiovascular and respiratory systems. Methoxyflurane is more potent (i.e., it has a lower minimal alveolar concentration) than halothane, as predicted from its higher oil:gas partition coefficient. Both result in considerably slower induction than nitrous oxide because their respective blood:gas partition coefficients are greater than that of nitrous oxide. Similarly, recovery from methoxyflurane is slower than that from halothane because its oil:gas partition coefficient is greater than that of halothane. An increase in ventilatory rate will make the onset of anesthesia more rapid for all inhalational anesthetics.

56. The answer is B. *(Cell biology; DNA and restriction enzymes)*
Restriction enzymes recognize specific base sequences in double-helical DNA and cleave both strands of the duplex at specific sites. Most of the cleavage sites contain a twofold rotational symmetry (the recognized sequence is palindromic). The cuts resulting from these enzymes may be either staggered or blunt. Restriction enzymes can cleave DNA molecules into a number of specific fragments. These enzymes are specific for DNA; they do not cleave RNA.

57. The answer is C. *(Behavioral science; physician–patient interactions)*
Regular, structured visits by the nurses can help to reassure a dependent and frightened patient and keep the nurses from feeling resentful. The patient's disease and disability have made him feel angry and out of control, and he is acting out his feelings by bothering the nurses. Punitive actions and indirect warfare with the patient will not remedy the situation.

58. The answer is C. *(Behavioral science; suicide risk)*
Elderly men have the highest suicide rate of any group, especially with the additional risk factors of widower-hood, alcohol abuse, chronic medical problems, and living alone. Although renal insufficiency, silent myocardial infarction, peripheral neuropathy, and pneumonia are valid concerns, suicide has the highest lethal potential and need for active monitoring.

59. The answer is C. *(Pharmacology; antibiotic action)*
Chloramphenicol is bacteriostatic and, therefore, was responsible for the leveling off of *curve A*. All of the agents listed, except chloramphenicol, are bactericidal. Cephalothin, methicillin, and vancomycin all interfere with cell wall synthesis, leading to bursting and to cell death. Polymyxin affects cell membrane function, causing irreversible loss of small molecules from the cell. Chloramphenicol inhibits protein synthesis and is bacteriostatic. Therefore, the cell number in the culture with chloramphenicol does not decrease, and the organisms are viable. Removal of chloramphenicol will result in growth.

60. The answer is C. *(Physiology; acid–base balance)*
According to the Henderson-Hasselbalch equation, the patient's pH is approximately 7.4 (normal), and his Pco_2 and $[HCO_3^-]$ are elevated. The elevation in Pco_2 (respiratory acidosis) has been compensated (i.e., normal pH) by a rise in $[HCO_3^-]$. This latter phenomenon is brought about by the kidneys excreting more acid and reabsorbing more HCO_3^-. Full compensation as in this example is most likely to be associated with chronic perturbations in acid–base balance. Such changes may be common in chronic obstructive pulmonary disease (COPD).

61. The answer is B. *(Physiology; Na^+ transport; adenosine triphosphate production)*
The ability of erythrocytes to pump Na^+ from the cytoplasm depends on a source of adenosine triphosphate (ATP). All of the erythrocyte's ATP is generated by glycolysis. The compound 1,3-diphosphoglycerate is a high-energy glycolytic intermediate that is converted to 3-phosphoglycerate with the concomitant phosphorylation of adenosine diphosphate (ADP) to ATP. This reaction is catalyzed by phosphoglycerate kinase. Pyruvate carboxylase and glucose 6-phosphatase are gluconeogenic enzymes and are not present in the erythrocyte. Malate dehydrogenase is a mitochondrial enzyme and is not present in the erythrocyte. Stearoyl coenzyme A (CoA) desaturase is an enzyme in β-oxidation and is not present in the erythrocyte.

62. The answer is B. *(Biostatistics; paired t-test)*
A paired t-test allows a comparison of mean K^+ values before and after treatment by comparing each patient's initial serum level with his or her repeat value.

63–64. The answers are: 63-D, 64-A. *(Microbiology; differential diagnosis of infectious mononucleosis)*
This patient presents with the classic picture of infectious mononucleosis caused by Epstein-Barr virus (EBV) infection. Extreme fatigue, difficulty concentrating, and fever are generalized systemic symptoms. Pharyngitis reflects the local immunologic response by T cells reactive against viral antigens on infected tonsillar B cells. Splenomegaly is also a consequence of immunologic response to EBV. Morphologic examination of lymphocytosis in the peripheral blood should reveal atypical lymphocytes, which are activated T cells with increased cytoplasm and less mature nuclear chromatin. Lymphocytes of infectious lymphocytosis and pertussis are morphologically normal, albeit increased in number; also pertussis is a disease of young children. Serum from this patient should yield a positive test for heterophile antibodies. The combination of pharyngitis and lymphadenopathy is characteristic of EBV-associated mononucleosis. Cytomegalovirus (CMV) mononucleosis lacks both of these features. Toxoplasmosis, a rare cause of mononucleosis, may have lymphadenopathy but not pharyngitis.

A not uncommon feature of infectious mononucleosis with EBV-mediated expansion of B cells is the development of antibodies to red cells, usually directed against the Ii antigen system. Most such antibodies are cold agglutinins; that is, they react with erythrocytes at temperatures less than 37°C. Cold agglutinins are usually of the immunoglobulin M (IgM) class, and a Coombs' test may or may not be positive. The virus-associated hemophagocytic syndrome has been seen in patients with EBV infections, although usually in immunocompromised patients. Direct infection of erythroid precursors is not a feature of EBV infection. Disseminated intravascular coagulation is a rare occurrence in infectious mononucleosis, and thrombocytopenia may cause petechiae but not hemorrhagic blood loss.

65. The answer is C. *(Microbiology; replication cycle of viruses)*
During the eclipse phase, it is impossible to recover the virus particles from infected cells. The eclipse phase of the virus replication cycle is the final stage of adsorption (during which the virus invades the cell, multiplies, kills, and lyses the cell) and the process of penetration and uncoating (during which the virus particles become engulfed by the cytoplasm of the host cell where virus particles are broken down and released).

66. The answer is E. *(Histology; cell function; organelles)*
Catalase is an enzyme that catalyzes the synthesis and degradation of hydrogen peroxide. Peroxisomes, also called microsomes, contain large amounts of catalase and, therefore, can be visualized after staining for catalase. Peroxisomes function in the metabolism of hydrogen peroxide, cholesterol, and lipids.

67. The answer is D. *(Immunology; delayed-type hypersensitivity reactions)*
The reaction observed was most likely caused by CD4+ T cells. It is a delayed reaction, demonstrating that the T cells are working fine; therefore, the patient could neither lack all T-cell–mediated immune function nor suffer from DiGeorge syndrome. Sensitization has already occurred; therefore, the secondary exposure would show symptoms faster than the primary reaction.

68–69. The answers are: 68-C, 69-C. *(Pathology, pharmacology; open-angle glaucoma)*
Primary open-angle glaucoma is a genetically determined disorder that is the most common form of glaucoma in the general population. In the patient described in the question, a decreased outflow facility resulted in an imbalance between aqueous humor inflow and outflow. Outflow of aqueous humor is accomplished primarily by filtration through the trabecular network to the canal of Schlemm and, to a lesser extent, via absorption into iris blood vessels (uveoscleral outflow).

Cholinomimetics contract the ciliary muscle, thereby reducing resistance of aqueous humor outflow through the trabecular mesh and canal of Schlemm. Accordingly, topical administration of pilocarpine is the agent of choice for this patient. Atropine is a muscarinic antagonist and may exacerbate this problem. Succinylcholine is a depolarizing muscle relaxant and may exacerbate this condition by acutely contracting the accessory striated muscles of the eye before its paralyzing effects. Dexamethasone is a glucocorticoid that may exacerbate primary open-angle glaucoma by further reducing aqueous outflow via the trabecular meshwork. Tubocurarine is a nondepolarizing muscle relaxant that has relatively little effect on muscarinic receptors of the ciliary muscle.

70. The answer is C. *(Physiology; mechanical ventilation)*
Hypoxemic or hypercarbic respiratory failure (or a combination of the two) can be an indication for mechanical ventilation. Both the assist-control and synchronized intermittent mandatory ventilation modes involve a backup respiratory rate. The difference is that only the assist-control mode provides mechanical support (providing a preset volume) to each breath that the patient takes (including breaths above the backup rate). Frequently, assist-control is the mode used initially for acute respiratory failure. Pressure support ventilation (PSV) is more frequently used to help wean patients off of a ventilator. One reason for this difference is that PSV does not initiate breaths for the patient, but controls only the airway pressure that is achieved for breaths that are initiated by the patient. Positive end-expiratory pressure can often decrease the number of collapsed alveoli and increase the arterial partial pressure of oxygen Po_2, but it may cause decreased oxygen delivery to the tissues because of a decrease in cardiac output. This lowering of cardiac output is due to the increased intrathoracic pressure, which reduces venous return to the heart. In any of the methods of mechanical ventilation, it is possible to set the oxygen concentration anywhere between room air and 100%. Tight control of this parameter is not possible with other methods, including a nasal cannula or a face mask, because they do not completely shut off access to room air as is done in mechanical ventilation.

71. The answer is C. *(Histopathology; peripheral nerve tumors)*
Schwannomas, such as neurilemomas, are solitary encapsulated tumors that form eccentric masses derived from peripheral nerves. The histologic appearance in the photomicrograph reveals Antoni A areas (*at right*), which are cellular regions with spindle cells that have elongated tapered nuclei. These nuclei may palisade to form a picket fence–like array called a Verocay body. The looser, edematous zones with hyalinized blood vessels are called Antoni B areas. In contrast, neurofibromas form unencapsulated, onion-like, bulbous expansions of the nerve and are composed of loose interlacing bands of spindle cells with wavy nuclei.

72. The answer is C. *(Physiology; gastrointestinal transport of fats)*
The formation of fatty acids and monoglyceride by pancreatic lipase is an important step in the digestive fate of triglycerides. Although there are gastric lipases, they have a relatively insignificant effect on ingested neutral fats. This is in contrast to a critical role for pancreatic lipase in the pancreatic juice. Neutral fats are emulsified by bile salts, and further agitation within the intestine makes their surface available for significant hydrolysis by the water-soluble pancreatic lipase. The products, fatty acids and 2-monoglyceride, would quickly convert back to fat if they were not made into micelles by bile salts. These bile salts ferry the micelles to the intestinal brush border where the hydrophobic fatty acid (and monoglyceride) rapidly diffuse passively through the lipid membrane.

73. The answer is A. *(Neuroanatomy; anterior spinocerebellar tract)*
The anterior spinocerebellar tract is thought to cross the spinal cord and ascend to the cerebellum where it crosses the spinal cord again. The spinal thalamic tract crosses the cord only once. The cuneocerebellar tract contains fibers that run from the nucleus gracilis and cuneatus to the ipsilateral cerebellar hemisphere. The vestibulospinal tract also remains ipsilateral.

74. The answer is B. *(Neurophysiology; epilepsy)*
The patient most likely has temporal lobe epilepsy, in which seizures are sometimes preceded by acoustic or olfactory hallucinations. Patients are also confused or anxious and sometimes perform complex and bizarre

behaviors with no recall of events after the attack. Klüver-Bucy syndrome results from bilateral destruction of the temporal lobes and manifests as loss of fear and anger as well as docility, increased appetite, and hypersexuality. Jacksonian seizures are the classic tonic–clonic convulsions due to focal activity in the primary motor cortex. Petit mal (or absence) seizures usually occur in children and involve brief myoclonic jerks, sudden loss in body tone with rapid recovery, or brief losses of consciousness during which the patient stares into space.

75. The answer is C. *(Microbiology; enteric infection by enterotoxigenic bacteria)*
The symptoms of cholera result from the attachment of *Vibrio cholerae* to the intestinal mucosa and production of cholera toxin. The infection is acute, and the bacteria remain extracellular. The action of cholera toxin involves elevation of intestinal cyclic adenosine monophosphate (cAMP) levels, which results in massive fluid loss (diarrhea).

76. The answer is C. *(Histology; cell cycle; organelles)*
Centrioles are made of nine tubular triplets, and they function in mitotic spindle formation and in the production of cilia and flagella. Centrioles are self-duplicated in the S (synthesis) phase of the cell cycle.

77. The answer is B. *(Biochemistry; energy storage and transfer)*
A high-energy bond is defined as a bond that, when hydrolyzed, will release a sufficient amount of energy to drive the synthesis of adenosine triphosphate (ATP) from adenosine diphosphate (ADP) and inorganic phosphate (P_i). This requires approximately 7.3 kcal/mol. There are two intermediates in glycolysis that are high-energy compounds: phosphoenolpyruvate and 1,3-bisphosphoglycerate. In the tricarboxylic acid (TCA) cycle, the conversion of succinyl coenzyme A (CoA) to succinate releases enough energy to synthesize guanosine triphosphate (GTP) from guanosine diphosphate (GDP) and P_i. In muscle tissue, phosphocreatine is a storage form of high energy. The hydrolysis of phosphate from phosphocreatine is coupled with the synthesis of ATP. A reaction that is exergonic is accompanied by a $\Delta G°$ that is < 0. The relationship between $\Delta G°$ and K_{eq} is $\Delta G° = -RT \ln K_{eq}$. For a reaction to proceed spontaneously, the K_{eq} must be > 1 and the $\Delta G°$ must be < 0.

78. The answer is B. *(Biochemistry; oxidative enzymes)*
The extraction of β-hydroxybutyrate from blood, and its oxidation to carbon dioxide and water, requires the participation of acetoacetate thiokinase and β-hydroxybutyrate dehydrogenase. All tissues except the liver use β-hydroxybutyrate as a metabolic fuel. The enzymes required for catabolism of the ketone bodies are localized in the mitochondria. These enzymes are β-hydroxybutyrate dehydrogenase, succinyl coenzyme A (CoA), acetoacetate acyltransferase, and acetoacetate thiokinase. 3-Hydroxy-3-methylglutaryl CoA (HMG CoA) lyase catalyzes a step in fatty acid oxidation that takes place in the kidneys or liver. HMG CoA lyase breaks down (*S*)-3-hydroxy-3-methylglutaryl CoA into acetyl CoA and acetoacetate.

79–81. The answers are: 79-B, 80-E, 81-B. *(Pharmacology; thiazide diuretic therapy)*
The thiazide diuretics, such as hydrochlorothiazide, primarily act in the early distal tubules by binding to a membrane protein that is a Na^+ and Cl^- cotransporter. Thus, both Na^+ and more importantly Cl^- reabsorption in the early distal tubules are blocked. The thiazide diuretics also have a small effect in the late proximal tubules.

Although most diuretics can cause all of the untoward effects listed in the question, the patient's neuromuscular dysfunction is most likely the result of hypokalemia, the most important and most serious side effect listed. Hypokalemia is produced because the diuretics cause a large amount of Na^+ to collect in the distal tubules, which leads to Na^+ reabsorption (sodium avidity) and a concomitant depletion of K^+. This Na^+–K^+ exchange site is a primary mechanism for renal control of K^+ homeostasis.

Because this patient is suffering from classic diuretic-induced K^+ loss, he should be supplemented with K^+. The physician may also prescribe a K^+-sparing diuretic, such as amiloride or spironolactone, to be used in combination with a reduced dosage of the thiazide diuretic to maintain K^+ balance. The altered blood K^+ would lead to an increased sensitivity to digitalis-related cardiovascular toxicity; therefore, digitalis should not be used to treat this patient's edema.

82. The answer is E. *(Microbiology; lac operon)*
A gene that is expressed at a constant, unregulated, and often low rate is said to be constitutively expressed. A mutation in either the operator sequence or the lac I gene, so that it produces an inactive repressor, results in an operon that cannot be regulated by the presence or absence of lactose and is therefore inactive. With an inactive repressor, the lac operon can still be regulated by catabolite repression. With a mutated repressor and no glucose, the expression of the lac operon would be high because there would be no catabolite repression by glucose. In the presence of glucose, it would be expressed, but at a low level. A mutated promoter that prevents RNA polymerase from binding leads to a complete inhibition of expression under all growth conditions. A missense mutation in the β-galactosidase gene is likely to reduce the activity of the enzyme but is not likely to affect its cellular levels. A mutated β-galactosidase has no effect on either of the other two enzyme products of the operon. A mutation in the catabolite activator protein (CAP) affects the lac operon's ability to be regulated by catabolite repression. The lac operon is not regulated by attenuation.

83. The answer is A. *(Behavioral science; psychotherapy management)*
The patient motorically and nonverbally expresses (acts out) his conflictual feelings and anxiety about the closeness he feels toward his physician by avoiding a scheduled appointment. There is some degree of repression of these feelings, but the motor behavior indicates that the patient is acting out. Suppression is a *conscious* decision to postpone something, but missing these appointments was not done consciously.

84. The answer is C. *(Biochemistry; disaccharide structure and function)*
The structure shown is that of the milk disaccharide lactose. Lactose is composed of 1 mol of galactose and 1 mol of glucose, which are joined by a β-galactosidic linkage. Lactose is the substrate for the intestinal enzyme lactase, which hydrolyzes the disaccharide. Therefore, lactose would not be digested or absorbed by a lactase-deficient child. Because galactosemia arises from an impaired ability to metabolize galactose, lactose would not be a good source of calories for a child with galactosemia. Additional galactose would augment the problem. Because the only requirement for a reducing sugar is an unsubstituted carbonyl group, the disaccharide would give a positive result in the Fehling-Benedict reducing sugar test. The anomeric carbon of the glucose residue is in equilibrium with the open chain structure, thereby providing an unsubstituted carbonyl group.

85. The answer is C. *(Microbiology; varicella-zoster virus)*
The lesions outside the dermatomal distribution are explained by depressed cell-mediated immunity. When varicella-zoster virus (VZV) goes outside a dermatomal distribution, it is because the affected person is immunosuppressed either from old age (> 65 years) or medication (in this case, chemotherapy). Thymidine kinase–negative mutants rarely occur, except in human immunodeficiency virus (HIV) patients on prolonged prophylaxis with acyclovir. Acyclovir blocks VZV thymidine kinase and does not alkylate DNA. Initial exposure to the infection always leads to viral latency of the dorsal ganglia. There is no evidence that VZV is oncogenic in breast cancer.

86. The answer is B. *(Histopathology; rheumatic fever)*
The photomicrograph of the heart shows an Aschoff body (*lower right*), which is pathognomonic of a history of rheumatic fever, and the mitral stenosis is also probably a consequence. Aschoff bodies constitute foci of fibrinoid necrosis surrounded by histiocytes, giant cells, and specialized histiocytes with linear chromatin called "caterpillar cells," which are seen with acute rheumatic fever and are eventually replaced by scar

tissue. Tissue affected by rheumatic heart disease usually shows pericardial adhesions, valvular deformities, and fusion and shortening of the chordae tendineae.

87. The answer is A. *(Behavioral science; personality assessment)*
The major projective instrument of personality assessment is the Rorschach test. The thematic apperception test, sentence completion test, and projective drawings all are projective tests, but they are less well studied and yield more limited information. The Minnesota Multiphasic Personality Inventory, which is the most frequently used personality test, is an objective instrument, not a projective test.

88. The answer is D. *(Microbiology; tuberculosis culture; diagnostic tests)*
Isolation of *Mycobacterium tuberculosis* is diagnostic of active tuberculosis. The tuberculin test can be positive in the absence of active disease. The clinical findings are not specifically pathognomonic for tuberculosis, nor is demonstration of acid-fast organisms.

89. The answer is B. *(Immunology; tumor)*
Antigens of physically induced tumors, such as those induced by chemical carcinogens, ultraviolet light, or x-rays, exhibit little or no antigenic cross-reactivity. Because random mutations are the most likely explanation for these types of tumors, each tumor displays distinct antigenic specificity. The cells of a given tumor arise from a single cell and are, therefore, antigenically similar.

90. The answer is A. *(Hematopoietic–lymphoreticular system)*
Reed-Sternberg cells are diagnostic for Hodgkin's lymphoma. The Philadelphia chromosome and decreased quantities of leukocyte alkaline phosphatase are commonly observed in chronic myelogenous leukemia. Auer rods are most often seen in increased numbers in acute myelogenous or myelomonocytic leukemia.

91. The answer is B. *(Neurology; normal age-related change)*
The selectivity of the deficit makes a supraforaminal lesion and a peripheral neuropathy impossible. Whether position sense is impaired has not been delineated. If it is impaired, the posterior column of the spinal cord becomes a possibility, but an isolated vibratory deficit can occur as a normal aging change. When diminished vibratory sensation is encountered, position sense must be tested carefully to make the branch point.

92. The answer is A. *(Pharmacology; autonomic pharmacology)*
Indirect-acting sympathomimetic agents, like amphetamine, are transported by the uptake 1 mechanism into nerve terminals where they displace norepinephrine to account for the pressor response. Because these agents lack hydroxyl groups on the catechol ring, they are without significant direct effects on synaptic receptors. Thus, their action is affected by the presence of other agents that modify adrenergic transmission. Reserpine depletes norepinephrine stores, and monoamine oxidase (MAO) inhibitors may potentiate norepinephrine levels. Therefore, the pressor response to amphetamine would be potentiated by an MAO inhibitor and decreased by reserpine. Imipramine interferes with uptake of amphetamine and reduces its effect in this and other ways. A hallmark of indirect-acting sympathomimetics is tolerance or tachyphylaxis. This is presumably secondary to depletion of endogenous norepinephrine pools after repetitive application of amphetamine.

93. The answer is C. *(Microbiology; nucleic acid transfer)*
Transduction is the technique whereby a virus, known as a bacteriophage, is used to introduce DNA into bacteria. Transformation uses high concentrations of calcium chloride to help DNA cross the bacterial plasma membrane. Conjugation refers to direct transfer of DNA between bacteria. Circular, or plasmid, DNA is the form of DNA most commonly used to transfer genes into bacteria via transformation.

94–100. The answers are: 94-D, 95-B, 96-E, 97-D, 98-C, 99-B, 100-C. *(Pharmacology; anatomy; properties of halothane; skeletal muscles)*

Unlike intravenous anesthetics (e.g., methohexital), inhalational anesthetics such as halothane do not possess notable excitatory effects on the central nervous system (CNS), and, therefore, do not lower seizure threshold. All anesthetics tend to depress cardiac function and respiratory drive. Halothane and other anesthetics may induce malignant hyperthermia in certain genetically susceptible individuals.

The anterior cruciate ligament (ACL) is important to the proper functioning of the knee joint. The ACL attaches the femur to the tibia. Damage to this ligament is usually sports-related and caused by rapid deceleration or torque. The ligament is essential to the stability of the knee joint, and surgery is necessary to prevent further injury.

Latin for "little vinegar saucer," the acetabulum is the rounded cavity on the external surface of the innominate bone that receives the head of the femur.

The epiphyseal plate lies between the epiphysis and diaphysis of long bones and is the area of highest mitotic activity. During bone growth, the epiphyseal plates migrate distally, finally becoming epiphyseal lines when growth is completed.

The cuboid is a tarsal bone. All of the other bones listed (i.e., capitate, trapezium, trapezoid) are carpal bones.

A haversian system, or osteon, is composed of osteocytes, lacunae, canaliculi, and concentric lamellae. It is the fundamental unit of compact bone. Compact bone is made up of lamellae, which are parallel bony columns that surround a central (haversian) canal; these canals are neurovascular channels and interconnect via Volkmann's canals. Osteocytes occupy lacunae and communicate with each other via gap junctions that are formed between tiny cytoplasmic projections found in canaliculi. Trabeculae are characteristic features of cancellous (spongy) bone.

101. The answer is C. *(Pathology; diagnostic tests)*

Lumbar puncture is absolutely contraindicated in patients with intracranial neoplasms because it may cause a rapid extrusion of brain tissue of the cerebral hemisphere through the tentorial notch or of the medulla and cerebellum through the foramen magnum. These tumors usually cause cerebrospinal fluid (CSF) pressure buildup, and lumbar puncture causes rapid depressurization of the fluid. Computed tomography (CT) with contrast medium, nuclear magnetic resonance (NMR), and x-ray are all useful tools in imaging brain tumors and do not cause the complications previously mentioned.

102. The answer is D. *(Pediatrics; croup and other respiratory infections)*

The age, timing of symptoms, fever, cough, and inspiratory stridor are typical of croup rather than bronchiolitis or epiglottitis. The etiology of croup is frequently parainfluenza virus types 1 and 2. Less likely causes are respiratory syncytial virus (RSV), other viral agents, and bacteria. However, RSV is the most common cause of bronchiolitis, which is more common in infants younger than 6 months old. Epiglottitis is frequently misdiagnosed as croup, but in this case the lack of drooling, slower onset (more than 1 day), and *Haemophilus influenzae* type b vaccination make epiglottitis less likely. However, intubation is the correct action in severe cases of epiglottitis. Temperature changes and cold air often improve the symptoms of croup for a brief period. Thus, they may not appear so severe when the patient arrives at the office. Children with croup should be put in a humidified room (although the benefit of this has not been proved). Oxygen, racemic epinephrine, and steroids are sometimes used in the treatment of croup.

103. The answer is A. *(Physiology; renal physiology)*

If glomerular filtration decreases, excessive reabsorption of Na^+ (and Cl^-) will occur in the ascending limb of the loop of Henle. The decrease in ion concentration within the distal tubules causes the release of renin from the juxtaglomerular cells (*1*), with subsequent formation of angiotensin II and vasoconstriction of the efferent arteriole (*2*) to help return filtration to normal values. In addition, there will be afferent arteriolar vasodilation to support glomerular filtration.

104. The answer is D. *(Microbiology; Gram stain; bacterial growth)*
Bacterial spores probably caused the decrease in the number of cells expected from the turbidity of the culture. Spores contribute to turbidity, but they do not stain in Gram's procedure.

105. The answer is C. *(Physiology; hemodynamics)*
Under the circumstances described in the question, the stroke volume is 100 ml. Cardiac output is the ratio of oxygen consumption to the arteriovenous difference. In this case, it is:

$$\frac{300 \text{ ml/min}}{20 \text{ ml/100 ml} - 15 \text{ ml/100 ml}} = 6000 \text{ ml/min}$$

Stroke volume is the ratio of cardiac output to heart rate:

$$\frac{6000 \text{ ml/min}}{60 \text{ min}} = 100 \text{ ml}$$

106. The answer is C. *(Microbiology; antiphagocytic virulence factors)*
Opsonizing antibodies promote phagocytosis and are often directed against the capsules of pathogens, including *Streptococcus pneumoniae*. The most important function of the *S. pneumoniae* capsule is to inhibit phagocytosis (until opsonizing antibodies are produced). The capsules of both *Haemophilus influenzae* type B and *Neisseria meningitidis* are polysaccharides that elicit a poor T-cell–dependent immune response. The existing DTP (diphtheria-tetanus-pertussis) vaccine contains killed whole *Bordetella pertussis* cells, not purified capsules.

107. The answer is D. *(Biochemistry; structure and function of proteins)*
The chemical properties of proteins are determined by the nature of the constituent amino acid side chains. There are no ionizing groups, physiologically speaking, on the side chain of serine to provide buffering capacity. Only those amino acids with aromatic side chains absorb significantly in the ultraviolet range. Both glutamic acid and aspartic acid have a pI of approximately 4.5, and only L-amino acids are incorporated into protein. The side chain of proline contains a cyclic ring that cannot bond hydrogen and, therefore, disrupts the α-helical structure.

108. The answer is A. *(Immunology; diagnosis of myelodysplastic syndrome)*
Clinically persistent and unexplained cytopenias associated with morphologically abnormal differentiation in bone marrow precursors define preleukemia, often referred to as the myelodysplastic syndrome. Many of these individuals will have bone marrow blast percentages of less than 5%, and patients suffer from complications of bone marrow failure such as bleeding, infection, and anemia. Others will show an increase in bone marrow blasts between 5% and 30% and have a higher propensity to develop frank acute myeloid leukemia, particularly at the higher levels. Bone marrow blasts greater than 30% define acute leukemia. Cytogenetic changes, if present in myelodysplastic syndrome, are similar to those observed with acute myeloid leukemia, such as an extra chromosome 8, loss of chromosome 5 or 7, or loss of the long arm of chromosome 5 or 7. Despite megaloblastoid morphologic changes, these patients do not resolve with treatment for megaloblastic anemia. It is rare for chronic myelogenous leukemia to present with a low white cell and platelet count and bone marrow dyspoiesis.

109. The answer is C. *(Pharmacology; histamine (H₂) receptor antagonists; toxicology therapy)*
Cimetidine, like most drugs, interacts with a specific receptor, the histamine (H_2) receptor. Mannitol is the osmotic diuretic used most frequently in the prevention and treatment of acute renal failure occurring in conditions such as cardiovascular surgery, trauma, and hemolytic transfusion reactions. Ethylenediaminetetra-acetic acid (EDTA) and dimercaprol chelate heavy metals but do not need to interact directly with any receptor for their pharmacologic actions.

110. The answer is D. *(Physiology; hemoglobin–oxygen interaction)*
The affinity of hemoglobin A_1 ($\alpha_2\beta_2$) for oxygen is decreased by an increase in H^+ concentration (a decrease in pH), by an increase in the P_{CO_2}, or by an increase in the concentration of 2,3-diphosphoglycerate (DPG). All of these conditions result in a shift of the oxygen saturation curve to the right. Fetal hemoglobin ($\alpha_2\gamma_2$) has a higher affinity for oxygen than does adult hemoglobin ($\alpha_2\beta_2$) and consequently becomes saturated at a lower P_{O_2}.

111. The answer is A. *(Anatomy: musculature of the oral cavity)*
During deglutition, the levator veli palatini muscle raises the soft palate to seal the nasopharynx. Contraction of the palatoglossus elevates the base of the tongue and, with help from the palatopharyngeus muscle, closes the oropharyngeal isthmus behind the food bolus. The superior constrictor muscle helps raise the posterior portion of the pharynx over the bolus.

112. The answer is C. *(Pharmacology; side effects of neuroleptics)*
Akathisia, an extrapyramidal side effect of neuroleptics, causes restlessness and an urge to keep moving. The agitation in the man presented in the question seems more motoric than psychic, making worsening psychosis less likely. Although hyperthyroidism causes hyperactivity, this patient has no other symptoms of thyroid disease. Restless legs syndrome is a sleep-related disorder, generally associated with nocturnal myoclonus. It is described as a creepy, crawly feeling in the legs at rest (especially when supine) that is relieved by walking.

113. The answer is B. *(Histology; extracellular matrix production and chondroblasts)*
Chondroblasts are cartilage cells located deep in the perichondrium, the dense connective capsule that surrounds cartilage. As chondroblasts secrete an extracellular matrix rich in type II collagen and cartilage proteoglycan, they become surrounded by their own extracellular matrix and differentiate into chondrocytes. Both chondroblasts and chondrocytes are capable of cell division by mitosis. The endosteum is a layer of osteoblasts in bone. The periosteum is the outer connective tissue covering of bone.

114. The answer is B. *(Pathophysiology; idiopathic thrombocytopenic purpura)*
Idiopathic thrombocytopenic purpura (ITP) is most common in young women, and the usual presentation is of isolated thrombocytopenia without associated illness. Amegakaryocytic thrombocytopenia can occur, but it is much less common, especially in this age-group. Drug-induced thrombocytopenia is also possible but is unlikely in a healthy woman who has no reason to take medications. Patients with thrombasthenia are not thrombocytopenic, and aleukemic leukemia is unlikely to occur without other cytopenias.

115–120. The answers are: 115-C, 116-B, 117-A, 118-E, 119-D, 120-A. *(Physiology; exocrine pancreatic function)*
Elevated serum amylase is the single most important diagnostic finding for confirmation of acute pancreatitis. A serum amylase level threefold higher than normal virtually confirms the diagnosis.
  Secretin is composed of 27 amino acids, is secreted by the mucosal cells of the duodenum, and promotes the secretion of pancreatic juice rich in electrolytes and water. Cholecystokinin is released by mucosal cells

in the upper small intestine in response to peptones and fats. It is absorbed into the bloodstream and stimulates the pancreas to secrete large quantities of digestive enzymes.

Although neuronal control of pancreatic exocrine function is secondary to hormonal control, parasympathetic stimulation of pancreatic secretory activity occurs via vagal fibers, which release acetylcholine (ACh).

Secretin and cholecystokinin are secreted by the mucosa of the small intestine into the bloodstream. They exert their effects after entering the pancreatic circulation. Secretin is stored in an inactive form in the S cells of the duodenum and is released and activated in response to acid. It causes the pancreas to secrete copious amounts of bicarbonate ion (HCO_3^-); but unlike cholecystokinin, which is secreted in response to food, secretin does not significantly affect pancreatic enzyme secretion. The proteolytic enzymes are synthesized as proenzymes, inactive precursors that must be processed before they are active. Many proenzymes, including chymotrypsinogen, procarboxypeptidase, and prophospholipase, are activated by trypsin. Trypsinogen is activated by enterokinase.

121. The answer is C. *(Immunology; complement fixation)*
The complement fixation test is composed of sheep red blood cells (SRBC), antibodies to SRBC, and complement. The concentration of complement is limiting, and any loss of complement is reflected by a decrease in the extent of SRBC lysis. This loss of complement could occur during preincubation of the complement with an antigen–antibody complex not related to the SRBC, which would cause fixation and activation of the cascade. All or most of the complement would be consumed so that the introduction of SRBC does not result in lysis. In this case, because lysis did occur, the patient's serum possesses no complement-fixable [immunoglobulin G (IgG)] anti-influenza type A antibodies. A cross-reactive antibody has no bearing on the complement fixation test.

122. The answer is D. *(Physiology; pulmonary mechanics)*
Inspiration is an active process brought about by contraction of the diaphragm. This contraction results in increased chest volume, thereby lowering pleural and alveolar pressure and creating a gradient for the movement of air. At the end of inspiration, flow is zero and alveolar pressure equals atmospheric pressure. The difference between alveolar and pleural pressure is the recoil pressure of the lung, which is always greatest at higher lung volumes and, thus, is greater at the end of inspiration. During expiration, inspiratory muscles relax, and the elastic forces of the lungs compress alveolar gas, which raises alveolar pressure to values greater than atmospheric pressure and creates a pressure gradient to expel gas from the lung.

123. The answer is A. *(Cell biology; RNA processing)*
RNA processing occurs in two locations within cells. The most common site is the cell nucleoplasm, where the majority of RNA transcribed in the nucleus is spliced, capped, and polyadenylated. The other site is the mitochondria, each of which contains a ring of DNA that codes for two ribosomal RNA (rRNA) molecules, proteins, and all the transfer RNA (tRNA) required to synthesize the encoded proteins.

124. The answer is C. *(Biochemistry; urea metabolism; amino acid enzymes)*
The pathway by which the α-amino groups of the amino acids are incorporated into urea involves a number of transaminases that transfer the amino group from the amino acids to α-ketoglutarate, with the concomitant formation of glutamate. The glutamate is converted back to α-ketoglutarate and ammonium by the mitochondrial enzyme glutamate dehydrogenase. The ammonium produced in the reaction is the substrate for carbamoyl phosphate synthesis. This reaction constitutes the first step in urea biosynthesis.

125. The answer is A. *(Physiology; control of respiration)*
The carotid bodies are the major sensors of hypoxia (the aortic bodies being much less sensitive), and the central chemoreceptors are the major sensors of hypercapnia. However, there is a synergistic effect of hypoxia

and hypercapnia on respiratory rate. The level of response to ventilatory stimuli is reduced during sleep because of decreased neural output and increased upper airway resistance (caused by the relaxation of dilator muscles). The Hering-Breuer reflex acts to terminate inspiration at tidal volumes greater than 1 L, and it is mediated through stretch receptors and vagal afferents. Peripheral chemoreceptors are the major mediator of the compensatory hyperventilation that occurs during metabolic acidosis. Individuals with increased elastic loads will compensate with short, rapid breaths, whereas people with increased resistive loads will generally take deeper breaths and decrease breathing frequency.

126. The answer is C. *(Histopathology; alcohol-induced acute liver damage)*
The liver biopsy shows the typical features of alcohol-induced acute liver injury, which include steatorrhea, acute inflammation, and Mallory bodies. Mallory bodies are intracellular filamentous material believed to be related to prekeratin, which is normally produced by the liver. This injury to the liver is a direct effect of alcohol.

127. The answer is A. *(Immunology; viral immunity)*
Antibodies cannot displace attached viruses from the host cell. The role of antibodies in preventing diseases caused by viruses is demonstrated by the effectiveness of the polio vaccine. For the poliovirus, and other viruses as well, antibodies bind to proteins on the surface of the viruses, which inhibits the virus from entering host cells. This attachment of immunoglobulins [most notably immunoglobulin G (IgG)] to the virus particle also leads to phagocytosis by attachment of the Fc portion of the antibody to macrophages. Attachment of the antibody to an infected host cell presenting viral antigens leads to complement-mediated lysis. Antibodies have been found that inhibit critical viral enzyme functions, such as neuraminidase of the influenza virus.

128. The answer is E. *(Biochemistry; cholesterol biosynthesis)*
The synthesis of cholesterol uses acetyl coenzyme A (CoA) as the sole source of carbon atoms and reduced nicotinamide-adenine dinucleotide phosphate (NADPH) as a source of reducing equivalents. The NADPH is supplied primarily through two reactions, which are catalyzed by a glucose 6-phosphate dehydrogenase and 6-phosphogluconate dehydrogenase. The formation of 3-hydroxy-3-methylglutaryl CoA (HMG CoA) results from the condensation of acetoacetyl CoA and acetyl CoA. The step that is committed to cholesterol synthesis is the conversion of HMG CoA to mevalonic acid. This step is catalyzed by HMG CoA reductase. HMG CoA is used to synthesize activated isoprenoid units, which are subsequently condensed to form squalene. Squalene is converted to lanosterol and then to cholesterol by a series of reactions that involve the addition of oxygen, cyclization to give the sterol ring structure, and elimination of three carbon atoms as carbon dioxide. Mevinolin is an inhibitor of HMG CoA reductase.

129. The answer is B. *(Physiology; blood pressure regulation)*
Angiotensin-converting enzyme (ACE) hydrolyzes the decapeptide angiotensin I to the vasoconstrictor octapeptide, angiotensin II. Inhibition of this enzyme by a number of competitive antagonists is a new and useful way to lower blood pressure in some individuals. In addition to reducing circulating levels of the endogenous angiotensin II peptide, inhibition of ACE may have central effects, including a decrease in the dipsogenic effect of angiotensin II. Furthermore, angiotensin II appears to facilitate neurotransmission in the central and peripheral sympathetic nervous systems. Although angiotensin II is a potent stimulator of aldosterone secretion in the zona glomerulosa of the adrenal cortex, and inhibition of this effect might be expected to reduce blood pressure (by enhancing Na^+ excretion by the kidneys), there usually is little change in aldosterone levels because other endogenous secretagogues, including steroids, K^+, and minimal levels of angiotensin II, can maintain aldosterone secretion. Nonetheless, there is little indication to believe that the aldosterone level would actually increase, and if it did, this would result in Na^+ reabsorption, water retention, and an increase in arterial blood pressure.

130. The answer is C. *(Histology; cell structure; membranes)*
The cell membrane is composed of a variety of proteins scattered within a phospholipid bilayer. The phospholipid molecules contain a hydrophilic head and a hydrophobic tail and, therefore, are amphipathic. The cell membrane readily allows the diffusion of molecules such as oxygen, carbon dioxide, nitrogen, and water; however, glucose does not diffuse through the cell readily, and entry into the cell is enhanced by carrier proteins (facilitated diffusion and active transport).

131. The answer is E. *(Physiology; sleep-disordered breathing)*
Sleep-disordered breathing is a condition that is often overlooked by medical professionals. Approximately 2% of women and 4% of men have clinically important conditions. The diagnostic criteria for obstructive sleep apnea syndrome include an apnea index greater than 5 with a persistent respiratory effort, as well as the complaint of daytime sleepiness. This condition is associated with increased risks of myocardial infarction, stroke, dysrhythmia, and motor vehicle accidents. Because hypothyroidism can be a factor in sleep-disordered breathing, it would be practical to first determine the level of thyroid-stimulating hormone. After diagnosis, behavioral therapy should be initiated to include weight loss (especially if obese), reduction of alcohol intake, cessation of smoking, and avoidance of the supine position. If these lifestyle modifications are ineffective, medical and surgical options do exist, including dental orthotics, tracheostomy, and uvulopalatopharyngoplasty.

132. The answer is C. *(Microbiology; prokaryotic and eukaryotic differences)*
Because shigellae are gram-negative prokaryotic bacteria, they have peptidoglycan-containing cell walls, lipopolysaccharide, 70S ribosomes, RNA, and DNA, but they do not have sterols in their plasma membranes. *Giardia* species are eukaryotic protozoa with 80S ribosomes, RNA, DNA, and sterol-containing plasma membranes.

133. The answer is D. *(Biochemistry; enzyme catalysis)*
The activation energy is the amount of energy required to pass into the transition state; the rate of the reaction depends on the number of molecules in the transition state. Increasing the activation energy lowers the reaction rate. Each enzyme has two kinetic parameters: V_{max} is an index of catalytic efficiency, and K_m is a measure of the affinity of the enzyme for the substrate. The binding of substrate to enzyme induces a conformational change in which the functional group that participates in catalysis is appropriately juxtaposed with the substrate bonds that are to be altered in the reaction. General acid–base catalysis is a catalytic mode frequently used by enzymes.

134. The answer is E. *(Physiology; respiratory failure)*
Adult respiratory distress syndrome (ARDS) is a model of acute alveolar injury with pulmonary edema and respiratory failure. A number of conditions can lead to ARDS, particularly if high concentrations of oxygen are used as supportive respiratory therapy. Focal atelectasis and alveolar collapse occur with the development of pulmonary edema; hyaline membranes appear, type II pneumocytes proliferate, and there is variable damage to the alveolar walls. The mechanisms of ARDS are not completely understood. The permeability of the endothelium of the pulmonary capillary and the epithelium of the alveolar wall is increased in ARDS, and it is responsible, in part, for the characteristics of the syndrome.

135. The answer is C. *(Anatomy; the respiratory system)*
Type II pneumonocytes cover less than 5% of the alveolar surface, but they form a reserve for replacement of damaged type I pneumonocytes. These multilamellar bodies are the source of the phospholipid-containing pulmonary surfactant. Defects in these cells contribute to infant and adult respiratory distress.

136. The answer is E. *(Biochemistry; cellular signal transduction)*
The nuclear oncogene product *c-fos* assists in the regulation of gene expression. Although its expression is affected by second messengers, it is not thought of as a second messenger, but rather as a more distal effector. Inositol 1,4,5-triphosphate (IP_3) and diacylglycerol (DAG) are important second messengers generated by phospholipase C from phosphatidylinositol bisphosphate. IP_3 causes the release of intracellular stores of Ca^{2+}, which is also an important second messenger, and DAG activates a Ca^{2+}-dependent protein kinase, protein kinase C. Cyclic adenosine monophosphate (cAMP) is synthesized by adenylate cyclase from adenosine triphosphate (ATP) and can act as a second messenger to activate enzymes such as cAMP-dependent protein kinase.

137. The answer is D. *(Anatomy; embolism)*
Thrombi from the left side of the heart to the parent vessels of the cerebral arteries all may embolize to occlude a cerebral artery; however, the abdominal aorta is beyond these vessels that lead to the brain and, thus, is unlikely to cause an embolism in the brain. Severe fracture of any long bone may result in a fat embolus to the cerebral arteries.

138. The answer is D. *(Physiology; pulmonary emboli)*
Diagnosis of pulmonary emboli is difficult but critical because pulmonary emboli may be life threatening. Pulmonary emboli present with a wide array of symptoms and are often asymptomatic. In addition, patients with pulmonary emboli may have a normal chest radiograph. Thus, other diagnostic tests are often required. Among these tests are ventilation/perfusion lung scans, venous ultrasonography, spiral computed tomography scan, and the "gold standard"—pulmonary angiography. The most common source of the thromboemboli are the deep veins of the leg (popliteal and femoral). Risk factors include indwelling catheters, sickle cell disease, surgery, and hypercoagulable states (including factor V Leiden mutation). Pulmonary emboli may affect both gas exchange and hemodynamics. These disruptions include an increase in pulmonary vascular resistance.

139. The answer is A. *(Biochemistry; RNA function)*
The synthesis of RNA in eukaryotes requires three different RNA polymerases: one each for the synthesis of messenger RNA (mRNA), ribosomal RNA (rRNA), and transfer RNA (tRNA). All of these RNAs are required for protein synthesis. The ribosome is a complex made up of approximately 75 proteins and several types of rRNA and is the site where mRNA and tRNAs come together to participate in protein synthesis. The triplet base codons for amino acids are contained in mRNA; tRNA contains a complementary anticodon, which promotes interaction between mRNA and tRNA during protein synthesis.

140. The answer is D. *(Anatomy: hormone receptors; Addison's disease)*
Addison's disease is caused by an overall atrophy of the adrenal cortex and is not related to an abnormality in hormone receptors. Many peptide hormone receptors are transmembrane proteins that may elicit their full biologic response when only a small fraction of the receptors are occupied by hormone. The specificity of the response of a particular cell or tissue is defined, at least in part, by the types of receptors localized on or in the cell. Some hormone receptors are desensitized by phosphorylation. Following phosphorylation, dissociation of the hormone from the receptor may occur without a corresponding decrease in the biologic response.

141. The answer is D. *(Neuroanatomy; subthalamus)*
The subthalamus is located (not surprisingly) below the thalamus. It is an exceedingly complex area of the brain connected to many areas to integrate motor control, but it is not connected with the cerebellum.

142–146. The answers are: 142-D, 143-B, 144-C, 145-C, 146-B. *(Embryology)*
Ectoderm gives rise to the nervous system, sensory epithelia, epidermis, mammary glands, and the pituitary gland. Melanocytes in the dermis arise from neuroectoderm. Mesoderm gives rise to cartilage, bone, connective tissue, muscles, the cardiovascular system, kidneys, gonads, spleen, and the adrenal cortex. Endoderm gives rise to gastrointestinal and respiratory mucosa, and the parenchyma of the tonsils, thyroid gland, parathyroid glands, thymus, liver, and pancreas.

147–149. The answers are: 147-C, 148-A, 149-B. *(Hepatic histology)*
This is a scanning electron micrograph of the liver. Liver parenchymal cells (*A*) secrete bile into the bile canaliculi (*B*) and blood proteins, such as serum albumin and transferrin, into the liver sinusoids (*C*). Liver sinusoids are modified fenestrated and discontinuous capillaries that receive blood from the portal vein and hepatic artery in the portal canals and carry it to the central veins.

150–154. The answers are: 150-E, 151-D, 152-C, 153-B, 154-A. *(Genetics, biochemistry; lipoproteins and genetic disorders)*
Lipoprotein lipase is an enzyme normally located within the capillary endothelium; it is involved in converting chylomicrons to chylomicron remnants. A deficiency in lipoprotein lipase leads to elevated circulating levels of chylomicrons. Chylomicron levels may also be elevated in systemic lupus erythematosus (SLE).

Familial hypercholesterolemia, caused by mutation within a single gene, is one of the most common human mendelian disorders. Low-density lipoprotein (LDL) levels are elevated in the serum because this disorder markedly decreases the number of high-affinity LDL receptors within the liver. LDL levels may also be elevated in nephrotic syndrome and hyperthyroidism.

Familial (type III) hyperlipoproteinemia has been traced to a single amino acid substitution within the receptor for apoprotein E. Because the apoprotein E receptor is required for the normal metabolism of both chylomicron remnants and intermediate-density lipoproteins (IDL), both of these molecules accumulate in the blood.

The biochemical defect underlying familial hypertriglyceridemia is unknown. In this disorder, serum levels of both very low-density lipoprotein (VLDL) and triglycerides are elevated. VLDL and triglyceride levels may also be elevated in diabetes mellitus and chronic alcoholism.

The defect underlying familial hyperlipidemia is unknown, although research suggests a deficiency in apoprotein CII. In this disorder, serum levels of VLDL and chylomicrons are elevated; alcoholism, diabetes mellitus, and oral contraceptives are also capable of elevating VLDL and chylomicron levels.

155–159. The answers are: 155-B, 156-C, 157-A, 158-D, 159-E. *(Neuroanatomy; neurotransmitters)*
Many neuroanatomic pathways now can be specified by their neurotransmitters. Thus, selective depletion of the neurotransmitters can be caused by sectioning the pathways or by destroying the perikarya that produce the neurotransmitter.

Destruction of interneurons of the spinal cord would deplete γ-aminobutyric acid (GABA) and glycine, inhibitory transmitters produced by interneurons. Dorsal root section would reduce substance P concentration in the dorsal horns. This neurotransmitter presumably transmits pain impulses from the small fibers in the lateral division of the dorsal roots. Destruction of the substantia nigra would deplete dopamine, the major neurotransmitter within the basal ganglia. Section of the medial forebrain bundle would destroy many of the axons that connect the catecholaminergic and serotoninergic nuclei of the brain stem with the cerebral cortex. Destruction of the medullary raphe would destroy the serotoninergic neurons of the medulla that project to the spinal cord.

Not only can the neurotransmitters be depleted by actual anatomic destruction of axonal pathways or the destruction of neuronal perikarya, but various drugs and chemicals can also selectively block neurotransmitters either by inhibiting their formation, inhibiting their release, or competing with binding sites on the postsynaptic membrane. By combining anatomic lesions with chemical blockade and direct chemical analysis, various lines of evidence can be developed to establish the transmitters involved in the various layers and regions of the cortex and the different nuclei of the central nervous system (CNS).

160–163. The answers are: 160-A, 161-C, 162-B, 163-E. *(Immunology; oncogenes; oncogenesis; signal transduction; growth factor receptors)*
Alteration of virtually any cellular signaling system has the potential for causing oncogenesis. The *ros* oncogene product is an activated insulin receptor. The homolog of one of the two subunits of the nerve growth factor (NGF) receptor is *trk*. The oncogene *erbB* has activated tyrosine kinase, which is also activated when epidermal growth factor (EGF) binds to the EGF receptor. The oncogenic homolog of the platelet-derived growth factor (PDGF) receptor is *kit*, whereas *sis* binds to the PDGF receptor. The nuclear oncogene *jun* is involved in the control of gene transcription.

164–169. The answers are: 164-E, 165-A, 166-C, 167-A, 168-D, 169-B. *(Microbiology; etiology of spirochetal diseases)*
Borrelia recurrentis is the etiologic agent of relapsing fever in humans. The disease occurs worldwide and is characterized by a febrile bacteremia. The disease name is derived from the fact that there can be 3–10 recurrences, apparently from the original infection. The disease is transmitted to humans from infected animals by ticks and from human to human by lice.

Bejel is nonvenereal, endemic syphilis caused by a variant of *Treponema pallidum*. The disease usually is seen in children in the Middle East and Africa. Transmission appears to be through the shared use of drinking and eating utensils; bejel is not transmitted sexually. The disease develops in primary, secondary, and tertiary stages.

Pinta is a tropical disease caused by *Treponema carateum*. It occurs primarily in Central and South America, where it appears to be spread by person-to-person contact. Unlike other treponemal diseases, the lesions of pinta remain localized in the skin.

The etiologic agent of syphilis is *T. pallidum*. Humans are the only natural host of the spirochete, and venereal transmission is the most common means of acquiring the infection. Congenital syphilis occurs when the fetus is infected transplacentally and survives to delivery. Accidental laboratory infections occasionally occur.

Fort Bragg fever is a localized name of pretibial fever caused by *Leptospira interrogans* serogroup *autumnalis*. The disease is characterized by a rash on the shins. Humans probably acquire the infection by contact with the urine of infected animals.

Treponema pertenue is the etiologic agent of yaws. The disease occurs primarily in children in tropical regions, where it appears to be transmitted by direct contact or by vectors such as flies. This potentially disfiguring disease has primary, secondary, and tertiary stages.

170–175. The answers are: 170-A, 171-C, 172-B, 173-B, 174-A, 175-A. *(Pathology; abnormal heart sounds)*
The first heart sound, S_1, is composed of the sounds of tricuspid and mitral valve closure. Mitral valve closure is normally almost silent, and S_1 is normally quieter than the second heart sound, S_2, which is the sound of the aortic and pulmonic valves closing. S_1 is better heard at the apex of the heart, and S_2 is better heard at the base of the heart. With mitral valve stenosis, the left ventricle is underfilled at the end of diastole, and its systolic contraction has force sufficient to cause the mitral valve leaflets to close audibly. During ventricular systole, the presence of aortic stenosis produces a high flow rate through the stenotic valve, which is appreciated as a pansystolic murmur. The sound is heard well at both the base and apex of the heart and is relatively unchanged by respiratory movements. In acute aortic regurgitation, the left ventricle is overfilled, and the ejection fraction is reduced. During ventricular systole, the pressure buildup is more sluggish than

normal due to the leaking aortic valve. The mitral valve closure becomes even quieter than normal; thus, S_1 is quieter than normal. In systemic hypertension, the higher than normal pressure within the aortic bulb at the end of systole causes the very forceful closure of the aortic valve, which produces an S_2 that is louder than usual. In cases of severe anemia or hyperthyroidism, the heart rate is increased along with cardiac output. The increase in heart rate causes the heart to spend a greater portion of its time in systole and less time in diastole. The reduction in diastolic time means that the left ventricle may be relatively underfilled at the beginning of systole. As stated above, the contraction of an underfilled ventricle allows the mitral valve to close with force sufficient to cause S_1 to be louder than S_2.

176–179. The answers are: 176-C, 177-D, 178-A, 179-B. *(Pathology; degenerative joint disease)*
Rheumatoid arthritis is a common chronic inflammatory disease affecting the joints. Initially, the small joints of the hands and feet are involved. The disease is strongly associated with genetic factors—over 75% of Caucasians affected have human leukocyte antigen DR4 (HLA-DR4).

Osteoarthritis is characterized by progressive deterioration of the articular cartilage of weight-bearing joints. Erosion of cartilage eventually leads to thickening of the underlying bone and to knobby protruding of the bone. These protrusions are called Heberden's nodes. They may break off the bone surface and form intra-articular bodies called ''joint mice.''

Lyme disease (Lyme arthritis) is caused by *Borrelia burgdorferi*, which is transmitted by ticks, whose reservoirs are field mice and deer. The disease has a spectrum of symptoms similar to those of rheumatoid arthritis, principally affecting the knees. Symptoms may last for a long period of time (months) and may lead to a chronic insidious polyarthritis.

Gout is manifested by hyperuricemia, arthritis (gouty arthritis), and the deposit of tophi (urate crystals) in and around the joints. The tophi are surrounded by histiocytes, giant cells, and fibroblasts, causing inflammation.

180. The answer is A. *(Physiology; action potentials)*
Voltage-sensitive sodium-ion (Na^+) and potassium-ion (K^+) channels distinct from the K^+–Na^+ leak channels underlie the molecular basis of the action potential, whereas the K^+–Na^+ leak channels underlie the molecular basis of the local potential. A local potential is a passive-graded response that decays. Compared to action potentials, local potentials have a small amplitude (0.1–10 mv) and a variable duration (5 seconds to several minutes).

Test V

QUESTIONS

DIRECTIONS: *Single best answer questions* consist of numbered items or incomplete statements followed by answers or by completions of the statement. Select the ONE lettered answer or completion that is BEST in each case.

Matching questions consist of a list of four to twenty-six lettered options (some of which may be in figures) followed by several numbered items. For each numbered item, select the ONE lettered option that is most closely associated with it. Each lettered option may be selected once, more than once, or not at all.

Questions 1–2

One week after bootcamp, an 18-year-old recruit comes to the infirmary with a fever, headache, stiff neck, and visual sensitivity to light. A lumbar puncture is performed, and meningitis is diagnosed. Several other recruits have since reported similar symptoms.

1. The most likely cause of this outbreak of meningitis is

(A) *Haemophilus influenzae* type B
(B) *Streptococcus pneumoniae*
(C) *Neisseria meningitidis*
(D) *Escherichia coli*
(E) *Streptococcus agalactiae*

2. All of the following are important virulence factors in meningococci EXCEPT

(A) polysaccharide capsule
(B) M protein
(C) endotoxin
(D) IgA protease

3. All of the following statements about polycythemia vera are true EXCEPT

(A) it is a polycythemia resulting from a decrease in plasma volume
(B) there is increased production of all myeloid elements
(C) it is rarely found in children or multiple members of a single family
(D) there is an increase in hemoglobin concentration
(E) it produces symptoms associated with increased blood viscosity
(F) it is characterized by splenomegaly

4. All of the following statements about essential thrombocytosis vera are true EXCEPT

(A) it is dominated clinically by a marked decrease in platelet count
(B) patients present with spontaneous bleeding
(C) bone marrow has large numbers of hyperploid megakaryocytes
(D) it is characterized by modest splenomegaly
(E) there is an abnormality in platelet aggregation in response to epinephrine

5. All of the following statements about glucagon are true EXCEPT

(A) it is secreted by the α-cells of the pancreatic islets
(B) it is a polypeptide hormone
(C) its action is anabolic, increasing fatty acid storage
(D) it increases glycogenolysis
(E) it increases gluconeogenesis

6. All of the following are inhibitors of glucagon secretion EXCEPT

(A) insulin
(B) hyperglycemia
(C) somatostatin
(D) catecholamines
(E) cortisol
(F) amino acids

7. All of the following are inhibitors of insulin secretion EXCEPT

(A) glucagon
(B) hypoglycemia
(C) somatostatin
(D) epinephrine
(E) prostaglandins

8. Which of the following statements describes the mechanism of action of amphetamine?

(A) It is mediated through the cellular release of stored catecholamines
(B) It blocks the reuptake of norepinephrine, serotonin, and dopamine by presynaptic fibers
(C) It blocks the ability of adrenergic neurons to transport norepinephrine from the cytoplasm into storage vesicles
(D) It blocks the release of stored norepinephrine
(E) It acts directly on α- or β-adrenergic receptors

9. Which of the following infectious diseases is caused by a spirochete?

(A) Lyme disease
(B) Yellow fever
(C) Typhus
(D) Dengue fever

10. All of the following statements regarding agnogenic myeloid metaplasia are true EXCEPT

(A) patients present with progressive splenomegaly
(B) there is gradual replacement of marrow elements with fibrosis
(C) it begins in late middle life and is gradual in onset and chronic
(D) peripheral blood smears show teardrop poikilocytes
(E) hepatomegaly can occur in the absence of splenomegaly
(F) almost all patients become anemic

11. The most common malignant childhood brain tumor is

(A) schwannoma
(B) medulloblastoma
(C) meningioma
(D) squamous cell carcinoma

12. All of the following statements regarding aplastic anemia are true EXCEPT

(A) patients have an acellular or markedly hypocellular bone marrow
(B) there is gradual replacement of marrow elements with fibrosis
(C) it is caused by an injury or destruction of a pluripotential stem cell
(D) an example of aplastic anemia is Fanconi's anemia
(E) infectious hepatitis can cause aplastic anemia
(F) peripheral blood smear usually shows pancytopenia

13. Bell's palsy is the most common ailment of which of the following cranial nerves (CN)?

(A) CN III (oculomotor)
(B) CN VII (facial)
(C) CN VI (abducens)
(D) CN VIII (acoustic)
(E) CN X (vagus)

14. The most common agent in narcotic endocarditis is

(A) *Streptococcus pneumoniae*
(B) *Staphylococcus aureus*
(C) gram-negative bacilli
(D) *Neisseria gonorrhoeae*

15. All of the following statements about pure red cell aplasia are true EXCEPT

(A) there is a selective failure of erythroid elements production in the bone marrow
(B) the patient presents with normal megakaryocytopoiesis
(C) an example of pure red cell aplasia is Blackfan-Diamond syndrome
(D) the patient presents with severe reticulocytopenia
(E) an acquired form of pure red cell aplasia is caused by thymomas
(F) the patient presents with suppressed granulopoiesis

16. All of the following are strong indications for splenectomy EXCEPT

(A) splenic abscess
(B) hereditary spherocytosis
(C) splenic neoplasia
(D) massive splenic trauma
(E) schistosomiasis

17. Which human herpes virus is implicated in the etiology of AIDS-associated non-Hodgkin's lymphoma?

(A) Herpes simplex virus type 1
(B) Herpes simplex virus type 2
(C) Epstein-Barr virus
(D) Cytomegalovirus

18. To withdraw cerebrospinal fluid (CSF) [i.e., perform a spinal tap], a needle tip must pass successively through the

(A) pia mater, dura mater, epidural space, and arachnoid membrane
(B) arachnoid membrane, epidural space, dura mater, and subdural space
(C) subdural space, dura mater, epidural space, and arachnoid membrane
(D) arachnoid membrane, subdural space, dura mater, and epidural space
(E) epidural space, dura mater, subdural space, and arachnoid membrane

19. Which of the following organisms extrude "sulfur granules" from a draining wound?

(A) *Francisella tularensis*
(B) *Pasteurella multocida*
(C) *Actinomyces israelii*
(D) *Yersinia pestis*

20. The accompanying graph shows the tubular loss of glucose (excretion rate) plotted against the rate at which glucose is filtered at the glomerulus (filtered load). Which lettered point on the curve corresponds to the Tm for glucose?

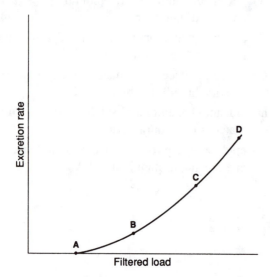

21. The most frequent type of primary brain tumor is

(A) meningioma
(B) glioma
(C) neural sheath tumor
(D) squamous cell carcinoma
(E) osteosarcoma

22. The accompanying micrograph depicts a section of distal lung. Which lettered structure is a cell that secretes surfactant?

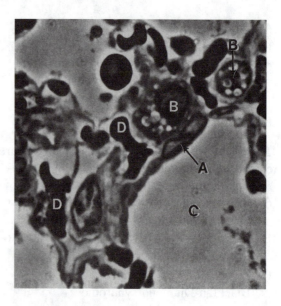

23. The most common cause of posttransfusion hepatitis is

(A) hepatitis A virus
(B) hepatitis B virus
(C) hepatitis C virus
(D) hepatitis D virus
(E) hepatitis E virus

24. In intravenous drug abusers, the valves most commonly affected in narcotic endocarditis are

(A) right-sided valves
(B) left-sided valves
(C) both right-sided and left-sided valves
(D) neither right- nor left-sided valves

25. Drugs used in multiple-drug therapies of choice for tuberculosis include

(A) isoniazid, rifampin, pyrazinamide, penicillin
(B) penicillin, rifampin, pyrazinamide, ethambutol
(C) isoniazid, penicillin, pyrazinamide, ethambutol
(D) isoniazid, rifampin, pyrazinamide, ethambutol
(E) isoniazid, rifampin, penicillin, ethambutol

Questions 26–27

A 34-year-old woman presents with intermittent dysesthesia, paresthesia, and hypesthesia in the middle digits of her right hand. Patient history, physical findings, and decreased nerve conduction velocity indicate that she is suffering from carpal tunnel syndrome.

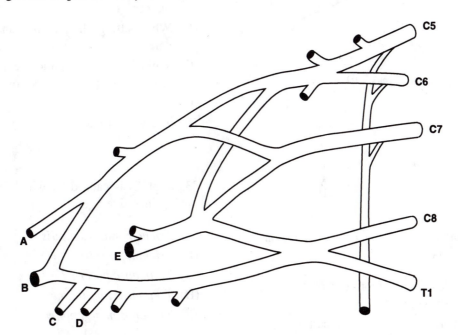

26. In the accompanying diagram of the brachial plexus, identify the nerve that is compressed in this syndrome.

27. All of the following may be used as treatment for carpal tunnel syndrome EXCEPT

(A) flexion exercises
(B) surgical section of the carpal ligament
(C) local adrenocorticosteroid injection
(D) use of a wrist splint

28. All of the following statements about action potentials are true EXCEPT

(A) the amplitude is large (70–110 mv)
(B) the duration is brief (1–10 msec)
(C) it has a graded response
(D) its propagation is active (self-propagating)
(E) the channels involved are voltage-gated sodium- and potassium-ion channels

29. In the accompanying diagram, which lettered point would provide the best point for auscultation of mitral stenosis?

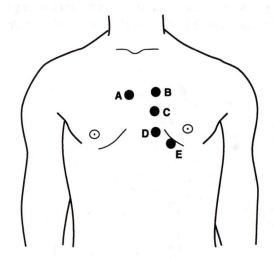

30. Which statement below is correct about the enzyme it describes?

(A) Aldolase cleaves a carbon–carbon bond to create a carboxyl group
(B) Dehydrogenase adds water to a carbon–carbon bond without breaking the bond or, conversely, removing water to create a double bond
(C) Hydrolase adds water to break a bond
(D) Isomerase hydrolyzes ester linkages to form an acid and an alcohol

31. Which of the following congenital immunodeficiencies involves only a T-cell deficiency?

(A) Thymic aplasia (DiGeorge's syndrome)
(B) Ataxia–telangiectasia
(C) X-linked hypogammaglobulinemia (Bruton's agammaglobulinemia)
(D) Chronic granulomatous disease
(E) Hereditary angioedema

32. Which of the following special maneuvers intensifies the murmur associated with aortic insufficiency?

(A) The patient rolls into the left lateral decubitus position
(B) While sitting, the patient leans forward, exhales, and holds his or her breath
(C) While sitting, the patient expires against a closed glottis (i.e., bears down)
(D) The patient stands
(E) The patient exercises briefly

33. Syphilis is caused by which one of the following infective agents?

(A) *Trichomonas vaginalis*
(B) *Trichinella spiralis*
(C) *Trypanosoma cruzi*
(D) *Treponema pallidum*
(E) *Trypanosoma gambiense*

34. Which of the following physical findings make up the classic triad in cardiac tamponade in patients with penetrating cardiac injuries, aortic dissection, or intrapericardial rupture of aortic or cardiac aneurysms?

(A) Hypotension, elevated systemic venous pressure, and small quiet heart
(B) Hypotension, elevated systemic venous pressure, and enlarged heart
(C) Hypotension, decreased systemic venous pressure, and small quiet heart
(D) Hypertension, elevated systemic venous pressure, and small quiet heart

35. A 72-year-old asthmatic man comes in for management of stable exertional angina that he has had for 2 years. Which of the following treatments for managing angina is contraindicated in this patient?

(A) Calcium-channel blockers
(B) Nitrates
(C) Noncardioselective β-blockers at low doses
(D) Cardioselective β-blockers at low doses

36. Which of the following congenital variable immunodeficiencies involves a combined B- and T-cell deficiency?

(A) Hyper-IgM syndrome
(B) Wiskott-Aldrich syndrome
(C) Chronic mucocutaneous candidiasis
(D) Chediak-Higashi syndrome
(E) Leukocyte adhesion deficiency syndrome

37. Which of the following vitamins can be synthesized by intestinal bacteria?

(A) Vitamin E
(B) Vitamin C
(C) Vitamin A
(D) Vitamin K
(E) Niacin

38. Reciprocal innervation is most accurately described as

(A) inhibition of flexor muscles during an extension
(B) activation of contralateral extensors during a flexion
(C) reduction of Ia fiber activity during a contraction
(D) simultaneous stimulation of alpha and gamma motoneurons
(E) inhibition of alpha motoneurons during a contraction

39. The region of the brain that is most involved in problem solving is the

(A) parietal lobe
(B) frontal lobe
(C) temporal lobe
(D) cerebellum
(E) occipital lobe

40. A hyperventilating patient is suffering from untreated diabetes. Over the past several days, he has experienced thirst, frequent urination, weight loss, and fatigue. Analysis of his blood reveals below normal pH, bicarbonate level, and partial pressure of carbon dioxide (P_{CO_2}) and above normal glucose level. The acid–base abnormalities of this patient can best be described as

(A) compensated respiratory acidosis with metabolic alkalosis

(B) compensated respiratory alkalosis with metabolic acidosis

(C) compensated metabolic acidosis with respiratory alkalosis

(D) compensated metabolic alkalosis with respiratory acidosis

(E) compensated metabolic acidosis with respiratory acidosis

41. Syphilis is treated with which one of the following antibiotics?

(A) Amphotericin B
(B) Ketoconazole
(C) Trimethoprim
(D) Rifampin
(E) Penicillin G

42. At normal pH, which of the following amino acids has a positively charged side chain?

(A) Glutamic acid
(B) Proline
(C) Aspartic acid
(D) Lysine
(E) Isoleucine

43. A renal allograft recipient presents with fever and adenopathy 3 months after engraftment. Serum studies show markedly elevated anti–Epstein-Barr virus (EBV) titers. A biopsy of the allograft is most likely to show

(A) fibrinoid necrosis of the small vessels

(B) vascular sclerosis

(C) interstitial fibrosis

(D) a dense lymphoplasmacytic interstitial infiltrate with cytologic atypia

(E) isometric vacuolar change in the tubular epithelial cells

44. All of the following statements regarding tumor necrosis factor (TNF) are true EXCEPT

(A) TNF is produced by macrophages in response to endotoxin

(B) TNF is structurally related to lymphotoxin

(C) TNF causes a cachectic state

(D) TNF stimulates lipoprotein lipase

45. All of the following statements regarding tumor growth factor-β are true EXCEPT

(A) it is synthesized as a larger inactive precursor protein

(B) it stimulates growth of epithelial and mesenchymal tissue

(C) it inhibits growth of immunologic cells

(D) a major source of tumor growth factor-β is platelets

46. All of the following statements about acidic and basic fibroblast growth factor are true EXCEPT

(A) acidic fibroblast growth factor is synthesized in many cells and tissues
(B) fibroblast growth factor is the major identified stimulator of angiogenesis
(C) both forms of fibroblast growth factor function via a single receptor
(D) they stimulate the growth of a variety of cells derived from the mesoderm and neuroectoderm

47. All of the following statements concerning platelet-derived growth factor (PDGF) are true EXCEPT

(A) PDGF is synthesized in megakaryocytes, endothelial, glial, and fibroblast cells
(B) PDGF stimulates growth of mesenchymal-derived cells, such as smooth muscle, glial, and fibroblasts
(C) PDGF acts via a monomer transmembrane receptor with intrinsic protein kinase activity
(D) PDGF is the major mitogen found in serum

48. All of the following statements regarding 1,25-$(OH)_2$D are true EXCEPT

(A) elevated parathyroid hormone (PTH) acts on renal tubules to increase the formation of 1,25-$(OH)_2$D
(B) 1,25-$(OH)_2$D is the biologically active form of vitamin D
(C) high levels of serum phosphate act on renal tubules to increase the formation of 1,25-$(OH)_2$D
(D) it increases the intestinal absorption of calcium and phosphate

49. All of the following statements regarding calcitonin are true EXCEPT

(A) calcitonin is synthesized in C cells located primarily in the thyroid gland
(B) calcitonin increases serum phosphate concentrations
(C) calcitonin lowers serum calcium concentrations
(D) calcitonin is synthesized as a large precursor protein

50. All of the following cranial nerves (CN) are commonly affected in tuberculous meningitis EXCEPT

(A) CN VI (abducens)
(B) CN X (vagus)
(C) CN III (oculomotor)
(D) CN XII (hypoglossal)

Questions 51–52

A 20-year-old disoriented woman presents to an emergency room with high fever, nausea, vomiting, watery diarrhea, hypotension, and diffuse erythema. A tentative diagnosis of toxic shock syndrome (TSS) is made.

51. Which of the following organisms is the etiologic agent of TSS?

(A) *Staphylococcus aureus*
(B) *S. epidermidis*
(C) *S. saprophyticus*
(D) *Pseudomonas aeruginosa*
(E) *Clostridium perfringens*

52. Which of the following conditions is the most likely complication of TSS?

(A) Kawasaki disease
(B) Toxic epidermal necrolysis
(C) Adult respiratory distress syndrome (ARDS)
(D) Infective endocarditis
(E) Thrombotic thrombocytopenic purpura

53. Which of the following drugs is a monoamine oxidase inhibitor?

(A) Trazodone
(B) Amitriptyline
(C) Phenelzine
(D) Fluoxetine
(E) Nortriptyline

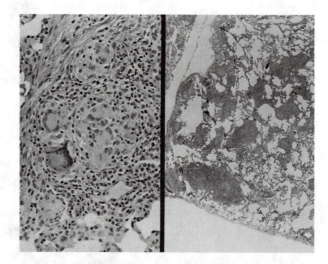

54. A 22-year-old man has shortness of breath and a cough. Chest radiographs (above) show mediastinal lymphadenopathy and bilateral pulmonary infiltrates. After bronchoalveolar lavage failed to grow microorganisms, a transbronchial biopsy was performed. The best diagnosis for this case is

(A) sarcoidosis
(B) Hodgkin's disease
(C) aspiration pneumonia
(D) alveolar proteinosis

55. Trypsin cleaves peptide bonds on the carboxyl side of which of the following amino acids?

(A) Arginine only
(B) Lysine only
(C) Either arginine or lysine
(D) Phenylalanine only
(E) Either phenylalanine or lysine

56. Which of the following is the drug of first choice in the treatment of absence seizures?

(A) Primidone
(B) Valproic acid
(C) Ethosuximide
(D) Phenytoin
(E) Carbamazepine

57. The primary screening method in the detection of AIDS carriers is

(A) virus isolation
(B) Western blot followed by immunoassay
(C) immunoassay followed by Western blot
(D) immunoassay for viral antigen
(E) DNA hybridization for viral RNA

58. If an area of the lung is not ventilated because of bronchial obstruction, the pulmonary capillary blood serving that area will have a Po_2 that is

(A) equal to atmospheric Po_2
(B) equal to mixed venous Po_2
(C) equal to normal systemic arterial Po_2
(D) higher than inspired Po_2
(E) lower than mixed venous Po_2

59. In a study designed to test the effect of a new knee brace on running speed, eight college athletes who wore the brace turned in the following times (in minutes) in a 1000-meter speed trial: 4, 2, 5, 2, 4, 5, 5, and 9. The mean finishing time for this group of subjects is

(A) 8.0 minutes
(B) 5.0 minutes
(C) 4.0 minutes
(D) 4.5 minutes
(E) none of the above

60. Which of the following statements describes the mechanism of action of lovastatin?

(A) It lowers serum cholesterol by causing an increase in uptake of low-density lipoprotein

(B) It strongly inhibits lipolysis in adipose tissue

(C) It causes a decrease in plasma triacylglycerol levels by increasing the activity of lipoprotein lipase

(D) It binds negatively charged bile acids in the small intestine

(E) It inhibits HMG CoA reductase, the enzyme controlling the rate-limiting step in cholesterol synthesis

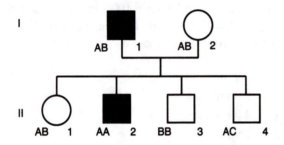

61. The accompanying figure shows the DNA typing for a family that has Huntington's disease (HD). I-1 has HD, as does his son II-2. Family members II-1, II-3, and II-4 want to know what their risk is of having inherited the abnormal gene. The family members have had DNA analysis with a marker approximately 2 million base pairs from the mutation causing HD. The risk for HD in II-1 is

(A) significantly increased

(B) significantly decreased

(C) mildly increased

(D) not changed because the markers are uninformative

(E) nonexistent

62. A hematologist is asked to see a 52-year-old man who has been hospitalized for 6 weeks because of various complications beginning with a bowel obstruction. The patient has had several operative procedures, one of which required transfusion of 3 units of packed red cells. He has been unable to eat and has been receiving broad-spectrum antibiotics almost continuously. Recently performed tests show a prolonged PT and PTT, which were corrected when the patient's plasma was mixed with an equal volume of normal plasma. Quantitative fibrinogen, thrombin time, and platelet count all are normal. The most likely cause of the coagulation abnormality is

(A) an acquired inhibitor

(B) dilution of coagulation factors secondary to transfusions

(C) vitamin K deficiency

(D) folate deficiency

(E) von Willebrand's disease

63. The anamnestic response is defined as

(A) a gradual rise in antibody titers

(B) true immunologic paralysis

(C) the prompt production of antibodies after a second exposure to antigen

(D) species-specific antibodies

(E) the lag in antibody production after initial antigen exposure

64. Which of the following drugs is a potassium-sparing diuretic?

(A) Furosemide

(B) Amiloride

(C) Acetazolamide

(D) Chlorothiazide

(E) Indapamide

	Respiratory Rate (breaths/min)	Tidal Volume (ml)	Change in Interpleural Pressure during Inspiration (cm H_2O)
Control	15	600	4
Experimental	25	600	10

65. Lung compliance in a 32-year-old female patient is studied. Data collected under control and experimental conditions are listed in the accompanying table. This patient's lung compliance during control and experimental conditions was

(A) unchanged
(B) 40 ml/breath and 24 ml/breath, respectively
(C) 150 ml/cm H_2O and 60 ml/cm H_2O, respectively
(D) 150 cm H_2O/ml and 60 cm H_2O/ml, respectively

66. A patient presenting with sweating, narrow pupils, a slow heart rate, and low blood pressure is most likely to have been poisoned with

(A) *Amanita muscaria*
(B) methyl alcohol
(C) chloroform
(D) heroin
(E) cocaine

67. A pediatrician wanted to determine the relationship between chronic otitis media in young children and parental history of such infections. From the records of a large pediatric practice, he identified 50 children between 1 and 3 years of age who had experienced at least three middle ear infections during the preceding year. Fifty children in the same age group, treated by the same practice for other illnesses, were also identified. The pediatrician interviewed the parents of subjects in both groups to determine their history of chronic otitis media as young children. Of the children with recurrent ear infections, 30 had a family history of chronic otitis media, compared with 20 of the children treated for other illnesses. This study is an example of

(A) a cross-sectional study
(B) a prospective cohort study
(C) a case–control study
(D) an experimental study
(E) a randomized controlled clinical trial

68. All of the following statements about somatostatin are true EXCEPT

(A) it is secreted by the hypothalamus
(B) it inhibits growth hormone release
(C) it inhibits thyroid-stimulating hormone
(D) it is secreted by the δ-pancreatic islet
(E) it stimulates the secretion of pepsin

69. All of the following statements about cortisol are true EXCEPT

(A) adrenocorticotropic hormone (ACTH) stimulates the synthesis and secretion of cortisol
(B) cortisol exerts positive feedback control on ACTH synthesis
(C) cortisol suppresses the formation of corticotropin-releasing hormone (CRH) in the hypothalamus
(D) secretion of cortisol exhibits a circadian rhythm

70. All of the following statements about eosinophils are true EXCEPT

(A) interleukin-5 directly stimulates the proliferation of eosinophils
(B) cells from the eosinophilic series are anucleated marrow cells
(C) eosinophils are found in the gastrointestinal tract
(D) eosinophils are found in the submucosa of the respiratory tract
(E) mature eosinophils contain major basic protein in large granules
(F) adrenal glucocorticoids cause a decrease in blood eosinophil levels

71. All of the following statements about basophils are true EXCEPT

(A) they are multilobed cells
(B) upon Wright's stain, they contain large metachromatic granules
(C) basophils are the least numerous of human white blood cells
(D) they are nucleated bone marrow cells
(E) they contain receptors for the Fc component of immunoglobulin A
(F) they contain the proteoglycan chondroitin sulfate

72. All of the following statements about mast cells are true EXCEPT

(A) upon Wright's stain, they contain large metachromatic granules
(B) mast cells contain the Charcot-Leyden crystal protein
(C) they are nucleated bone marrow cells
(D) they contain receptors for the Fc component of immunoglobulin E
(E) they contain the proteoglycan chondroitin sulfate

73. All of the following statements about natural killer cells are true EXCEPT

(A) they lyse targets on first contact without prior antigen sensitization
(B) they are descended from the lymphoid stem cells giving rise to T lymphocytes
(C) natural killer cells do not require thymic processing
(D) natural killer cells represent less than 10% of circulating blood lymphocytes
(E) they do not express surface T-cell antigen receptors

Color Plates (Use for questions 79-109 in Test V.)

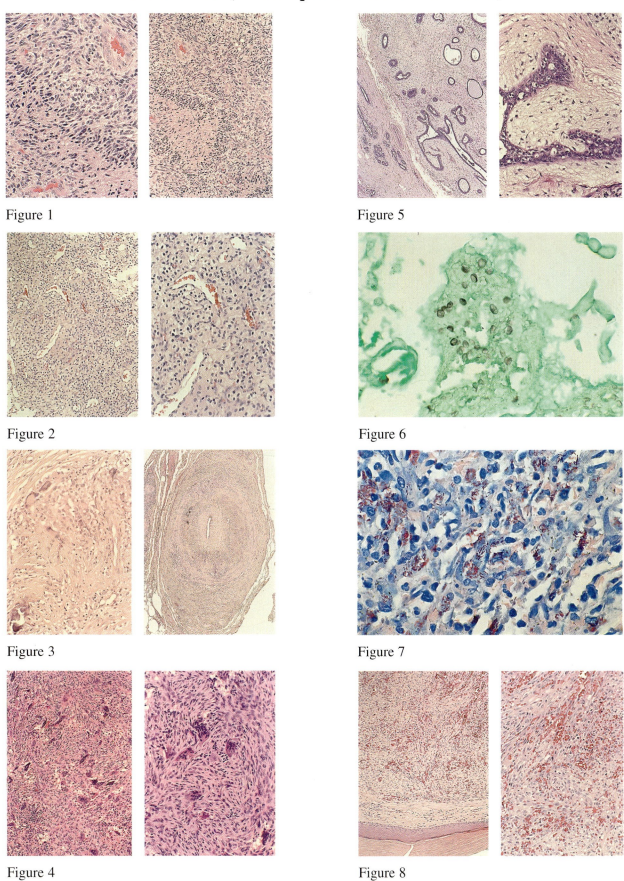

Figure 1

Figure 2

Figure 3

Figure 4

Figure 5

Figure 6

Figure 7

Figure 8

Color Plates (Use for questions 79-180 in Test V.)

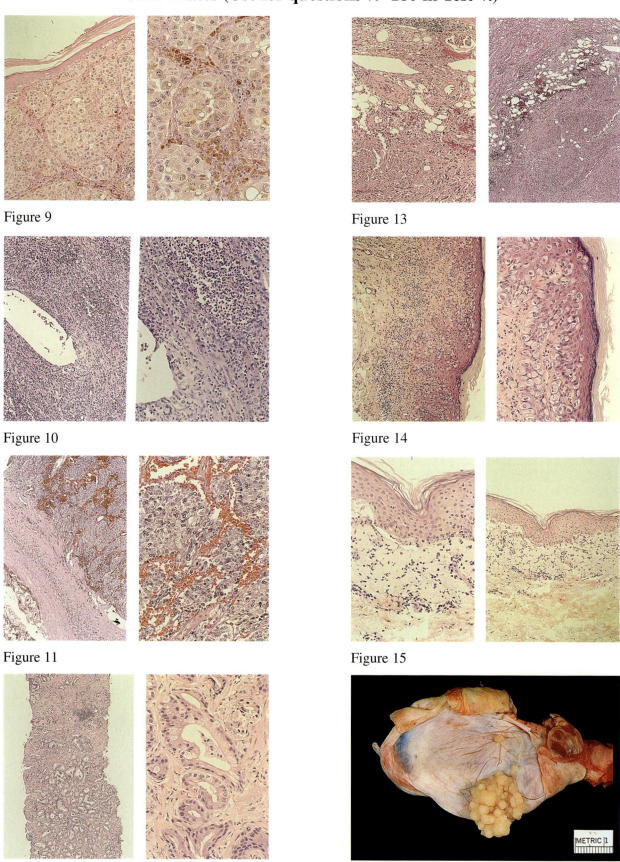

Figure 9

Figure 10

Figure 11

Figure 12

Figure 13

Figure 14

Figure 15

Figure 16

Color Plates (Use for questions 79-180 in Test V.)

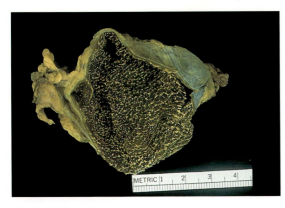

Figure 17

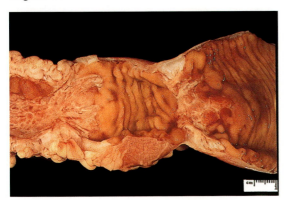

Figure 18

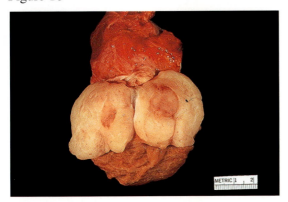

Figure 19

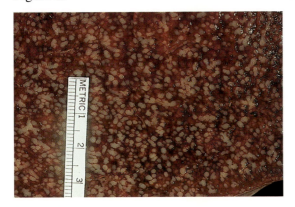

Figure 20

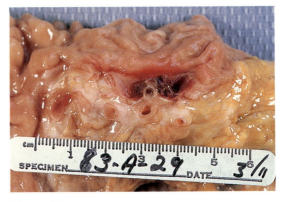

Figure 21

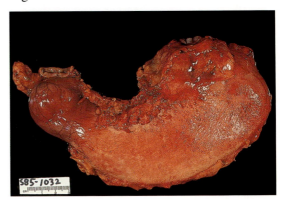

Figure 22

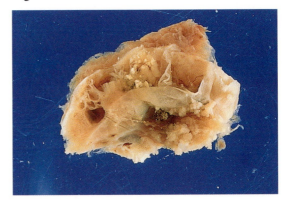

Figure 23

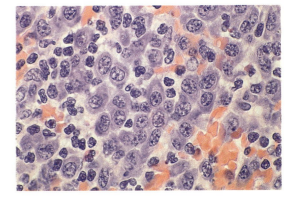

Figure 24

Color Plates (Use for questions 79-180 in Test V.)

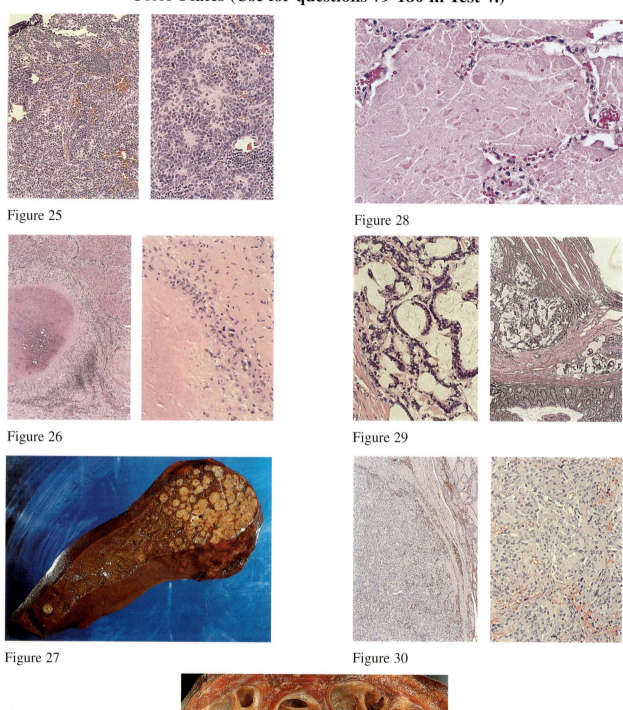

Figure 25

Figure 28

Figure 26

Figure 29

Figure 27

Figure 30

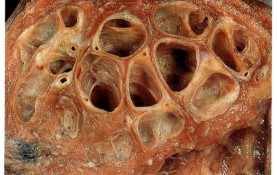

Figure 31

Color Plates (Use for questions 166-180 in Test V.)

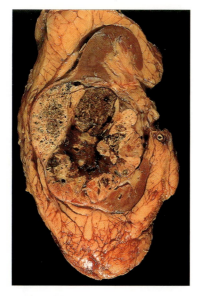

Figure 32

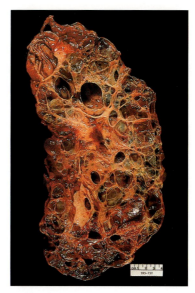

Figure 33

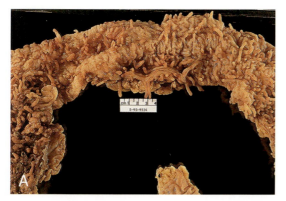

Figure 34A

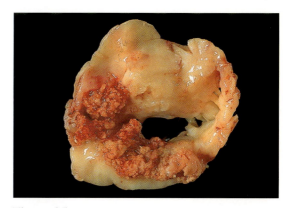

Figure 35

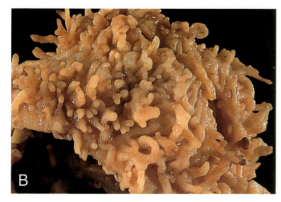

Figure 34B

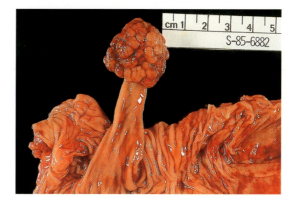

Figure 36

Color Plates (Use for questions 166-180 in Test V.)

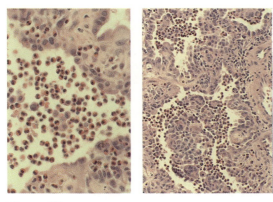

Figure 37

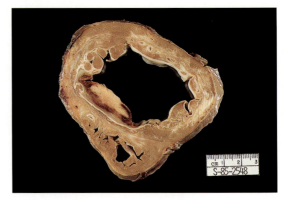

Figure 40

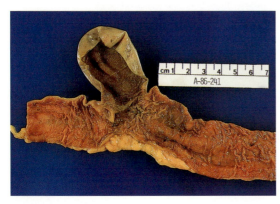

Figure 38

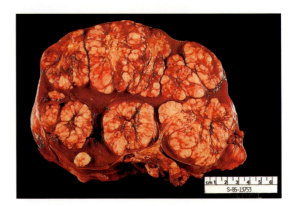

Figure 41

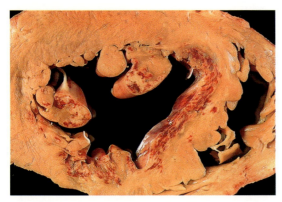

Figure 39

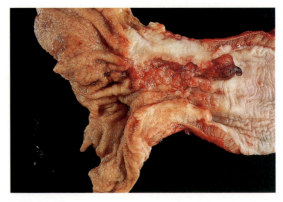

Figure 42

Color Plates (Use for questions 166-180 in Test V.)

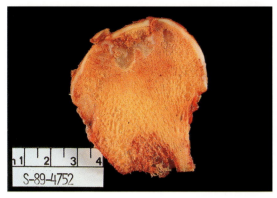

Figure 43

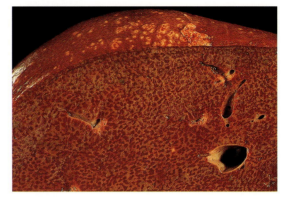

Figure 45

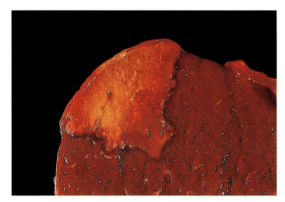

Figure 44

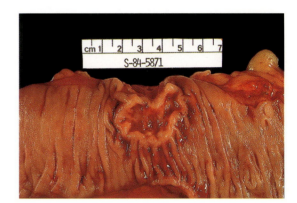

Figure 46

74. All of the following statements about the semicircular canals of the vestibuloacoustic apparatus are true EXCEPT

(A) semicircular canals contain endolymph, which is rich in potassium and low in sodium
(B) endolymph is separated from the perilymph by a continuous membrane
(C) the three semicircular canals are at 45-degree angles to one another
(D) loss of function of a canal can be compensated for by the respective paired canals

75. Which of the following glycogen storage diseases is caused by deficiency of an enzyme involved in glycogen synthesis?

(A) Type I: von Gierke's disease
(B) Type II: Pompe's disease
(C) Type III: Cori's disease
(D) Type IV: Andersen's disease
(E) Type V: McArdle's disease

76. The graded dose–response for drug *X* is depicted by *curve B* in the accompanying graph. The curve that best describes the response of the drug in the presence of a noncompetitive antagonist is

(A) *curve A*
(B) *curve C*
(C) *curve D*
(D) *curve E*

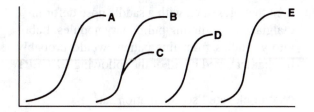

77. Chronic renal allograft rejection involves all of the following EXCEPT

(A) vascular sclerosis
(B) interstitial fibrosis
(C) tubular atrophy
(D) glomerulosclerosis
(E) tubulitis

78. All of the following are important functions of glutathione EXCEPT

(A) oxidation of hydrogen peroxide
(B) protection of lipids against auto-oxidation
(C) amino acid transport in the γ-glutamyl cycle
(D) reduction of lipids

Questions 79–109

Questions 79–109 refer to the color plates section in this test.

79. Figure 1 depicts a soft, hemorrhagic brain lesion that crosses the corpus callosum. Which of the following classifications best describes this lesion?

(A) Anaplastic astrocytoma
(B) Oligodendroglioma
(C) Meningioma
(D) Glioblastoma multiforme

80. The cerebellar tumor depicted in Figure 2 is frequently associated with which of the following conditions?

(A) Von Hippel-Lindau disease
(B) Pancreatic cysts
(C) Renal cell carcinoma
(D) Adenoma sebaceum

81. A patient presents with a throbbing right frontal headache. A cord-like, subcutaneous abnormality in the right side of the head is biopsied, and the tissue is depicted in Figure 3. The correct diagnosis is

(A) wallerian degeneration of a nerve
(B) temporal arteritis
(C) helminthic infection (i.e., cutaneous larval migrans)
(D) ganglion cysts

82. The multicystic tumor depicted in Figure 4 arose in the epiphysis of the femur and was associated with bone pain. The correct diagnosis is

(A) osteosarcoma
(B) chondroblastoma
(C) giant cell tumor
(D) chondromyxoid fibroma

83. The well circumscribed, 3-cm tumor of the breast depicted in Figure 5 bulged from the plane of cutting and had a gray, glistening appearance. The correct diagnosis is

(A) infiltrating ductal adenocarcinoma
(B) infiltrating lobular adenocarcinoma
(C) tubular adenoma
(D) fibroadenoma

84. A bone marrow transplant recipient developed progressive alveolar infiltrates visible on chest radiographs, and a lung biopsy was performed. The biopsied tissue, treated with silver stain, is depicted in Figure 6. The agent responsible for this infection is most likely

(A) *Pneumocystis carinii*
(B) *Cryptococcus neoformans*
(C) *Histoplasma capsulatum*
(D) *Nocardia asteroides*

85. The stain demonstrating the mycobacterial organisms depicted in Figure 7 is best classified as a

(A) Gram stain
(B) acid-fast stain
(C) silver stain
(D) mucicarmine stain

86. Figure 8 depicts tissue taken from a skin lesion of a 35-year-old homosexual man. Grossly, the lesion had a purple appearance. The correct diagnosis is

(A) Kaposi's sarcoma
(B) hemangiopericytoma
(C) bacillary angiomatosis
(D) arteriovenous malformation

87. Figure 9 depicts tissue biopsied from a raised brown nodule on the skin of a patient. The slide depicts cells containing

(A) iron
(B) lipofuscin
(C) melanin
(D) glycogen

88. Figure 10 depicts tissue biopsied from a patient that presented with a saddle nose deformity, otalgia, and cavitating pulmonary nodules. Laboratory studies from this patient would probably be characterized by all of the following EXCEPT

(A) an elevated sedimentation rate
(B) antineutrophil antibodies
(C) hematuria
(D) antimitochondrial antibodies

89. Which of the following statements does NOT describe the epidemiology of the adrenal neoplasm pictured in Figure 11?

(A) 10% are malignant
(B) 10% are pigmented
(C) 10% are bilateral
(D) 10% are familial

90. Figure 12 depicts tissue from a needle biopsy of the prostate. Which of the following conditions is demonstrated?

(A) Adenosis
(B) Nodular hyperplasia
(C) Adenocarcinoma
(D) Chronic prostatitis with glandular atrophy

91. The kidney tumor depicted in Figure 13 is sometimes associated with which one of the following conditions?

(A) Adrenal cortical carcinoma
(B) Tuberous sclerosis
(C) Seminomas of the testes
(D) Erythrocythemia

92. An elderly woman presented with an area of persistent ulceration of the nipple of the breast. The ulceration was unresponsive to multiple topical steroid creams, and a biopsy was performed. The biopsied tissue, depicted in Figure 14, is characteristic of which one of the following conditions?

(A) Seborrheic keratosis
(B) Verruca vulgaris
(C) Paget's disease
(D) Neurodermatitis

93. The skin lesion depicted in Figure 15 is characteristically associated with

(A) exposure to drugs
(B) vulvar abnormalities
(C) pruritus
(D) microabscesses

94. The cystic ovary depicted in Figure 16 exuded a clear yellow fluid upon opening. The inner lining demonstrates which one of the following conditions?

(A) Teratoma
(B) Serous intermediate tumor
(C) Tubal pregnancy
(D) High grade ovarian carcinoma

95. The gallbladder depicted in Figure 17 demonstrates which one of the following conditions?

(A) Vasculitis
(B) Invasive carcinoma
(C) Choledocholithiasis
(D) Cholesterolosis

96. Which of the following inflammatory bowel diseases is most likely represented in Figure 18?

(A) Crohn's disease
(B) Ulcerative colitis
(C) Ischemic colitis
(D) Pseudomembranous colitis

97. The testis depicted in Figure 19 demonstrates which one of the following conditions?

(A) Embryonal carcinoma
(B) Teratoma
(C) Seminoma
(D) Epidermal inclusion cyst

98. The section of spleen depicted in Figure 20 demonstrates which one of the following conditions?

(A) Gaucher's disease
(B) Acute myelogenous leukemia
(C) Hereditary spherocytosis
(D) Malignant lymphoma

99. The patient whose small intestine is depicted in Figure 21 most likely did NOT present with which one of the following symptoms?

(A) Stomach pain
(B) Malabsorption
(C) Heme-positive stools
(D) Hematemesis

100. The "leather bottle" stomach depicted in Figure 22 reflects involvement by

(A) Ménétrier's disease
(B) adenomatous polyps
(C) reflux esophagitis
(D) signet ring adenocarcinoma

101. The primary thyroid malignancy depicted in Figure 23 is best classified as

(A) papillary carcinoma
(B) follicular carcinoma
(C) medullary carcinoma
(D) insular carcinoma

102. The bone tumor depicted in Figure 24 is probably associated with which one of the following conditions?

(A) Von Willebrand's disease
(B) Von Hippel-Lindau disease
(C) Multiple myeloma
(D) Multiple osteochondromatosis

103. The kidney tumor depicted in Figure 25 is best classified as

(A) Wilms' tumor
(B) teratoma
(C) neuroblastoma
(D) hamartoma

104. The section of heart and valve depicted in Figure 26 demonstrates a histologic change that is typically associated with a clinical history of all of the following EXCEPT

(A) pancarditis
(B) chorea
(C) erythema multiforme
(D) migratory polyarthritis

105. The primary liver tumor depicted in Figure 27 is which one of the following?

(A) Hepatocellular carcinoma
(B) Epithelioid hemangioendothelioma
(C) Hepatic adenoma
(D) Cholangiocarcinoma
(E) None of the above

106. The lung depicted in Figure 28 is filled with eosinophilic granular material. This lung is most likely affected by which one of the following conditions?

(A) Pulmonary edema
(B) Bronchioloalveolar adenocarcinoma
(C) Alveolar proteinosis
(D) Aspirated food

107. Which one of the following classifications describes the annular lesion affecting the rectum that is depicted in Figure 29?

(A) Signet ring adenocarcinoma
(B) Mucinous adenocarcinoma
(C) Leiomyoma
(D) Solitary rectal ulcer syndrome with cystic change

108. The thyroid neoplasm depicted in Figure 30 is most likely associated with which one of the following conditions?

(A) Giant cell tumors of bone
(B) Wernicke's encephalopathy
(C) Pheochromocytoma
(D) Renal cysts

109. The hereditary lung disease depicted in Figure 31 is best classified as

(A) diffuse interstitial fibrosis, familial type
(B) cystic adenomatoid malformation
(C) cystic fibrosis
(D) congenital emphysema (alpha-1-antitrypsin deficiency)

110. Turner syndrome shows all of the following characteristics EXCEPT

(A) absence of menses
(B) numerous ovarian follicles
(C) webbed neck
(D) sterility
(E) 45, X karyotype

111. Renal agenesis can be associated with all of the following causes or clinical features EXCEPT

(A) abnormal allantoic regression
(B) failure of inductive interaction between the ureteric bud and the metanephric blastema
(C) an absence of symptoms
(D) oligohydramnios
(E) death soon after birth

112. All of the following statements correctly characterize the drug neostigmine EXCEPT

(A) it reversibly inhibits acetylcholinesterase
(B) it enters the central nervous system
(C) it is used to stimulate the bladder and gastrointestinal tract in order to prevent postoperative abdominal distention and urinary retention
(D) it is used as an antidote for tubocurarine poisoning
(E) it is used in the symptomatic treatment of myasthenia gravis

Questions 113–117

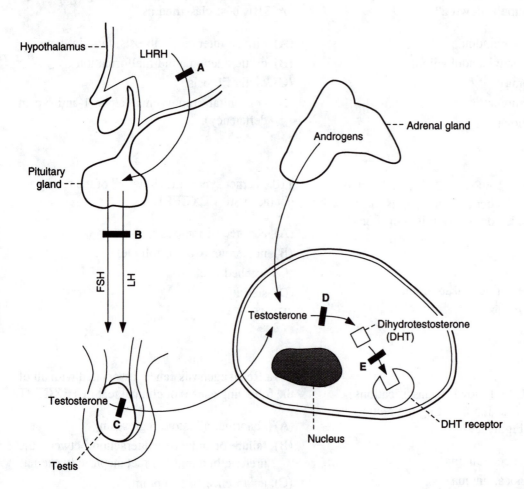

A 67-year-old man presents with urinary frequency, hesitancy in voiding, urinary retention, and nocturia. Digital rectal examination of this patient reveals an indurated nodule within the prostate; needle biopsy of this region verifies that the patient has carcinoma of the prostate. Computed tomographic evidence and pelvic lymph node biopsy sampling confirm the presence of metastatic disease. The patient receives androgen ablation therapy for management of the disease. The diagram represents potential pathways for pharmacologic intervention. Match the following pharmacologic agents with the appropriate lettered pathways they inhibit.

113. Leuprolide

114. Ketoconazole

115. Flutamide

116. Diethylstilbestrol

117. Cyproterone acetate

Questions 118–122

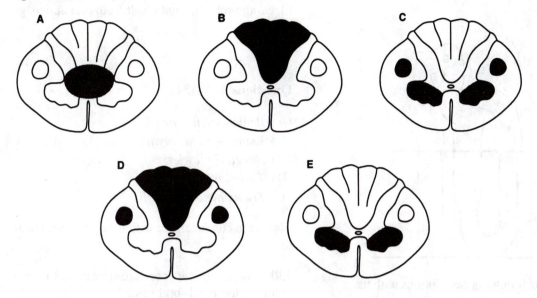

Match each of the depicted lesions (*gray areas*) of the spinal cord with the associated disorder.

118. Amyotrophic lateral sclerosis

119. Syringomyelia

120. Tabes dorsalis

121. Polio

122. Pernicious anemia

Questions 123–125

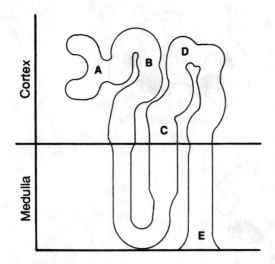

Match each of the following descriptions with the most appropriate lettered region of the nephron pictured.

123. Tubular fluid always is hyposmotic at this site

124. The TF/P ratio for glucose is 1:0 at this site

125. The urea concentration is highest at this site

Questions 126–129

(A) Warfarin
(B) Tissue-type plasminogen activator
(C) Vitamin K
(D) Erythropoietin
(E) Aspirin

Match the following descriptions with the appropriate pharmacologic agent that affects blood.

126. A coumarin anticoagulant that owes its action to its ability to antagonize the cofactor functions of vitamin K

127. A serine protease used to treat myocardial infarction by dissolving clots

128. A glycoprotein, normally produced by the kidney, that regulates red cell proliferation and differentiation in bone marrow

129. A compound that is administered to stem bleeding problems that result from oral anticoagulants

Questions 130–131

(A) *Pneumocystis carinii*
(B) *Entamoeba histolytica*
(C) *Naegleria fowleri*
(D) *Toxoplasma gondii*
(E) *Trichomonas vaginalis*

Match the characteristic with the appropriate protozoan.

130. Oocysts in cat feces are transmitted to humans by the fecal–oral route

131. Etiologic agent of fulminant meningoencephalitis causing death in 3–5 days

Questions 132–139

(A) Metabolic acidosis with normal anion gap
(B) Metabolic acidosis with increased anion gap
(C) Metabolic alkalosis
(D) Respiratory acidosis
(E) Respiratory alkalosis

Match each of the following conditions with the appropriate cause of acid–base disorder.

132. Vomiting

133. Diarrhea

134. Chronic renal failure

135. Diuretics

136. Narcotics

137. Methanol poisoning

138. Pulmonary fibrosis

139. Carbonic anhydrase inhibitors

140. All of the following are true statements about gonadotropins EXCEPT

(A) luteinizing hormone (LH) and follicle-stimulating hormone (FSH) are produced in the posterior lobe of the pituitary gland

(B) LH is released in pulses as a consequence of gonadotropin-releasing hormone (GnRH) stimulation

(C) Kallman's syndrome is characterized by defective GnRH production

(D) LH, FSH, or both are present in gonadotrophs

(E) serum LH and FSH are degraded and cleared by the liver and kidney

141. All of the following are clinical findings of an upper motor neuron lesion EXCEPT

(A) positive Babinski sign

(B) spasticity

(C) hyperreflexia

(D) fasciculations and fibrillations

(E) paralysis

Questions 142–143

(A) Coombs' test

(B) Ham's test

(C) Osmotic fragility test

(D) Heinz bodies test

(E) Donath-Landsteiner antibody test

For each of the hematologic disorders presented below, select the diagnostic test by which it can be identified.

142. Autoimmune hemolytic anemia with warm-type antibody

143. Glucose-6-phosphate dehydrogenase (G6PD) deficiency, Mediterranean type

Questions 144–145

(A) Allelic heterogeneity

(B) Variable expressivity

(C) Nonpenetrance

(D) Consanguinity

(E) Locus heterogeneity

Match each condition described below with the term of inheritance that best defines it.

144. A man shows no detectable signs of Marfan syndrome (an autosomal dominant disorder of connective tissue), although his father and two daughters are affected

145. In a family with myotonic dystrophy, the father has frontal balding, severe weakness, and cardiac arrhythmia; his sister has early-onset cataracts; and his child has electromyographic abnormalities

Questions 146–147

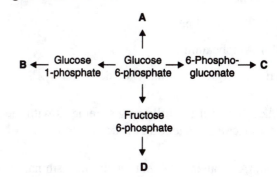

In the accompanying diagram, each letter represents a different metabolite that is derived from glucose 6-phosphate (G6P). Match each compound listed with the correct letter.

146. Glycogen

147. Pyruvate

Questions 148–149

(A) Liver diverticulum

(B) Midgut

(C) Dorsal pancreatic rudiment

(D) Cloaca

(E) Vitelline duct

Match each of the descriptions below with the embryonic structure that it best describes.

148. This structure forms the ileum and ascending colon

149. This structure forms endocrine and exocrine tissue as it grows into the septum transversum

Questions 150–154

(A) Doxapram

(B) Phencyclidine

(C) Theophylline

(D) Amphetamine

(E) Lysergic acid diethylamide

Match each of the following statements with the pharmacologic agent that it describes.

150. A popular treatment for chronic asthma, especially when asthmatic symptoms cannot be controlled with adrenergic agents

151. A weak inhibitor of monoamine oxidase (MAO). Its peripheral actions are mediated primarily by the cellular release of stored catecholamines

152. A respiratory stimulant used to treat acute ventilatory failure resulting from an overdose of central nervous system depressants such as barbiturates

153. A drug that shows serotonin agonist activity at presynaptic receptors in the midbrain

154. An inhibitor of the reuptake of dopamine, serotonin, and norepinephrine, and an analog of ketamine

Questions 155–159

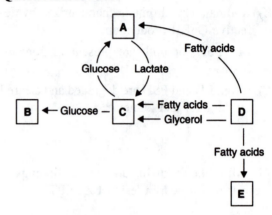

In this figure, the letters in each box correspond to organs or tissues in the postabsorptive state. Match the listed organs and tissues to the correct letter in each box in the figure.

155. Liver

156. Brain

157. Skeletal muscle

158. Heart muscle

159. Adipose tissue

Questions 160–162

(A) Cyclophosphamide

(B) 5-Fluorouracil

(C) Cytarabine

(D) Vincristine

(E) Mitomycin

Match each statement about drug action with the drug that is most likely to be associated with it.

160. In addition to being a natural product, this drug is an alkylating agent because it is reduced intracellularly and alkylates DNA.

161. This drug inhibits DNA polymerase and can be incorporated into DNA and RNA.

162. This drug is a phase-specific agent, producing metaphase arrest.

Questions 163–165

(A) Tuberoinfundibular tract
(B) Nigrostriatal tract
(C) Mesolimbic tract
(D) Medullary periventricular tract
(E) Incertohypothalamic tract

Neuroleptic drugs have been shown to block postsynaptic dopamine 2 (D_2) receptors. For each effect of neuroleptic drugs, select the dopaminergic tract thought to underlie the action.

163. Lactation

164. Parkinsonism

165. Antipsychotic effects

Questions 166–180

Questions 166–180 refer to the color plates section in this test.

166. The renal tumor shown in Figure 32 is associated with

(A) hypotension
(B) polycythemia
(C) cerebellar glioblastomas
(D) chromosome 12 abnormalities
(E) chromosome 17 abnormalities

167. The renal disease shown in Figure 33 is associated with which one of the following conditions?

(A) Angiomyolipomas of the kidney
(B) Transitional cell carcinoma of the urinary bladder
(C) Glioblastomas
(D) Intracranial berry aneurysms

168. The chronic inflammatory bowel disease shown in Figure 34 is best classified as

(A) ulcerative colitis
(B) collagenous colitis
(C) Crohn's disease
(D) ischemic colitis

169. The resected mitral valve in Figure 35 shows which one of the following?

(A) Calcific deposits
(B) Vegetations
(C) Mural thrombi
(D) Perforation

170. The lesion affecting the large intestine in Figure 36 is most likely a

(A) hyperplastic polyp
(B) tubular adenoma
(C) villous adenoma
(D) polypoid adenocarcinoma

171. Which one of the following conditions is represented in Figure 37, a photomicrograph of the lung?

(A) Asthma
(B) Klebsiella infections
(C) Cystic fibrosis
(D) Thermophilic actinomyces
(E) Pulmonary neoplasia

172. The best diagnosis for the process shown in Figure 38, which occurs approximately 30 cm from the ileocecal valve, is

(A) Meckel's diverticulum
(B) mucocoele
(C) intestinal reduplication
(D) false diverticulum

173. The change in Figure 39, a cross section of the heart, is

(A) artifactual
(B) 2 days old
(C) 6 days old
(D) 14 days old
(E) 48 days old
(F) 1 year old

174. The patient with the transversely transected heart at autopsy shown in Figure 40 most likely presented with which one of the following conditions?

(A) Pulmonary emboli
(B) Metastatic carcinoma
(C) Cerebral infarct
(D) Cardiac tamponade

175. The most likely cause of these abnormalities in the spleen shown in Figure 41 is

(A) histoplasmosis
(B) infarct
(C) lymphoma
(D) chronic congestion

176. This distal constricting lesion at the gastro-esophageal junction shown in Figure 42 is most likely caused by

(A) impacted food stuffs
(B) varices
(C) Barrett's esophagus
(D) Crohn's disease

177. The bony abnormality seen in the femur shown in Figure 43 is caused by which one of the following conditions?

(A) Metastatic carcinoma
(B) Sickle cell disease
(C) Gout
(D) Fracture
(E) Asthma

178. The spleen shown in Figure 44 demonstrates which one of the following abnormalities?

(A) Infarct
(B) Granuloma
(C) Angiosarcoma
(D) Hemangioma

179. The gross abnormality shown in the liver in Figure 45 most likely is caused by which one of the following conditions?

(A) Kaposi's sarcoma
(B) Massive hepatic necrosis
(C) Viral hepatitis
(D) Chronic congestion
(E) Testicular neoplasia

180. The most likely origin for the abnormality of the large intestine shown in Figure 46 is which one of the following conditions?

(A) Volvulus
(B) Prolapse
(C) Ulcerative colitis
(D) Colonic polyps

ANSWER KEY

1-C	31-A	61-D	91-B	121-E
2-B	32-B	62-C	92-C	122-D
3-A	33-D	63-C	93-A	123-C
4-A	34-A	64-B	94-B	124-A
5-C	35-C	65-C	95-D	125-E
6-F	36-C	66-A	96-A	126-A
7-A	37-D	67-C	97-C	127-B
8-A	38-A	68-E	98-D	128-D
9-A	39-B	69-B	99-B	129-C
10-E	40-C	70-B	100-D	130-D
11-B	41-E	71-E	101-A	131-C
12-B	42-D	72-E	102-C	132-C
13-B	43-D	73-B	103-C	133-A
14-B	44-D	74-C	104-C	134-B
15-F	45-B	75-D	105-D	135-C
16-E	46-A	76-B	106-C	136-D
17-C	47-C	77-E	107-B	137-B
18-E	48-C	78-D	108-C	138-D
19-C	49-B	79-D	109-C	139-A
20-B	50-B	80-A	110-B	140-A
21-B	51-A	81-B	111-A	141-D
22-B	52-C	82-C	112-B	142-A
23-C	53-C	83-D	113-B	143-D
24-A	54-A	84-A	114-C	144-C
25-D	55-C	85-B	115-E	145-B
26-B	56-C	86-A	116-A	146-B
27-A	57-C	87-C	117-E	147-D
28-C	58-B	88-D	118-C	148-B
29-E	59-D	89-B	119-A	149-A
30-C	60-E	90-C	120-B	150-C

151-D	157-A	163-A	169-B	175-C
152-A	158-E	164-B	170-B	176-C
153-E	159-D	165-C	171-A	177-B
154-B	160-E	166-B	172-A	178-A
155-C	161-C	167-D	173-B	179-D
156-B	162-D	168-A	174-C	180-D

ANSWERS AND EXPLANATIONS

1. The answer is C. *(Microbiology; Neisseria meningitidis)*
Neisseria meningitidis is the most common cause of meningitis in adolescents and young adults, and is the most likely cause of epidemics of meningitis. *Haemophilus influenzae* type B is responsible for 70% of cases of bacterial meningitis in children between the ages of 2 months and 5 years. *Escherichia coli* and *Streptococcus agalactiae* cause meningitis in neonates who acquire the infection during passage through the birth canal. *S. pneumoniae* predominates in adults over 40 years of age, in the very young, and in trauma patients.

2. The answer is B. *(Microbiology; Neisseria meningitidis)*
M protein is an antiphagocytic surface component that is not produced by meningococci. Virulence factors produced by meningococci include the polysaccharide capsule, which enables the organism to resist phagocytosis by leukocytes; endotoxin, which causes fever, shock, and other pathophysiologic changes; and IgA protease, which cleaves secretory IgA, allowing the bacteria to attach to the membranes of the upper respiratory tract.

3. The answer is A. *(Hematology; myeloproliferative disorders)*
Polycythemia vera is distinct from spurious (relative) polycythemia, which results from a decrease in the plasma volume rather than a true increase in red blood cell mass. Polycythemia vera is characterized by splenomegaly and an increased production of all myeloid elements. Polycythemia vera is generally dominated by an increase in hemoglobin concentration and produces symptoms associated with increased blood volume and blood viscosity. The hematocrit and total blood volume may become markedly elevated, which is a consequence of the sharply increased red blood cell mass.

4. The answer is A. *(Hematology; myeloproliferative disorders)*
Essential thrombocytosis is dominated clinically by a markedly elevated platelet count. Patients with essential thrombocytosis may present with erythromyalgia, venous or arterial thromboses, or spontaneous bleeding. Splenomegaly is seen in two-thirds of the patients but is generally modest. In vitro platelet function tests typically reveal an abnormality in platelet aggregation in response to epinephrine. Bone marrow examination reveals large numbers of hyperploid megakaryocytes.

5. The answer is C. *(Physiology; endocrine system)*
The action of glucagon is catabolic, decreasing glucose, fatty acid, and amino acid storage. Glucagon is a polypeptide hormone secreted by the α-cells of the pancreatic islets. It activates glycogen phosphorylase via cyclic adenosine monophosphate (cAMP) to increase glycogenolysis and gluconeogenesis.

6. The answer is F. *(Physiology; endocrine system)*
Amino acids stimulate glucagon secretion. The effects of glucose on glucagon secretion are reciprocal to those of insulin secretion in that hyperglycemia suppresses the secretion of glucagon. Insulin is a potent inhibitor of glucagon secretion and acts within the pancreatic islet. Catecholamines and glucocorticoids, such as cortisol, inhibit glucagon secretion. Somatostatin is secreted by the δ-pancreatic islet and inhibits secretion by the other three pancreatic islets, including the α-pancreatic islets, which secrete glucagon.

7. The answer is A. *(Physiology; endocrine system)*
Glucagon stimulates insulin secretion and acts within the pancreatic islet. The effects of glucose on insulin secretion are reciprocal to those of glucagon secretion in that hypoglycemia suppresses the secretion of insulin. Somatostatin is secreted by the δ-pancreatic islet and inhibits secretion by the other three pancreatic islets, including the β-pancreatic islets, which secrete insulin. Sympathetic stimulation via the splanchnic nerve inhibits insulin release as can be seen by the administration of epinephrine, which inhibits insulin release. Salicylates are effective hypoglycemic agents because they inhibit the conversion of arachidonic acid to prostaglandins, which have been shown to inhibit insulin release.

8. The answer is A. *(Pharmacology; central nervous system stimulants)*
Amphetamine's mechanism of action is mediated through the cellular release of stored catecholamines. Cocaine blocks the reuptake of norepinephrine, serotonin, and dopamine by presynaptic fibers. Reserpine blocks the ability of adrenergic neurons to transport norepinephrine from the cytoplasm into storage vesicles. Guanethidine blocks the release of stored norepinephrine. Isoproterenol acts directly on α- or β-adrenergic receptors, producing effects similar to those that occur following stimulation of sympathetic nerves. Unlike isoproterenol, amphetamine's agonist activity is indirect.

9. The answer is A. *(Microbiology; spirochete,* Borrelia burgdorferi)
Three genera of spirochetes can cause human infections: *Treponema,* which causes syphilis; *Leptospira,* which causes leptospirosis; and *Borrelia*, which causes a number of tick-borne diseases. Lyme disease is caused by the *Borrelia burgdorferi* spirochete. Upon Giemsa stain, *B. burgdorferi* appear as large, loosely coiled organisms. Lyme disease is treated with tetracycline or amoxicillin for acute infections, and penicillin for chronic infections. Dengue fever is caused by the dengue virus, and yellow fever is caused by the yellow fever virus; both of these viruses are transmitted by the *Aedes aegypti* mosquito. Typhus is caused by the bacteria *Rickettsia typhi* and is transmitted by flea bites.

10. The answer is E. *(Hematology; myeloproliferative disorders)*
Enlargement of the liver resulting from agnogenic myeloid metaplasia does not occur in the absence of splenomegaly. Agnogenic myeloid metaplasia is characterized by the tendency of the neoplastic stem cells to lodge and grow in multiple sites outside the marrow. Typically, there is progressive splenomegaly, the gradual replacement of marrow elements by fibrosis, progressive anemia, and variable changes in the number of granulocytes and platelets. The peripheral blood smear usually shows dramatic changes in red blood cell and platelet morphology. Basophilic stippling is prominent, and bizarre red cells (including teardrop poikilocytes, fragmented cells, and nucleated red cells) are common, as are giant platelet forms.

11. The answer is B. *(Pathology; cancer; medulloblastoma)*
Medulloblastoma is the most common malignant tumor of the brain in children. Its most frequent site of occurrence is the cerebellum. Meningioma is a primary brain tumor arising from the meninges. It is the second most common primary intracranial neoplasm. Squamous cell carcinoma is a tumor composed of cells that resemble cells of the squamous layer of the epidermis. Schwannoma is a neural sheath tumor. Its most frequent site of occurrence is the eighth cranial nerve, and it is the third most common primary intracranial neoplasm.

12. The answer is B. *(Hematology; primary bone marrow disorders)*
Myelophthisic anemia suppresses erythropoiesis because the marrow is infiltrated with tumor, granulomas, or fibrosis. The term aplastic anemia should be restricted to conditions in which an acellular or markedly hypocellular bone marrow results in pancytopenia. A peripheral blood smear usually demonstrates pancytopenia. Aplastic anemia is thought to be caused by injury or destruction of a common pluripotential stem cell affecting all subsequent cell populations. Fanconi's anemia, the most common constitutional aplastic anemia, is an autosomal recessively inherited disease usually appearing in childhood. Several cases of aplastic anemia have been reported following infectious hepatitis.

13. The answer is B. *(Pathology; neuroanatomy; Bell's palsy)*
Bell's palsy is a demyelinating viral inflammatory disease that is the most common ailment of cranial nerve (CN) VII. Onset usually is preceded by viral prodrome and is acute. Duration is approximately 5 days. Findings are unilateral, and can involve loss of facial expression, widened palpebral fissure, diminished taste, difficulty in chewing, hypesthesia in one or more branches of CN V, and hyperacusis.

14. The answer is B. *(Pathology; microbiology; infective endocarditis)*
While *Streptococcus pneumoniae* is the most common cause of infective endocarditis in general (65% of cases), *Staphylococcus aureus* is the most common agent in narcotic endocarditis (more than 50% of cases).

15. The answer is F. *(Hematology; primary bone marrow disorders)*
In pure red cell anemia, granulopoiesis and megakaryocytopoiesis remain normal. Pure red cell anemia involves a selective failure in the production of erythroid elements in the bone marrow. Severe reticulocytopenia exists, and the bone marrow is characterized by an absence of any erythroid precursors in otherwise normal cellular elements. Blackfan-Diamond syndrome, a rare chronic constitutional red blood cell aplasia, may appear in infants from the time of birth to the age of 2 years. In the rare acquired form of pure red cell anemia, one-third of the patients have thymomas.

16. The answer is E. *(Pathology; anatomy; splenic disorders)*
Splenectomy is indicated for a number of disorders such as primary splenic tumors (rare), metastatic disease (particularly Hodgkin's and non-Hodgkin's lymphoma), splenic abscesses (rare), hereditary spherocytosis, bleeding esophageal varices that are caused by splenic vein thrombosis, and massive splenic trauma. (Attempts should be made to salvage the spleen from minor trauma.) A number of other conditions are relative indications for splenectomy, such as hemolytic anemias, idiopathic thrombocytopenic purpura that is refractory to steroid treatment, and thrombotic thrombocytopenic purpura. Hereditary spherocytosis is always treated with splenectomy because the spleen is the only site of destruction of these abnormal red blood cells. Hereditary spherocytosis is a genetic disorder that is transmitted in an autosomal dominant fashion and is characterized by thick and rigid erythrocyte cell membranes. These cells are sequestered in the splenic pulp, leading to glucose deprivation, adenoxyltransferase depletion, and cell lysis. Splenectomy in these patients is curative, and postsplenectomy blood smears characteristically demonstrate the presence of Howell-Jolly bodies (nuclear remnants of red blood cells). Schistosomiasis may cause splenic rupture due to secondary splenomegaly, but splenectomy is not indicated. Rather, therapy for schistosomiasis is directed toward eradication of the fluke (e.g., praziquantel treatment).

17. The answer is C. *(Microbiology; herpes virus)*
Epstein-Barr virus is present in about half of AIDS-associated non-Hodgkin's lymphomas; tumor cells carry Epstein-Barr virus DNA and express viral proteins. Herpes simplex virus type 1 can cause gingivostomatitis, recurrent herpes labialis, keratoconjunctivitis, and encephalitis. Herpes simplex virus type 2 causes genital herpes, neonatal herpes, and aseptic meningitis. Cytomegalovirus causes cytomegalic inclusion disease in neonates and can cause pneumonia in immunocompromised patients. Neither type of herpes simplex viruses nor cytomegalovirus have been implicated in the etiology of AIDS-associated non-Hodgkin's lymphoma.

18. The answer is E. *(Neuroanatomy; spinal tap)*
The physician can insert a needle into the subarachnoid space to withdraw cerebrospinal fluid (CSF) for diagnostic analysis. The needle tip passes successively through the epidural space, the dura mater, the subdural space, and the arachnoid membrane. The CSF is between the arachnoid membrane and the pia mater, the innermost of the three meningeal sheaths.

19. The answer is C. *(Microbiology;* Actinomyces israelii)
Actinomyces israelii is an anaerobe that is a part of the normal flora of the oral cavity. It may invade tissues after local trauma, forming filaments surrounded by areas of inflammation. Hard, yellow granules, called ''sulfur granules,'' are formed in pus in the area of infection. *Yersinia pestis* causes plague. The most common form of plague is bubonic plague, also known as black plague. *Pasteurella multocida* causes wound infections associated with cat and dog bites. *Francisella tularensis* causes tularemia. None of these organisms are associated with the extrusion of ''sulfur granules'' from a draining wound.

20. The answer is B. *(Biochemistry; tubular loss of glucose)*
When the filtered load of a substance exceeds the Tm for that substance, the excess is not reabsorbed, and, thus, proportionately more of the substance is excreted. In this example, the Tm for glucose (*B* on the curve) is determined by extrapolation of the linear portion of the curve (from *C* to *D*) to the abscissa (filtered load). The splay of the curve (from *A* to *C*) indicates that all of the tubules are not uniform in length, number of glucose transporters, or renal threshold.

21. The answer is B. *(Pathology; brain tumor)*
Most primary brain tumors can be divided into three classes: gliomas, meningiomas, and neural sheath tumors. Gliomas are the most frequent type of primary brain tumor and include astrocytomas, ependymomas, oligodendrogliomas, and medulloblastomas. Meningiomas are the next most common type of primary brain tumor. Neural sheath tumors are less common. Squamous cell carcinoma is a tumor composed of cells that resemble cells of the squamous layer of the epidermis. It is the second most common skin cancer. Osteosarcoma arises from primitive mesenchymal cells and is a malignant primary bone tumor. Neither osteosarcoma nor squamous cell carcinoma are a type of primary brain tumor.

22. The answer is B. *(Histology; distal lung components)*
Alveoli (*C*) in the lungs are lined by an epithelium that contains type I cells and type II cells. Type I cells (*A*) are extremely attenuated squamous cells specialized for gas exchange. Type II cells (*B*) are rounded cells containing phospholipid-rich multilamellar bodies of secretion product (surfactant). Alveoli are adjacent to capillaries, which are filled with erythrocytes (*D*). Macrophages are abundant in alveoli, where they phagocytose and destroy inspired debris such as bacteria.

23. The answer is C. *(Microbiology; hepatitis)*
Hepatitis C virus is the most common cause of post-transfusion hepatitis. Hepatitis A is easily spread by the oral/fecal route and is often called infectious hepatitis. Hepatitis B is contracted by contact with blood or other bodily secretions from infected individuals and is often called serum hepatitis. Hepatitis D requires hepatitis B surface antigen (HBsAg) to become pathogenic, and transmission is closely linked with the transmission of the hepatitis B virus. Hepatitis E is a major cause of enterically transmitted hepatitis. It is the most common cause of water-borne epidemics in Asia, Africa, India, and Mexico but is uncommon in the United States.

24. The answer is A. *(Pathology; microbiology; infective endocarditis)*
Intravenous drug abuse–associated infective endocarditis usually has vegetation that is acute and is located on right-sided valves. Most other cases of infective endocarditis are associated with left-sided valves.

25. The answer is D. *(Pharmacology; pulmonary tuberculosis)*
Multiple-drug therapy is used to prevent the emergence of drug-resistant mutants during the 6–9 month duration of treatment. Isoniazid (a bactericidal drug), rifampin, and pyrazinamide are the drugs used to treat most patients with pulmonary tuberculosis. Ethambutol is added initially for those who have AIDS with central nervous system involvement, dissemination, or suspected isoniazid resistance. Penicillin is not effective against the tubercle bacillus.

26–27. The answers are: 26-B, 27-A. *(Neuroanatomy; carpal tunnel syndrome)*
Carpal tunnel syndrome results from compression of the median nerve as it passes deep within tissue to the flexor retinaculum. The median nerve originates in the brachial plexus by the joining of the lateral and medial cords. The nerves labeled *A, C, D,* and *E* are the musculocutaneous nerve, medial cutaneous nerve of the forearm, ulnar nerve, and radial nerve, respectively.

Carpal tunnel syndrome can be managed by wrist splinting and local injection of a long-acting adrenocorticosteroid preparation. Severe or persistent disease, however, may necessitate surgical section of the carpal ligament. Forced flexion of the wrist is contraindicated as therapy, but it is useful for diagnosis because it exacerbates the condition (i.e., Tinel sign).

28. The answer is C. *(Physiology; action potentials)*
An action potential is a self-propagating spike response (all-or-none response) unique to excitable tissues. Voltage-sensitive sodium-ion (Na^+) and potassium-ion (K^+) channels distinct from the K^+–Na^+ leak channels underlie the molecular basis of the action potential. Compared to local potentials, action potentials have a large amplitude (70–110 mv) and a brief duration (1–10 msec).

29. The answer is E. *(Anatomy; auscultation of heart sounds)*
When routinely auscultating the heart, one should listen in the second intercostal space along the right sternal border, in the second through the fifth intercostal spaces along the left sternal border, and at the apex. Locations for auscultations of heart valve sounds are: aortic valve (*point A*), pulmonary valve (*point B*), tricuspid valve (*points C and D*), and mitral valve (*point E*).

30. The answer is C. *(Biochemistry; enzymes)*
Hydrolase adds water to break a bond. This is called hydrolysis. Aldolase cleaves a carbon–carbon bond to create an aldehyde group. Dehydrogenase removes hydrogen atoms from its substrate. Hydratase adds water to a carbon–carbon bond without breaking the bond or, conversely, removing water to create a double bond. Isomerase converts between *cis* and *trans* isomers, D and L isomers, or aldose and ketose. Esterase hydrolyzes ester linkages to form an acid and an alcohol.

31. The answer is A. *(Immunology; congenital immunodeficiencies)*
Thymic aplasia (DiGeorge's syndrome) involves a T-cell deficiency caused by failure of both the thymus and parathyroids to develop properly because of a defect in the third and fourth pharyngeal pouches. Ataxia–telangiectasia is an autosomal recessive disease that appears by 2 years of age and involves a combined B- and T-cell deficiency. X-linked hypogammaglobulinemia (Bruton's agammaglobulinemia) is a B-cell deficiency caused by a mutation in the gene encoding a tyrosine kinase. Hereditary angioedema is a complement deficiency caused by an uncommon autosomal dominant disease that results from a deficiency of C1 esterase inhibitor. Chronic granulomatous disease is a phagocyte deficiency caused by an X-linked disease in most cases (in some patients the disease is autosomal) that appears by the age of 2 years.

32. The answer is B. *(Physiology; aortic insufficiency)*
Aortic insufficiency (regurgitation) is accentuated by leaning forward while seated, exhaling completely, and holding one's breath. The Valsalva maneuver, in which the patient expires against a closed glottis while seated, is useful for diagnosing mitral valve prolapse. Having the patient roll into the left lateral decubitis position aids diagnosis of mitral stenosis, as does brief exercise. Standing decreases ventricular filling and increases the murmurs associated with mitral valve prolapse and idiopathic hypertrophic subaortic stenosis (IHSS). Squatting increases the murmurs associated with mitral and aortic valve insufficiencies.

33. The answer is D. *(Microbiology; syphilis)*
Treponema pallidum causes syphilis. This organism multiplies at the site of inoculation and then spreads widely via the bloodstream. No toxins or virulence factors are known for this organism. *Trichomonas vaginalis* causes trichomoniasis, *Trichinella spiralis* causes trichinosis, *Trypanosoma cruzi* causes Chagas disease, and *Trypanosoma gambiense* causes sleeping sickness.

34. The answer is A. *(Pathology; cardiac tamponade)*
Hypotension, elevated systemic venous pressure, and small quiet heart make up the classic triad of physical findings in cardiac tamponade in patients with penetrating cardiac injuries, aortic dissection, or intrapericardial rupture of aortic or cardiac aneurysms. These are uncommon causes today. The most common causes of cardiac tamponade are currently neoplastic disease and idiopathic pericarditis, followed by acute myocardial infarction and uremia.

35. The answer is C. *(Pharmacology; antianginal drugs)*
This patient has two medical problems: asthma and chronic stable angina. Available antianginal drugs are classified as (1) nitrates, (2) β-blockers, and 3) calcium-channel blockers. The presence of asthma constitutes a contraindication for the use of noncardioselective β-blockers. β-adrenergic antagonists can induce acute episodes of asthma, and regularly produce airway obstruction in asthmatics. Even the selective β-adrenergic antagonists do this, particularly at high doses. At low doses, cardioselective β-blockers may be used with caution. Calcium-channel blockers and nitrates can also be used to treat this patient.

36. The answer is B. *(Immunology; congenital immunodeficiencies)*
Hyper-IgM syndrome and chronic mucocutaneous candidiasis also involve T-cell deficiency. Hyper-IgM syndrome results from a defect in helper T cells in a surface protein that interacts with the CD40 antigen on the B-cell surface. Chronic mucocutaneous candidiasis results from a T-cell deficiency specifically for *Candida albicans;* other T- and B-cell functions are normal. Wiskott-Aldrich syndrome also involves a combined B- and T-cell deficiency where B cell numbers are normal but antibody responses to polysaccharide antigens are absent and T-cell deficiencies are variable. Chediak-Higashi syndrome and leukocyte adhesion deficiency syndrome are phagocyte deficiencies. Chediak-Higashi syndrome is an autosomal recessive disease while leukocyte adhesion deficiency syndrome is caused by a defective adhesion (LFA-1) protein on the surface of their phagocytes.

37. The answer is D. *(Biochemistry; vitamins)*
Intestinal bacteria synthesize vitamin K. The main dietary source of vitamin K is green leafy vegetables. Vitamin E, vitamin A, vitamin C, and niacin are not synthesized by intestinal bacteria. The main dietary source for vitamin E is vegetable oils. The main dietary sources for vitamin C are fresh fruit and vegetables. The main dietary sources for vitamin A are liver, whole milk, fish oils, and eggs. The main dietary sources for niacin are meat and nuts.

38. The answer is A. *(Neuroanatomy; reciprocal innervation)*
Reciprocal innervation is most accurately described as inhibition of the antagonist muscle when the agonist muscle is activated. For example, flexor muscles are inhibited during an extension. Reciprocal innervation allows extensor contraction to occur without interference from the flexor muscles that are being stretched during the movement. Under normal circumstances, stretching the flexors will elicit a stretch reflex leading to contraction of the flexor muscles. Inhibiting the alpha motoneurons that innervate the flexor muscles prevents the stretch reflex from interfering with the extension. Reciprocal innervation characterizes all movements, not just extension.

39. The answer is B. *(Neuroanatomy; areas of the brain)*
Although the pathology in many parts of the central nervous system (CNS) can impair problem solving, damage to the frontal lobes is the major cause of dysfunctional intellectual processes. The frontal lobe is the area of the brain that is most involved with the ability to solve problems.

40. The answer is C. *(Biochemistry; acid–base disorders)*
Metabolic acidosis is defined as a below normal level of serum bicarbonate. Respiratory alkalosis is defined as a below normal partial pressure of carbon dioxide (P_{CO_2}). The respiratory alkalosis represents an attempt by the lungs to compensate for the metabolic acidosis. If the lungs do not compensate, the blood pH is even lower.

41. The answer is E. *(Pharmacology; syphilis)*
Treponema pallidum, which causes syphilis, is susceptible to penicillin G. Amphotericin B and ketoconazole have antifungal activity and do not affect *T. pallidum.* Rifampin inhibits mRNA synthesis, and trimethoprim inhibits nucleotide synthesis. Neither of these drugs is needed to treat syphilis.

42. The answer is D. *(Biochemistry, protein structure)*
Lysine is a basic amino acid that is positively charged at normal pH. Glutamic acid and aspartic acid are acidic amino acids that are negatively charged at normal pH. Proline and isoleucine are amino acids with nonpolar side chains. They have no net charge at normal pH.

43. The answer is D. *(Pathology; renal transplant)*
Transplant recipients are at risk for a variety of opportunistic infections. Epstein-Barr virus (EBV) infection with posttransplant lymphoproliferative disorder (PTLD) is one such complication. In PTLD, the immunosuppressed host suffers from primary or reactivated infection. EBV exerts a proliferative pressure on the B cells. In the absence of regulatory T-cell control, B cells may expand and develop clonal populations (i.e., lymphoma).

44. The answer is D. *(Immunology; tumor necrosis factor)*
Tumor necrosis factor (TNF) is a growth inhibitor that inhibits lipoprotein lipase, induction of interferon-β_2, and stimulation of fibroblast growth. It is produced by macrophages in response to endotoxin and is structurally related to lymphotoxin. TNF also causes a cachectic, or wasting, state and causes necrosis in tumors, hence its name.

45. The answer is B. *(Biochemistry; growth factors)*
Tumor growth factor-β inhibits the growth of epithelial, mesenchymal, and immunologic cells. It is synthesized from a larger inactive precursor and must be activated by release from this latent complex. The major source of tumor growth factor-β is platelets, although it is synthesized by other cells as well.

46. The answer is A. *(Biochemistry; growth factors)*
In contrast to the ubiquitous nature of basic fibroblast growth factor, acidic fibroblast growth factor is synthesized in the brain and retina, not in many cells and tissues. Fibroblast growth factor is the major identified stimulator of angiogenesis, and it stimulates the growth of a variety of cells derived from the mesoderm and neuroectoderm. Also, both basic and acidic fibroblast growth factor function via a single receptor.

47. The answer is C. *(Biochemistry; growth factors)*
Platelet-derived growth factor (PDGF) binds to and causes PDGF receptors, which have intrinsic protein kinase activity, to dimerize; thus, PDGF acts through a dimerized transmembrane receptor and not a monomer. PDGF is synthesized in megakaryocytes, as well as endothelial, glial, and fibroblast cells. It stimulates growth of mesenchymal-derived cells, such as smooth muscle, glial cells, and fibroblasts. PDGF is also the major mitogen found in serum. It is stored in α-granules in platelets and is released during platelet release action.

48. The answer is C. *(Physiology; endocrinology; mineral metabolism)*
Low serum phosphate levels and elevated parathyroid hormone (PTH) act on renal tubules to increase the formation of 1,25-$(OH)_2$D (dihydroxyvitamin D). Dihydroxyvitamin D is the biologically active form of vitamin D, and the last enzymatic step in its formation is the principal site of regulation. This biologically active form of vitamin D also causes an increase in the intestinal absorption of calcium and phosphate so that serum calcium concentrations return to normal.

49. The answer is B. *(Physiology; endocrinology; mineral metabolism)*
Calcitonin's two major biologic effects are to lower both serum calcium and serum phosphate concentrations. Calcitonin is synthesized in C cells of neuroendocrine origin, which are located primarily in the thyroid gland and, to a lesser extent, in the thymus.

50. The answer is B. *(Microbiology; tuberculous meningitis)*
Cranial nerves (CN) III, VI, VII, and VIII are the cranial nerves most commonly affected in tuberculous meningitis, and not CN X. CN III and VI functions are involved in moving the eye, constricting the pupils, and accommodation. CN VII functions are involved in moving the face, tasting, salivation, and crying. CN XII functions are involved in moving the tongue.

51–52. The answers are: 51-A, 52-C. *(Microbiology; toxic shock syndrome)*
Toxic shock syndrome (TSS) is caused by a toxin [toxic shock syndrome toxin-1, (TSST-1)] produced by *Staphylococcus aureus*. Although this disease is usually associated with tampon use in menstruating women, it can be associated with nonmenstruating women and men (most frequently as a postoperative wound infection). Recurrent episodes may occur in menstruating women with a frequency of up to 30%.

Treatment consists of administration of a β-lactamase–resistant antistaphylococcal agent, in conjunction with management of shock and renal failure. The death rate from the disease is about 3%, and death most frequently results from refractory hypotension associated with adult respiratory distress syndrome (ARDS), with or without the concomitant occurrence of disseminated intravascular coagulation. Differential diagnosis for TSS includes Kawasaki syndrome, toxic epidermal necrolysis, Rocky Mountain spotted fever, meningococcemia, streptococcal scarlet fever, leptospirosis, and rubella.

53. The answer is C. *(Pharmacology; antidepressants)*
All clinically useful antidepressant drugs potentiate, either directly or indirectly, the actions of norepinephrine, dopamine, and serotonin in the brain. Phenelzine is a monoamine oxidase inhibitor. Trazodone and fluoxetine are serotonin uptake inhibitors. Amitriptyline and nortriptyline are tricyclic antidepressants that block norepinephrine, dopamine, and serotonin uptake into the neuron. All tricyclic antidepressants have similar therapeutic efficacy, and the choice of drug depends on the patient's tolerance of side effects and on the duration of action required.

54. The answer is A. *(Pathology; sarcoidosis)*
The clinical presentation in this case is characteristic of sarcoidosis—a young individual, often African American, with persistent symptoms and lymph node enlargement (''potato nodes'') with lung infiltrates. Fever, skin nodules, or iritis is often coexistent. The figure shows small nodules in the lung parenchyma (*left*), which at higher magnification are shown to be small non-necrotizing granulomas (*right*). There granulomas are composed of giant cells, epithelioid histocytes, and lymphocytes (usually T cells).

55. The answer is C. *(Biochemistry; peptidases)*
Trypsin cleaves peptide bonds on the carboxyl side of either arginine or lysine. The fragments produced are called tryptic peptides. Chymotrypsins can cleave peptide bonds on the carboxyl side of phenylalanine, tyrosine, tryptophan, and other bulky residues. Trypsin and chymotrypsin are both pancreatic enzymes.

56. The answer is C. *(Pharmacology; anti-epileptics)*
Ethosuximide is the drug of first choice in the treatment of absence seizures. Primidone is used in the treatment of partial and tonic–clonic seizures. Although valproic acid diminishes absence seizures, it is the drug of second choice because of its hepatotoxic potential. Phenytoin is not effective for absence seizures. In fact, seizures may worsen if a patient with absence seizures is treated with this drug. Carbamazepine is highly effective for all partial seizures and is often the drug of first choice for partial seizures.

57. The answer is C. *(Microbiology; AIDS screening)*
The current method of screening patients for evidence of infection by human immune deficiency virus (HIV) is to perform an immunoassay on their serum to detect the presence of antibodies to HIV. Immunoassay-positive sera are retested using a Western blot to confirm that the reactive antibodies are HIV specific. Currently, the direct detection of the HIV virus itself either by cultivation or by immunoassay is not reliable. The detection of viral RNA in blood looks promising in some cases but is still not enough to be anything more than a research tool.

58. The answer is B. *(Physiology; respiration)*
If an area of lung is not ventilated, there can be no gas exchange in that region. The pulmonary capillary blood serving that region will not equilibrate with alveolar Po_2, but will have a Po_2 equal to that of mixed venous blood.

59. The answer is D. *(Statistics)*
The mean finishing time ($\overline{Y}$) for this group of eight subjects is the arithmetic average of their individual times:

$$\overline{Y} = \Sigma \ Y_i/n$$
$$= 36/8$$
$$= 4.5 \ \text{minutes}$$

60. The answer is E. *(Pharmacology; antihyperlipidemic drugs)*
Lovastatin's mechanism of action is to inhibit HMG CoA reductase, the enzyme that controls the rate-limiting step in cholesterol synthesis. Probucol lowers serum cholesterol by causing an increase in the uptake of low-density lipoprotein. Niacin acts to reduce plasma cholesterol by strongly inhibiting lipolysis in adipose tissue. Clofibrate causes a decrease in plasma triacylglycerol levels by increasing the activity of lipoprotein lipase. Cholestyramine and colestipol reduce serum cholesterol by binding negatively charged bile acids in the small intestine.

61. The answer is D. *(Genetics; DNA typing for Huntington's disease)*
Evidently, the gene causing Huntington's disease (HD) in this family is inherited together with the A marker. However, II-1 has AB markers, and it is impossible to know whether she has inherited the A or the B marker from the affected father; therefore, her risk of having inherited the HD gene has not changed.

62. The answer is C. *(Hematology; coagulation abnormality)*
This patient's coagulation abnormality most likely is the result of vitamin K deficiency. A prolonged period of malnutrition with administration of broad-spectrum antibiotics is a common combination that frequently results in vitamin K deficiency. Correction of the prothrombin time (PT) and partial thromboplastin time (PTT) in the mixing test excludes the possibility of an acquired inhibitor. Coagulation factors would not have been diluted by the transfusion of 3 units of packed red cells; only massive transfusions might cause

this effect. Folate deficiency is not associated with abnormalities of the coagulation cascade, and von Willebrand's disease does not affect the PT.

63. The answer is C. *(Immunology; anamnestic response)*

The anamnestic response, or anamnesis, is also called the booster response, memory response, or secondary immune response. It is characterized by the prompt production of high levels of antibody (i.e., a rapid rise in antibody titers) following secondary exposure to antigen. Anamnesis is caused by the presence of B and T memory cells that were induced during the primary immune response. Immune paralysis is the inability to mount a response to a normally immunogenic substance.

64. The answer is B. *(Pharmacology; diuretics)*

Potassium-sparing diuretics act in the distal tubule to inhibit sodium reabsorption, potassium secretion, and hydrogen secretion. Amiloride blocks sodium transport channels, resulting in a decrease in sodium–potassium exchange, and, as a result, acts as a potassium-sparing diuretic. Furosemide is one of the loop diuretics; their major site of action is the ascending loop of Henle. Acetazolamide is a carbonic anhydrase inhibitor that acts in the proximal tubular epithelial cells. Chlorothiazide and indapamide are thiazide diuretics that act on the distal tubule.

65. The answer is C. (Physiology; lung compliance)

Lung compliance is calculated as the change in volume per unit change in distending pressure. Because alveolar pressure is zero at the beginning and end of inspiration, the transmural (distending) pressure for the lung is zero minus the interpleural pressure. Only the change in interpleural pressure between the beginning and end of inspiration is given. This difference divided into the tidal volume gives the lung compliance during dynamic conditions, or 150 and 60 ml/cm H_2O. Note that compliance is expressed as volume/pressure.

66. The answer is A. *(Pharmacology;* Amanita muscaria *poisoning)*

The mushroom *Amanita muscaria* causes muscarinic effects on the nervous system (i.e., sweating, narrow pupils, a slow heart rate, and low blood pressure); however, in contrast to poisoning with *Amanita phalloides*, patients usually recover without more severe problems. Methyl alcohol may cause blindness, and chloroform causes liver toxicity, which would not produce this patient's symptoms. Nasal bleeding secondary to perforation is a common presentation of cocaine sniffers. In heroin overdose, shortness of breath due to pulmonary edema is often seen.

67. The answer is C. *(Biostatistics; case–control study)*

This study uses a case–control study design; that is, it begins with the selection of cases of the disease in question (chronic otitis media) and disease-free controls. Both groups are then followed backward in time to determine exposure to the putative risk factor (parental history of ear infections).

68. The answer is E. *(Physiology; endocrine system)*

Somatostatin has been shown to occur throughout the gastrointestinal tract and acts as an inhibitor of many gastrointestinal functions, such as pepsin release. Somatostatin is secreted by the δ-pancreatic islet and inhibits secretion by the other three pancreatic islets, including the β-pancreatic islets, which secrete insulin, and the α-pancreatic islet, which secretes glucagon. Somatostatin is a tetradecapeptide that is secreted by the hypothalamus, and it is a potent inhibitor of the release of growth hormone and thyroid-stimulating hormone from the pituitary gland.

69. The answer is B. *(Physiology; endocrine system)*

Cortisol (but not other adrenal steroids) exerts negative feedback control on the synthesis of adrenocorticotropic hormone (ACTH). Cortisol does this by suppressing transcription of the ACTH gene in the pituitary and by suppressing the formation of corticotropin-releasing hormone (CRH) in the hypothalamus. Production of cortisol and androgen precursors is controlled by ACTH. Secretion of ACTH and of cortisol exhibits a circadian rhythm, with the highest rate occurring in the morning upon awakening.

70. The answer is B. *(Hematology; eosinophils)*
Cells from the eosinophilic series are nucleated marrow cells that mature in the bone marrow. The cytokine interleukin-5 directly stimulates the proliferation and maturation of eosinophils. Mature eosinophils are primarily found in the skin, and the respiratory, gastrointestinal, and genitourinary tracts. A material called major basic protein (MBP) makes up approximately 50% of the mass of the large granules found in eosinophils. Administration of adrenal glucocorticoids causes eosinophil levels to fall within 2 hours.

71. The answer is E. *(Hematology; basophils)*
The basophil surface membrane contains receptors for the Fc fragment of immunoglobulin E (IgE). In acute allergic reactions, a specific antigen reacts with IgE bound to basophils, and the basophils release their granule contents, which include histamines. Basophils are multilobed cells that on Wright's stain contain large metachromatic granules. They are the least numerous of human white blood cells, comprising only 0.1% of nucleated bone marrow cells. Basophils also contain the proteoglycan chondroitin sulfate; however, its function within the basophil is not known presently.

72. The answer is E. *(Hematology; mast cells)*
Mast cells contain the proteoglycan heparin, not the proteoglycan chondroitin sulfate. The mast cells' surface membrane contains receptors for the Fc fragment of immunoglobulin E (IgE). In immediate hypersensitivity reactions, a specific antigen reacts with IgE bound to mast cells, and the mast cells release their granule contents, which include histamines, prostaglandins, and other inflammatory agents. Mast cells are round and, on Wright's stain, contain large metachromatic granules.

73. The answer is B. *(Hematology; natural killer cells)*
The ontogeny of natural killer cells is unclear, but it is known from bone marrow transplant studies that they do not descend from lymphoid stem cells giving rise to T and B lymphocytes. Unlike cytotoxic T cells, natural killer cells lyse targets on first contact without prior antigen sensitization. Natural killer cells also do not require thymic processing and do not express surface T-cell antigen receptors. These cells represent less than 10% of circulating blood lymphocytes.

74. The answer is C. *(Physiology; semicircular canals)*
Each semicircular canal constitutes a circular "mill race" in one plane, and the three planes are at right angles to one another, not 45-degree angles. Semicircular canals also contain endolymph, which is rich in potassium and low in sodium. The endolymph is separated from the perilymph by a continuous membrane. If for any reason the function of one canal is lost, the respective paired canal apparently furnishes enough information for central integration processes in the brain stem to compensate for that loss.

75. The answer is D. *(Biochemistry; glycogen storage disease)*
Type IV glycogen storage disease (Andersen's disease) is caused by a deficiency of glycosyl 4:6 transferase. This enzyme creates branches in glycogen by transferring a chain of 5–8 glucosyl residues from the nonreducing end of the glycogen chain (breaking an α-1,4 bond) to another residue on the chain, attaching the two by an α-1,6 linkage. The resulting new nonreducing end—as well as the old reducing end from which the chain came—can now be further elongated by glycogen synthase.

Pompe's disease is caused by a deficiency of lysosomal α-glucosidase enzyme. McArdle's disease is caused by a deficiency of skeletal muscle glycogen phosphorylase. Cori's disease is caused by amylo-1,6-glucosidase deficiency. Von Gierke's disease is caused by a deficiency of glucose-6-phosphatase. All of these enzymes are involved in glycogen degradation.

76. The answer is B. *(Pharmacology; pharmacokinetics)*
A noncompetitive antagonist changes the maximal response at high concentration, represented by *curve C*. *Curve A* represents a shift of the dose–response curve to the left, indicating an apparent increase in the potency of drug *X*, which would not occur in the presence of a noncompetitive antagonist. *Curve D* represents the effects of a partial agonist on the drug's dose response. A partial agonist causes less of a response than does a full agonist by itself and acts as a weak competitive antagonist, shifting the dose–response curve to the right. *Curve E* represents a shift of dose response to the right, which occurs in the presence of a competitive antagonist.

77. The answer is E. *(Immunology; chronic renal allograft rejection)*
Active lymphocytic inflammation in tubules ("tubulitis") is a feature of acute cellular rejection. Chronic rejection of the kidney is represented by sclerosing pathology. In the vessels, chronic rejection shows vascular sclerosis; in the interstitium, fibrosis and tubular atrophy; and in the glomerular compartment, glomerulosclerosis.

78. The answer is D. *(Biochemistry; enzymes; glutathione)*
Glutathione is a tripeptide-thiol that is present at high concentrations in most cells. Glutathione and glutathione reductase participate in the formation of the correct disulfide bonds of many proteins and polypeptide hormones. Also, a number of potentially toxic electrophilic xenobiotics are conjugated to the nucleophilic glutathione. Glutathione is therefore an important defense mechanism against certain toxic compounds. Another important function of glutathione is the oxidation of hydrogen peroxide. Glutathione also protects lipids against auto-oxidation, but it does not reduce lipids. Glutathione is important in amino acid transport in the γ-glutamyl cycle.

79. The answer is D. *(Pathology; gliomas of the brain)*
Gliomas of the brain are divided into low grade (e.g., benign astrocytoma), intermediate grade (e.g., anaplastic astrocytoma), and high grade variants. The most aggressive form is glioblastoma multiforme. Glioblastomas characteristically involve the cerebral hemispheres. They frequently cross the corpus callosum, and they present with progressive neurologic defects. Glioblastomas are characterized by a variegated gross appearance with zones of yellow necrosis, hemorrhage, and cystic change. Microscopically, the characteristic features of glioblastoma include cellular anaplasia, necrosis with pseudopalisading, and a dramatic endothelial proliferation, in which small clusters of capillaries called "glomeruli" are formed. These tumors are extremely aggressive. Mortality within the first year after diagnosis is high.

80. The answer is A. *(Pathology; cerebellar tumors)*
Hemangioblastomas are well circumscribed, frequently cystic lesions that classically involve the cerebellar hemispheres. A tumor is characterized by an anastomosing network of capillary-sized vessels associated with a proliferation of stromal cells—large, polygonal cells with abundant pale cytoplasm rich in fat. The nuclei of these cells are small but display significant pleomorphism. The histogenesis of these cells is uncertain. Many researchers believe they are related to endothelial cells and pericytes. Others believe they derive from precursors of macrophages and monocytes.

81. The answer is B. *(Pathology; vasculitis)*
This slide shows the classic histologic features of temporal arteritis. The cylindrical structure is a large artery with focal areas of granulomatous inflammation in its wall. Giant cells are visible surrounding fragments of the mural elastic lamina. It is important to recognize temporal arteritis because it may be associated with coexistent involvment of the retinal artery and may lead to blindness if not treated appropriately.

82. The answer is C. *(Pathology; bone neoplasms)*
Giant cell tumors of bone classically involve the epiphysis of the long bones and are associated with a lytic, expansile lesion occasionally associated with bone sclerosis. Grossly, these tumors are hemorrhagic. Microscopically, as shown in this photograph, they are characterized by two main cellular components: stromal cells and giant cells. The stromal cells probably are the neoplastic component. These tumors may be locally aggressive, and metastasis is rare. If completely excised or curetted, however, they usually have a benign clinical course.

83. The answer is D. *(Pathology; breast tumors)*
Fibroadenomas of the breast are a common benign lesion affecting the breast of young to middle-aged women. They are characterized by a proliferation of stromal cells associated with a similar proliferation of ductal cells. Visible at low magnification are slit-like spaces, some having a leaf-like configuration, that are lined by hyperplastic ductal epithelium with a surrounding cellular stroma. Malignant lesions that mimic fibroadenomas include phyllodes tumors.

84. The answer is A. *(Microbiology; pneumocystis pneumonia)*
Silver stains are used in tissue sections to identify fungi and some protozoa. This silver stain demonstrates black cysts of *Pneumocystis carinii* with a green background counterstain. Infection by *P. carinii* is characterized by cup-shaped cysts, 4–7 mm in diameter, frequently with a dot-like, black accentuation of the cyst wall visible upon silver staining. These cysts resemble schistocytes in red blood cell smears. Pneumocystis pneumonia is characterized by alveolar filling by a frothy, honeycomb exudate, and silver staining highlights the cysts present within this proteinaceous matrix. Recent studies suggest *Pneumocystis* species are more closely related to fungi than protozoa.

85. The answer is B. *(Microbiology; staining techniques)*
Acid-fast stains are used to demonstrate mycobacteria. They characteristically stain the mycolic acids within the cell wall of the mycobacteria, resulting in a red, beaded appearance of the bacillary forms. This has led to the colloquial designation of mycobacterial agents as "red snappers." Acid-fast stain morphology of the bacteria cannot discriminate between different species. Variations of this stain can also demonstrate *Nocardia* and *Rhodococcus* species.

86. The answer is A. *(Pathology; vascular sarcomas)*
Kaposi's sarcoma is a presumed neoplasm that occurs frequently in the HIV-positive homosexual population. It is characterized by a proliferation of spindle cells thought to be of endothelial derivation. The spindle cell proliferation is associated with abundant extravasated red blood cells, which account for the purple discoloration of the overlying skin. Sporadic forms of Kaposi's sarcoma do occur on the distal extremities of non–HIV-positive patients, particularly older individuals.

87. The answer is C. *(Histology; melanoma)*
This slide demonstrates the classic morphology of a nodular melanoma. There is a proliferation of malignant cells with nuclei of variable size. Several of these nuclei have intranuclear cytoplasmic invaginations, and most of the nuclei have prominent eosinophilic nucleoli, a characteristic of malignant melanoma. The most

striking aspect of this neoplastic proliferation is the presence of brown pigment within the cytoplasm of the cells and within melanophages in the adjacent stroma. This pigment is melanin that is produced by the neoplastic cells themselves. It accounts for the brown appearance of these nodules in the skin, and also accounts for the brown appearance of metastatic lesions in the viscera.

88. The answer is D. *(Pathology; Wegener's granulomatosis)*
This case history is classic for Wegener's granulomatosis, which, in its typical presentation, combines necrotizing granulomas and vasculitis of the upper and lower respiratory tracts with glomerulonephritis. The slide demonstrates areas of necrosis with a palisaded histiocytic reaction and a segmental vasculitis. This triad of histologic abnormalities characterizes Wegener's granulomatosis. The presence of cytoplasmic antineutrophil antibodies has recently been noted to be very sensitive for the diagnosis of Wegener's granulomatosis. These autoantibodies are directed at proteinase 3, which is a serine protease.

89. The answer is B. *(Pathology; pheochromocytoma)*
This slide demonstrates classic features of a pheochromocytoma, a neoplasm derived from the cells of the adrenal medulla. Pheochromocytoma is frequently accompanied by a history of facial flushing and systemic hypertension. These clinical symptoms are caused by the production of norepinephrine by the tumor cells. Pheochromocytomas are almost always brown or mahogany-colored neoplasms. They have been labeled the ''10% tumor''—roughly 10% are malignant, 10% are bilateral, 10% are familial, and 10% are extra-adrenal. Histologically, they are characterized by a grape-like clustering of the neoplastic cells, accompanied by a delicate, branching vascular network. The cells contain granular cytoplasmic contents that correspond to neurosecretory granules containing norepinephrine.

90. The answer is C. *(Pathology; prostatic adenocarcinoma)*
The histologic appearance of prostatic adenocarcinoma is characterized by small glands in a tightly compact architectural configuration. The glands are lined by a single cell, and the cells contain large nuclei with eosinophilic nucleoli. Occasional intraluminal crystalloids are also seen. Prostatic adenocarcinomas are frequently associated with elevation of serum prostate-specific antigen and prostatic acid phosphatase.

91. The answer is B. *(Pathology; renal neoplasm)*
This slide shows a rare renal neoplasm called an angiomyolipoma. Angiomyolipomas contain adipose tissue, a vascular component composed of tortuous blood vessels that frequently lack elastic laminae, and a smooth muscle component that consists of spindle-shaped smooth muscle cells that exhibit pleomorphism and mitotic activity. The presence of fat and the prominent vascularity make the tumor readily recognizable on ultrasonographic and computed tomography (CT) scan examination. In approximately one third of patients, neurologic and/or cutaneous findings suggestive of tuberous sclerosis are also present. These tumors can cause massive and sometimes fatal hemorrhage and may be locally aggressive. For the most part, however, they behave in a benign fashion.

92. The answer is C. *(Pathology; Paget's disease)*
This slide shows a proliferation of pleomorphic malignant cells along the dermal–epidermal junction. These neoplastic cells have abundant clear cytoplasm and contain cytoplasmic mucin. They derive from the apocrine sweat glands of the breast, or may derive from intraductal carcinomas of the breast whose cells have migrated up the major ducts to involve the overlying skin. Paget's disease of the nipple is a common cause of nonhealing ulcers of the nipple, and clinical concern for this malignant condition should precipitate biopsy.

93. The answer is A. *(Pathology; drug-induced disease)*
The skin biopsy shows features of erythema multiforme, which frequently manifests as a generalized vesicobullous disease. Vesicobullous lesions are evaluated microscopically by observing the level of the plane of separation of the epidermis and by identifying the type of cellular infiltrates. This slide demonstrates a subepidermal split between the epidermis and dermis, which raises three major histologic differential diagnoses: bullous pemphigoid, dermatitis herpetiformis, and erythema multiforme. The features most characteristic of erythema multiforme are subepidermal edema, abundant nuclear dust in the dermis, and a superficial perivascular lymphoplasmacytic infiltrate. It is frequently associated with exposure to drugs and is presumably a result of immune complexes depositing along the basement membrane.

94. The answer is B. *(Pathology; ovarian tumors)*
Serous intermediate tumors of the ovary are characterized grossly by a cauliflower-like proliferation of cytologically bland cuboidal cells, frequently accompanied by psammoma bodies. These papillary lesions are noninvasive and have an excellent prognosis in contrast to invasive serous carcinomas of the ovary. They occur in young women and may recur in the abdomen, causing small bowel obstruction.

95. The answer is D. *(Pathology; biliary/hepatic pathology)*
The gross appearance of this gallbladder, indicative of cholesterolosis, is characteristic of the so-called "strawberry gallbladder." This term derives from the mixture of bile-stained epithelium, which appears green in the slide, admixed with biliary epithelium that overlies submucosal aggregates of fat-laden macrophages. These aggregated macrophages impart the yellow reticulated appearance to the gallbladder mucosa. Cholesterolosis is frequently associated with gallstones and is common in individuals who are obese or have hypercholesterolemia.

96. The answer is A. *(Pathology; Crohn's disease)*
Crohn's disease is characterized by segmental involvement of the bowel, which contrasts with diffuse involvement of the bowel characteristic of ulcerative colitis. In this photograph, two strictures surrounding apparently normal mucosa are identifiable. These strictures account for the frequent presence of fistulae between portions of the small and large bowel and reflect the transmural thickening and inflammation of the bowel wall, a common feature in Crohn's disease.

97. The answer is C. *(Pathology; testicular/germ cell tumor)*
This testis contains a gray, well-circumscribed fleshy tumor nodule. The differential diagnosis of such white or gray tumor nodules in the testes is limited to two possibilities: seminoma and malignant lymphoma. Seminomas tend to be sharply circumscribed, whereas lymphomas are diffuse infiltrative neoplasms. The sharp circumscription of this lesion should lead to a diagnosis of seminoma. The absence of hemorrhage and necrosis argues against embryonal carcinoma.

98. The answer is D. *(Pathology; lymphomas involving the spleen)*
Malignant lymphomas that involve the splenic parenchyma characteristically cause either large white tumor nodules or small, pinpoint white tumor nodules. In most instances, low grade malignant lymphomas cause small (2–4 mm in diameter) white nodules, such as those depicted in this slide. These nodules replace the normal malpighian bodies of the spleen. Low grade lymphomas include small cleaved cell lymphoma and small lymphocytic lymphoma. As a general rule, large white nodules in the spleen represent either Hodgkin disease or high grade large cell lymphoma.

99. The answer is B. *(Pathology; duodenal ulcer)*
This photograph shows the classic features of a duodenal ulcer, which has eroded into an artery. This resulted in massive gastric bleeding and hematemesis. Exsanguination occurred and this specimen was obtained at autopsy. The gross features are those of a well-circumscribed ulcer with a sharp margin and a hemorrhagic base. In the base, the hemorrhagic exudate appears to be eroding into a small blood vessel that contains a brown thrombus.

100. The answer is D. *(Pathology; adenocarcinoma of the stomach)*
The gross appearance of a "leather bottle" stomach is caused by a diffuse infiltration of the wall of the stomach by a poorly differentiated adenocarcinoma, usually a signet ring adenocarcinoma. This accounts for the gray, plaque-like thickening of the stomach wall apparent in this photograph. The adjacent prepyloric stomach appears to have a a glistening serosal surface. Signet ring adenocarcinomas diffusely infiltrate through the wall of the stomach, invade the serosal adipose tissue and omentum, and have a very poor prognosis.

101. The answer is A. *(Pathology; papillary carcinoma)*
This portion of thyroid demonstrates multiple cysts containing a papillary proliferation of cellular elements. This papillary architecture is characteristic of a form of adenocarcinoma of the thyroid gland termed papillary carcinoma. In this neoplastic proliferation, cuboidal cells line fibrovascular cores and are associated with psammomatous calcifications. These tumors are usually cystic and exude an oily hemorrhagic fluid.

102. The answer is C. *(Pathology; bone tumor)*
This bone tumor is characterized by a proliferation of cells with a cartwheel-like arrangement of chromatin and abundant eccentric cytoplasm. Adjacent to the nucleus is a clear space, called a hof, that corresponds to the Golgi apparatus. This histologic appearance is characteristic of a plasma cell tumor of bone. Plasmacytomas of bone are frequently associated with systemic plasma cell disorders such as multiple myeloma. Systemic involvement can be confirmed by demonstrating a monoclonal spike in serum protein electrophoresis or by identifying multiple lytic bone lesions by radiographic study.

103. The answer is C. *(Pathology; neuroblastoma)*
Neuroblastomas are among the most frequent tumors of early childhood. They are derived from neural crest cells, and neoplastic cells may produce epinephrine or norepinephrine. The neoplastic cells have a salt-and-pepper chromatin and frequently form rosettes, with the background matrix having a fibrillary or a reticular appearance. This appearance derives from the tendency of these cells to produce abortive neurites or dendritic connections.

104. The answer is C. *(Pathology; rheumatic carditis)*
This section of heart shows the characteristic Aschoff nodule of rheumatic carditis. These nodules have a central region of degenerated collagen surrounded by histiocytes. Many of these histiocytes are multinucleated or have central stripes of chromatin within their nucleus (hence the term "caterpillar cells"). Rheumatic endocarditis is typically associated with pancarditis, chorea, erythema marginatum, and migratory polyarthritis.

105. The answer is D. *(Pathology; hepatic neoplasm)*
This primary liver tumor is characterized by multiple white nodules involving the right lobe of the liver. Cholangiocarcinomas, which are adenocarcinomas derived from the bile ducts, tend to track along the normal biliary system of the liver, forming multiple nodules along the arborizing biliary network. The white nodules visible in this slide reflect this propensity. These tumors are extremely aggressive neoplasms and frequently cause patients to present with obstructive jaundice.

106. The answer is C. *(Pathology; pulmonary alveolar proteinosis)*
Pulmonary alveolar proteinosis is a condition associated with an inherited or acquired defect in macrophage function. The failure of alveolar macrophages to phagocytose surfactant produced by alveolar pneumocytes results in accumulation of eosinophilic granular material within the lung parenchyma. This material stains strongly with periodic acid–Schiff (PAS) stains and contains fat and lipoprotein. Treatment of patients with idiopathic alveolar proteinosis includes whole lung lavage.

107. The answer is B. *(Pathology; adenocarcinoma of the large intestine)*
This section of the large intestine shows an infiltrating adenocarcinoma, with neoplastic cells arranged in cords and glands. They are free floating within large pools of mucin, which is produced by the neoplastic cells. By definition, adenocarcinomas either form glandular structures or produce neutral mucin. They are the most common form of carcinoma affecting the large intestine. Tumors that produce abundant amounts of mucin (colloid carcinomas) have an especially poor prognosis. The cord-like and tube-like arrangement of the neoplastic cells in this mucinous adenocarcinoma contrasts with the vacuoles and displaced nucleus typical of signet ring adenocarcinoma.

108. The answer is C. *(Pathology; multiple endocrine neoplasia)*
This thyroid proliferation consists of nests of cells with abundant eosinophilic cytoplasm and round-to-uniform nuclei with salt-and-pepper chromatin. This morphology is characteristic of a medullary carcinoma of the thyroid gland, which is a neuroendocrine carcinoma derived from the thyroid C cells. Medullary carcinoma is often a component of the multiple endocrine neoplasia (MEN) syndromes, in particular MEN 2 (Sipple's syndrome) or MEN 3 (mucosal neuroma syndrome). These syndromes frequently have associated parathyroid hyperplasia and may or may not be associated with adenomas of the pancreas and pituitary glands. Recent research has identified an association of MEN syndromes with the *RET* proto-oncogene on chromosome 10.

109. The answer is C. *(Pathology; cystic fibrosis)*
Cystic fibrosis is a disease characterized by production of abnormal mucin. This mucin tends to accumulate within the pulmonary tracheobronchial tree, causing extreme dilatation of the airways. This gross picture shows dilated airways with hyperplastic smooth muscle in their walls, resulting in a trabeculated appearance. This is a classic example of bronchiectasis, which causes pulmonary insufficiency in cystic fibrosis patients.

110. The answer is B. *(Genetics; Turner syndrome)*
Turner syndrome is an example of gonadal dysgenesis. A patient with Turner syndrome has a 45, X karyotype. As a result of this genetic anomaly, normal ovaries fail to form. The abnormal ovaries that do form have no follicles in them. Therefore, secondary sexual characteristics, which are normally induced by follicular steroids, are also lacking. Sterility, lack of menses, and a webbed neck are all characteristics of patients with Turner syndrome.

111. The answer is A. *(Embryology; renal agenesis)*
Normally, a reciprocal inductive interaction between the ureteric bud and the metanephric blastema leads to the development of the definitive adult kidney. Failure in this inductive system leads to renal agenesis. Failure of allantoic degeneration leads to urinary bladder fistula or to cysts in the umbilical region.

Renal agenesis can be unilateral or bilateral. Unilateral renal agenesis is often asymptomatic and is compatible with a normal life because of compensatory hypertrophy of the single normal kidney. Bilateral renal agenesis is associated with oligohydramnios (decreased volume of amniotic fluid) because of an absence of fetal urine production. A newborn infant with complete renal agenesis can be born normally at term because of the maternal elimination of fetal nitrogenous wastes by way of the placenta, but the infant will die soon after birth.

112. The answer is B. *(Pharmacology; anticholinesterases)*
Neostigmine, an anticholinesterase, does not enter the central nervous system. Anticholinesterases indirectly cause a cholinergic effect by binding to acetylcholinesterase, thereby reversibly inhibiting the hydrolysis of acetylcholine produced endogenously at the cholinergic nerve endings. This results in the accumulation of acetylcholine in the synaptic space. Neostigmine reversibly inhibits acetylcholinesterase. Because neostigmine stimulates the bladder and gastrointestinal tract, it is administered to prevent postoperative abdominal distention and urinary retention. It is an antidote for tubocurarine poisoning and is used in the symptomatic treatment of myasthenia gravis.

113–117. The answers are: 113-B, 114-C, 115-E, 116-A, 117-E. *(Pharmacology; endocrinology)*
Androgen ablation therapy is the mainstay for prostatic carcinoma, which is presently the most commonly diagnosed malignancy and the second-leading cause of cancer death among American males. Estrogens, such as diethylstilbestrol, act by suppressing leuteinizing hormone–releasing hormone (LHRH) release from the hypothalamus. Estrogen therapy, however, produces serious complications, including cardiovascular and thromboembolic side effects.

LHRH agonists, such as leuprolide, produce an initial short-term increase in serum testosterone levels, followed by long-term receptor desensitization and subsequent decreased release of follicle-stimulating hormone (FSH) and leuteinizing hormone (LH).

To reduce the incidence of tumor flare caused by these LHRH agonists, antiandrogens, such as flutamide and cyproterone acetate, are used to inhibit dihydrotestosterone (DHT) binding to receptors.

Ketoconazole inhibits adrenal and testicular cytochrome P-450–dependent enzymes and produces castrate levels of testosterone within several hours. However, hepatotoxicity limits the use of ketoconazole to acutely ill patients only.

Finasteride, a 5α-reductase inhibitor, blocks the intracellular conversion of testosterone to DHT. It is currently under investigation for use in prostate cancer and is presently used to treat benign prostatic hyperplasia.

118–122. The answers are: 118-C, 119-A, 120-B, 121-E, 122-D. *(Neuroanatomy; spinal cord lesions)*
Amyotrophic lateral sclerosis is an idiopathic disease characterized by disappearance of both corticospinal tract and anterior horn cells. This results in combined signs of upper and lower motor neuron defects including muscle atrophy, fibrillation, fasciculations, and hyperreflexia; the sensory system remains intact.

Syringomyelia involves progressive cavitation of the central spinal cord or lower brain stem, classically resulting in loss of pain and temperature sensations. This loss of sensation is caused by the destruction of decussating pain fibers in the anterior white commissure.

Tabes dorsalis (locomotor ataxia) is a neurologic manifestation of tertiary syphilis and is associated with the degeneration of the posterior columns. Clinical findings in tabes dorsalis include the progressive loss of peripheral reflexes, loss of joint position (ataxia), and presence of "lightning pain" in the extremities. Other neurologic manifestations of tertiary syphilis include chronic meningitis (meningitic neurosyphilis) and cerebral atrophy, which causes progressive dementia (paretic neurosyphilis).

Poliomyelitis virus causes degeneration of the anterior horn cells, which results in symptoms of lower motor neuron defects (i.e., flaccid paralysis, fasciculations and fibrillations, muscle atrophy, and hyporeflexia).

Pernicious anemia (vitamin B_{12} deficiency) causes degeneration of the posterior columns and of the corticospinal tracts, causing proprioceptive loss and upper motor neuron defects, respectively.

123–125. The answers are: 123-C, 124-A, 125-E. *(Biochemistry; nephrons)*
The solute concentration in the ascending limb of the loop of Henle (*C*) is less than that in any segment of the descending limb. The tubular fluid leaves the ascending limb at a lower concentration than it had when it entered the descending limb. Thus, the fluid presented to the distal tubule always is hyposmotic, regardless of the body's state of hydration.

Ultrafiltration separates water and nonprotein constituents (the crystalloids) of plasma from the blood cells and protein macromolecules (the colloids). Except for proteins and lipids, the concentrations of crystalloids (e.g., Na^+, glucose) in the plasma and in Bowman's space (*A*) are nearly the same.

The wall of the ascending limb of the loop of Henle is relatively impermeable to water. Therefore, sodium chloride in this segment is reabsorbed to the virtual exclusion of water, a process that renders the medullary and papillary interstitium hyperosmotic to plasma. The medullary interstitial osmolality is higher in antidiuresis than diuresis, due largely to urea. Thus, the highest osmolality exists in the papillary interstitium. With continued reabsorption of water, urea becomes even more concentrated at the terminals of the collecting ducts (*E*).

126–129. The answers are: 126-A, 127-B, 128-D, and 129-C. *(Pharmacology; drugs that affect blood)*
Warfarin is employed clinically as an oral anticoagulant. Its major adverse effect is hemorrhage. Therefore, it is important to monitor the effects of the drug.

Tissue-type plasminogen activator (t-PA) is a thrombolytic drug that activates the conversion of plasminogen to plasmin. Bleeding complications may occur upon administration. Heparin is therefore administered simultaneously with t-PA to enhance reperfusion and decrease the rate of formation of secondary thrombi.

Intravenous administration of vitamin K can stem bleeding problems resulting from oral anticoagulants. It should be administered slowly to avoid dyspnea, chest pain, and possibly death. The response to vitamin K is also slow, requiring about 24 hours.

Human erythropoietin, made by recombinant DNA technology, is effective in the treatment of anemia caused by end-stage renal disease.

Aspirin is a platelet aggregation inhibitor that decreases the formation of chemicals that promote platelet aggegation. Specifically, aspirin blocks the synthesis of thromboxane A_2 from arachidonic acid in platelets by irreversibly acetylating, and thus inhibiting, cyclooxygenase, a key enzyme in prostaglandin synthesis.

130–131. The answers are: 130-D, 131-C. *(Microbiology; characteristics of protozoa)*
Domestic cats and other felines are the primary definitive hosts of *Toxoplasma gondii*. Infectious oocysts are excreted in the feces of these animals, and humans become infected by the fecal–oral route.

Naegleria fowleri is the etiologic agent of primary amoebic meningoencephalitis. This fulminant disease typically causes death in 3–5 days. The free-living amoeba appears to be acquired from water and dust by the respiratory route.

Trichomonas vaginalis is the etiologic agent of a sexually transmitted disease frequently seen in women. It is estimated that 3 million women acquire the disease annually in the United States. Men who acquire the infection tend to be asymptomatic.

Entamoeba histolytica is the etiologic agent of amoebic dysentery; the disease usually occurs in debilitated people and during pregnancy. It is characterized by abdominal pain, fever, and profuse bloody stools. Hepatic abscess is seen in approximately 5% of patients with clinically overt amoebiasis caused by *E. histolytica*.

Pneumocystis carinii is the etiologic agent of pneumonia in immunosuppressed people. The disease generally is rare, but it has become an important cause of fatalities in AIDS patients.

132–139. The answers are: 132-C, 133-A, 134-B, 135-C, 136-D, 137-B, 138-D, 139-A. *(Physiology; acid–base disorders)*
Acid–base disorders are clinically common and are classified as either acidosis or alkalosis. Determination of blood pH, Pco_2, and HCO_3^- is crucial for the investigation of acid–base disorders. In approaching acid–base disorders it is first necessary to establish whether the disorder is an acidosis (i.e., pH < 7.37) or an alkalosis (i.e., pH > 7.44); then, to determine if the disturbance is metabolic or respiratory by interpretation of Pco_2 and HCO_3^- as follows:

Acid–Base Disorder	Metabolic or Respiratory	P_{CO_2}	HCO_3^-
Acidosis	Metabolic	↓	↓
	Respiratory	↑	↑
Alkalosis	Metabolic	↑	↑
	Respiratory	↓	↓

Metabolic acidosis is characterized by a loss of HCO_3^- and a decrease in P_{CO_2}, which results from a compensatory increased rate of respiration. Metabolic acidosis can be subdivided based upon the anion gap, which is defined as:

$$\text{anion gap} = [Na^+] - ([Cl^-] + [HCO_3^-])$$

The normal range for the anion gap is 8–12 mmol/L. An anion gap greater than 12 mmol/L is increased and is caused by the accumulation of acids. Metabolic acidosis with an increased anion gap has either exogenous or endogenous causes. Exogenous causes include ingestion of salicylates, methanol, paraldehyde, or ethylene glycol (antifreeze). Endogenous causes include lactic acidosis, ketoacidosis (diabetic, starvation-induced, or alcoholic), or renal failure. In contrast, metabolic acidosis with a normal anion gap is reflective of gastrointestinal problems (diarrhea, pancreatic fistula) or kidney problems (renal tubular acidosis). Iatrogenic causes of metabolic acidosis with a normal anion gap include the use of carbonic anhydrase inhibitors, rapid intravenous hydration, and hyperalimentation. Finally, a low anion gap may occur as a result of decreased concentrations of unmeasured anions (hypoalbuminemia) or increased concentrations of unmeasured cations (hypercalcemia, hypermagnesemia).

Metabolic alkalosis is characterized by an increase in HCO_3^- and an increase in P_{CO_2}, which results from a compensatory decreased rate of respiration. The increase in HCO_3^- occurs following a loss of acid that may be primary or secondary due to hypokalemia (with a lowered potassium concentration, the kidneys exchange H^+ for Na^+, causing a loss of acid in the urine). Common causes of metabolic alkalosis include gastrointestinal loss of H^+ (vomiting, excessive nasogastric suctioning) or renal loss of H^+ (diuretics). It also occurs in patients with cystic fibrosis, Cushing's syndrome, Conn's syndrome, and Bartter's syndrome.

Respiratory acidosis is characterized by a primary increase in P_{CO_2}, with a compensatory increase in HCO_3^-. The increased P_{CO_2} occurs as a result of decreased alveolar gas exchange. This decreased gas exchange may occur by decreased ventilation (iatrogenic, narcotic use, cerebrovascular accidents, muscular dystrophy, myasthenia gravis), airway obstructions (chronic obstructive pulmonary disease, tumor, acute asthma attack), and decreased gas diffusion (pulmonary fibrosis, massive pulmonary edema, severe pneumonia, pleural effusions).

Respiratory alkalosis is characterized by a primary decrease in P_{CO_2}, with a compensatory decrease in HCO_3^-. The decreased P_{CO_2} occurs from increased ventilation from either central or peripheral causes, as well as from iatrogenic overventilation. Central causes of hyperventilation include head trauma, cerebrovascular accidents, pain, anxiety, fever (sepsis), and tumors. Peripheral causes include congestive heart failure, pulmonary embolism, mild pulmonary edema, high altitude, and hypoxemia.

In each acid–base imbalance, rectifying the underlying cause of the disturbance is key to resolution of the disorder.

140. The answer is A. *(Physiology; gonadotropins)*
Luteinizing hormone (LH) and follicle-stimulating hormone (FSH) are synthesized by gonadotrophs in the anterior lobe of the pituitary gland, which are degraded and cleared by the liver and kidney. Immunohisto-chemical studies have shown that both LH and FSH are present in most gonadotrophs, although a minority

of cells contain one form of the gonadotropins. Pituitary LH is released in pulses as a consequence of intermittent GnRH stimulation. Kallman's syndrome, a genetic disorder characterized by defective hypothalamic GnRH production, can be treated with GnRH replacement therapy.

141. The answer is D. *(Neuroanatomy; motor neuron lesions)*
Upper and lower motor neuron lesions each cause paralysis; however, other clinical findings are not shared by these conditions. Upper motor neuron lesions are associated with spastic paralysis, hyperreflexia, and a positive Babinski reflex (i.e., dorsiflexion of great toe accompanied by fanning of other toes in response to stroking of the lateral aspects of the sole of the foot). In contrast, the Babinski reflex is absent in lower motor neuron lesions. These lesions are characterized by the presence of a flaccid paralysis, fasciculations and fibrillations, significant muscle atrophy, and hyporeflexia. Atrophy, fasciculations, and fibrillations are absent in upper motor neuron lesions.

142–143. The answers are: 142-A, 143-D. *(Hematology; testing for hematologic disorders)*
Although the indirect Coombs' test may give positive results in two thirds of patients with autoimmune hemolytic anemia, the direct Coombs' test will demonstrate the presence of autoantibodies, complement, or both on the red cell surface. The indirect Coombs' test demonstrates antibodies in the serum, and they are specific to antigens in the donor red cells, causing a delayed hemolytic transfusion reaction.

The formation of Heinz bodies (unstable hemoglobin precipitates) can be seen on crystal violet stain in glucose-6-phosphate dehydrogenase (G6PD) deficiency during episodes of hemolysis. Although the test is nonspecific, diagnosis is made by transiently assaying enzyme levels in red cells during the stable phase.

144–145. The answers are: 144-C, 145-B. *(Genetics; inherited disorders)*
A disorder is said to be nonpenetrant when there is no clinical evidence of a mutant allele in an individual known to have inherited the gene. When the gene is expressed, the form of expression may be highly variable, with some family members being severely affected and others having few signs of the disorder. This is common with autosomal disorders and is called variable expression. Different mutations of either the same gene (i.e., at the same locus) or different genes may give a similar clinical picture. Consanguineous individuals have a proportion of their genes in common by inheritance from a common ancestor. In some villages originated by a few settlers, disease alleles may be in higher frequencies, and a particular recessive disorder may be more common in that community.

146–147. The answers are: 146-B, 147-D. *(Biochemistry; glucose 6-phosphate metabolites)*
Glucose 1-phosphate, which is formed from glucose 6-phosphate (G6P), is the precursor for glycogen formation. Conversion of G6P to fructose 6-phosphate occurs in the glycolytic pathway. Subsequent reactions yield pyruvate, which is the end product of glycolysis. Conversion of G6P to 6-phosphogluconate is the first step in the pentose phosphate pathway, which yields ribose 5-phosphate as a product. In gluconeogenic tissues, such as the liver, G6P may be dephosphorylated to directly form glucose.

148–149. The answers are: 148-B, 149-A. *(Embryology; embryonic structures)*
The site where the liver diverticulum (A) and the pancreatic buds (C) arise is the boundary between the foregut and the midgut. The liver diverticulum (A) forms the epithelial parenchymal cells, which have both an endocrine and an exocrine function. The pancreatic buds (C) form part of the pancreas, including the islets of Langerhans. The midgut (B) forms the distal small intestine, including most of the duodenum, all of the jejunum, and all of the ileum, as well as the ascending and proximal transverse colon. The cloaca (D) is a hindgut derivative that receives the excurrent ducts of the urinary and reproductive systems. The vitelline duct (E) is a midgut diverticulum that projects into the umbilicus and serves as the axis of rotation of the midgut loop along with the superior mesenteric artery.

150–154. The answers are: 150-C, 151-D, 152-A, 153-E, 154-B. *(Pharmacology; central nervous system stimulants)*
Drugs that primarily stimulate the central nervous system (CNS) can be divided into three basic groups: (1) psychomotor stimulants, such as theophylline and amphetamine; (2) convulsant and respiratory stimulants, such as doxapram; and (3) hallucinogens, such as lysergic acid diethylamide and phencyclidine. Psychomotor stimulants cause excitement and euphoria, decreased feelings of fatigue, and increased motor activity. Convulsants and respiratory stimulants have minimal effects on mental functions, but do produce exaggerated reflex responses, increased activity in respiratory and vasomotor centers, and can cause convulsions at high doses. Hallucinogens produce extreme changes in thought and mood patterns with little effect on the spinal cord or brain stem.

155–159. The answers are: 155-C, 156-B, 157-A, 158-E, 159-D. *(Biochemistry; organs and tissues in the postabsorptive state)*
The flow of metabolites shown in the figure occurs during the postabsorptive state, several hours after a meal. The adipose tissue releases fatty acids, which are used by the heart, skeletal muscle, and liver for fuel. Glycerol, which is taken up by the liver and converted to glucose, is also released by adipose tissue. The liver releases glucose into the blood. The glucose, which is derived from glycogenolysis and gluconeogenesis, is taken up and used for fuel by the brain and skeletal muscle. The skeletal muscle releases lactate, formed from glucose via pyruvate, which is taken up by the liver and used as a substrate for gluconeogenesis.

160–162. The answers are: 160-E, 161-C, 162-D. *(Pharmacology; drug action)*
Mitomycin is both a natural product and an alkylating agent. Isolated from a *Streptomyces* species, mitomycin C is reduced by a reduced nicotinamide adenine dinucleotide phosphate (NADPH)–dependent reductase and alkylates DNA. Cytarabine inhibits DNA polymerase and, thus, kills cells in S phase. Cytarabine nucleotides can be incorporated into DNA and RNA, but the significance of this is not known. Vincristine, a natural product, is an M-phase–specific agent, blocking proliferating cells as they enter metaphase.

163–165. The answers are: 163-A, 164-B, 165-C. *(Pharmacology; effects of neuroleptic drugs)*
Lactation (via the tuberoinfundibular tract) and parkinsonism (via the nigrostriatal tract) both are associated with the effects of neuroleptic drugs on postsynaptic dopamine 2 (D_2) receptors. Some of the antipsychotic effects are also thought to be mediated by dopaminergic blockade, but the brain tracts involved are believed to be the mesolimbic and possibly the mesocortical pathways. There is little evidence that the nigrostriatal and tuberoinfundibular tracts are important in the direct antipsychotic effects of neuroleptics. However, other neurotransmitter systems probably are involved in the neuroleptic effects.

166. The answer is B. *(Pathology; renal neoplasia)*
This renal tumor is a classic renal cell carcinoma reflected in its parenchymal location and deep golden appearance (due to abundant cytoplasmic fat). Patients with renal cell carcinomas often present with costovertebral pain, hematuria, and a palpable abdominal mass; polycythemia, hypercalcemia, and Cushing's syndrome among other endocrinopathies also may be associated. Polycythemia results from abnormal production of erythropoietin-like hormones by the tumor. These tumors arise from proximal tubular epithelium and may appear in patients with von Hippel-Lindau syndrome, which is associated with chromosome 3 abnormalities. These individuals also have a risk for cerebellar hemangioblastomas.

167. The answer is D. *(Pathology; renal disease)*
This resection specimen shows a kidney affected by multiple, variably sized cysts, some with recent hemorrhage. This diffuse process is diagnostic of adult polycystic kidney disease, an autosomal dominant disease with high penetrance that usually manifests in adulthood. The disease is bilateral, progressive, and ultimately

requires dialysis or transplantation. There is often cystic disease affecting other organs including liver, spleen, pancreas, and lungs. Berry aneurysms are present in 10%–30% of patients and may be a cause of subarachnoid hemorrhage. A slight risk for the development of renal cell carcinoma exists with this condition.

168. The answer is A. *(Pathology; inflammation of bowel)*
This diffuse, nonsegmental process is characterized by dramatic needle-like polyps projecting from the mucosal surface. Such pseudopolyps are features of chronic ulcerative colitis, in which zones of hyperplasia alternate with areas of mucosal flattening and atrophy. Crohn's disease is a segmental process, as is ischemic colitis, and it is not associated with such pronounced pseudopolyps. Collagenous colitis, which is a microscopic disease with thickening of the basement membrane of the colonic mucosa, shows a grossly normal mucosa.

169. The answer is B. *(Pathology; cardiovascular system, microbiology)*
The polypoid hemorrhage tissue adherent to this white fibrotic and stenotic valve is characteristic of bacterial vegetations associated with endocarditis. These vegetations derive from bacterial seeding of defective or congenitally abnormal valves. In this case, the white fibrosis thickening of the valve cusps was associated with stenosis. Vegetations may be associated with bacteria of low virulence (e.g., streptococcus) or those that are highly aggressive and destructive (e.g., staphylococcus). They may cause valve perforation and insufficiency, or they may embolize, causing infarction and secondary infection.

170. The answer is B. *(Pathology; gastrointestinal tract)*
This gross picture shows a pedunculated polyp with a cauliflower-like neoplasm attached to the colonic mucosa by a thin stalk. These neoplastic polyps contain dysplastic colonic glands and may be precursors to colonic adenocarcinomas. Malignant transformation is related to the size, severity of dysplasia, and amount of villous architecture on histologic examination. Hyperplastic polyps are small, sessile proliferations of hyperplastic epithelium. They lack stalks and are smooth, hemispheric mucosal protrusions. Villous adenomas are sessile-based tumors with a finger-like brushy surface resembling a sea anenome.

171. The answer is A. *(Pathology; pulmonary disease)*
The photomicrograph shows consolidation of air spaces by bilobed leukocytes—eosinophils. This pattern is diagnostic of eosinophilic pneumonia, which is an allergic reaction mediated by immunoglobulin E. This condition occurs in asthmatic patients and is accompanied by peripheral air space consolidation and peripheral blood eosinophilia. Known causes include drug reactions, filarial infections, and some fungal diseases (e.g., Coccidioides, Aspergillus). Klebsiella infections are bacterial pneumonias with multilobate neutrophils, not eosinophils. Thermophilic actinomyces cause a type IV immune reaction mediated by lymphocytes and histiocytes that results in the histopathology associated with hypersensitivity pneumonitis.

172. The answer is A. *(Pathology; gastrointestinal tract)*
A small sac or outpouching occurring at this site (30–70 cm from the ileocecal valve) is most likely a Meckel's diverticulum. These true diverticula are vestiges of the vitelline duct, and they are usually less than 6 cm long. Meckel's diverticula are present in 2% of the population. Interestingly, the intestinal mucosa of the Meckel's diverticulum may show heterotopic rests of gastric mucosa in 50% of cases. The production of acid by this mucosa may lead to peptic ulceration distal to the diverticulum and possibly perforation.

173. The answer is B. *(Pathology; myocardial infarct)*
This gross specimen shows the classic appearance of a recent (2–4 days old) subendocardial infarct. Early after vascular occlusion, the most distal myocardium—the subendocardial zone—undergoes coagulative necrosis. This is accompanied by vasospasm and extravasation of red blood cells. The gross appearance is

one of subendocardial hemorrhage and edema. Over time, red cells lyse, macrophages phagocytose debris, and myocardial fibers degenerate; this later stage (6–14 days) has a pale gray appearance. In time, white fibrosis scar tissue replaces necrotic muscle fibers.

174. The answer is C. *(Pathology; cardiology)*
The heart shows extensive replacement of myocardium by dense white fibrous scars, the consequence of previous infarcts. Adherent to the endocardium is a white mural thrombus. Portions of the thrombus ejected from the left ventricle can cause distal infarcts, including those in the brain. Cerebral infarcts are a common cause of such thromboembolic events. No tumor nodules are seen in this case, and no evidence of rupture is seen, although this may be noted in patients with large infarcts.

175. The answer is C. *(Pathology; neoplasia)*
The spleen is affected by large white nodules having a fleshy appearance and central hemorrhage and necrosis. The most common cause of large nodular masses in the spleen is malignant lymphoma. Large nodules (larger than 5 mm) are usually attributed to large cell lymphoma or Hodgkin's disease, whereas small nodules usually result from low-grade, non-Hodgkin's lymphomas (i.e., small lymphocytic, follicular center cell). Infarcts of the spleen are wedge shaped and capsule based. Histoplasmosis can cause a granulomatous splenitis, but the granulomas are usually small (size of millet seed) and calcified. Chronic congestion of the spleen causes a diffuse brownish discoloration because of hemosiderin-laden macrophages with white fibrous plaques along the capsular surface.

176. The answer is C. *(Pathology; gastrointestinal neoplasia)*
This gross photomicrograph shows an annular, ulcerating, and infiltrating carcinoma arising at the gastro-esophageal junction. Most distal esophageal carcinomas are gland-forming tumors, so-called adenocarcinomas. Their constrictive growth results in dysphagia and chest discomfort. Many adenocarcinomas occur in association with Barrett's esophagus—a metaplastic phenomenon in which glandular mucosa replaces the normal squamous epithelium of the esophagus—and the most common cause of this change is reflux esophagitis. The only other consideration is Crohn's disease, which may affect the esophagus and stomach where it induces zones of stenosis. This would be extremely unusual at the cardioesophageal junction, and this inflammatory process lacks the infiltrative quality of the specimen shown.

177. The answer is B. *(Pathology; hematology)*
The bone shows a wedge-shaped subcortical infarct, so-called avascular necrosis of the femoral head. As an end organ with a single vascular supply, bone infarcts tend to be pyramidal in shape, abut on the cortical surface, and are sharply defined. The causes of bone infarcts are usually related to thromboembolic events. Patients with sickle cell disease are predisposed to vaso-occlusive events and avascular necrosis of bones. Patients with metastatic carcinoma often have multiple well-circumscribed white nodules within the medulla. Fractures tend to be hemorrhagic, irregular, and jagged, not well defined and triangular. Gout usually affects the synovium as grainy, chalk-gray deposits. Asthma is not associated with bony abnormalities.

178. The answer is A. *(Pathology; spleen)*
The spleen in this case shows a wedge-shaped zone of hemorrhage and consolidation that abuts the capsular surface and has its apex pointing toward the center of the organ. The circulation to the spleen occurs through progressive branching of the splenic artery, forming arcades that feed pyramidal-shaped zones with their bases at the capsule. Occlusion of the arteries—usually through thromboembolic events or progressive atherosclerosis—results in initial hemorrhage and then, after red cell lysis and mononuclear cell infiltration, a pale "white" infarct. Granulomas of the spleen are round, white, and have central necrosis. These granulomas do not rest adjacent to the splenic capsule. Angiosarcoma and hemangiomas form tumor nodules, with hemorrhage and necrosis. A sponge-like quality is seen with well-differentiated endothelial processes.

179. The answer is D. *(Pathology; liver)*
This gross photograph displays the classic changes of chronic congestion, resulting in the prototypic "nutmeg liver." Regions of reddish discoloration reflect the presence of sinusoidal congestion around the central veins of the hepatic lobule. Chronic congestion is most often caused by congestive heart failure, but it may result from many conditions that cause hepatic vein congestion, including heart failure and obstruction to the inferior vena cava or hepatic veins (Budd-Chiari syndrome). Kaposi's sarcoma is a localized lesion in the liver, not a diffuse process, and massive hepatic necrosis would not have this repetitive reticulated pattern. Instead, necrosis would be diffuse and uniformly brown in color.

180. The answer is D. *(Pathology; intestines)*
This gross photo shows an ulcerating lesion with heaped-up, rolled edges, which is a classic appearance for carcinomas of the large intestine. Such tumors in the proximal colon tend to present as polypoid fungating masses, whereas those in the distal colon (as in this case) form annular, encircling lesions that produce napkin-ring constrictions of the bowel. These carcinomas are thought to arise in colonic polyps in which progressive molecular perturbations result in malignant transformation. Most colonic carcinomas are adeno-carcinomas, and prognosis depends on the extent of the tumor at the time of diagnosis. The most widely used classifications focus on the depth of invasion of the colonic wall and the presence of lymph node metastases (Dukes classification, Astler Coller classification).

Test VI

QUESTIONS

DIRECTIONS: *Single best answer questions* consist of numbered items or incomplete statements followed by answers or by completions of the statement. Select the ONE lettered answer or completion that is BEST in each case.

Matching questions consist of a list of four to twenty-six lettered options (some of which may be in figures) followed by several numbered items. For each numbered item, select the ONE lettered option that is most closely associated with it. Each lettered option may be selected once, more than once, or not at all.

1. All of the following factors indicate a poor prognosis in hypertension EXCEPT

(A) persistent diastolic pressure greater than 115 mm Hg
(B) hypercholesterolemia
(C) diabetes mellitus
(D) female gender

2. All of the following statements about the use of ketone bodies as a fuel by the body are true EXCEPT

(A) ketone bodies are soluble in aqueous solution and therefore do not require carriers in the body
(B) ketone bodies are produced in response to elevated levels of fatty acids in the liver, when the amount of acetyl CoA exceeds the oxidative capacity of the liver
(C) acetone is not used by the body as a fuel
(D) the liver oxidizes ketone bodies for energy when their plasma levels are elevated

3. All of the following are associated with alcohol withdrawal EXCEPT

(A) tremulousness
(B) alcoholic hallucinosis
(C) petit mal seizures
(D) delirium tremens

4. All of the following laboratory data support a diagnosis of liver disease owing to chronic alcohol abuse EXCEPT

(A) elevation in gamma-glutamyl transpeptidase (GGT)
(B) SGOT:SGPT ratio greater than or equal to 2:1
(C) hyperalbuminemia
(D) prolonged prothrombin time
(E) thrombocytopenia

5. All of the following statements about erythromycin are correct EXCEPT

(A) it is mainly concentrated and excreted in an active form in the bile
(B) it binds irreversibly to the 50s ribosomal subunit
(C) it is bactericidal
(D) it is contraindicated in patients with hepatic dysfunction
(E) it is used as a penicillin substitute

Questions 6–7

The accompanying figure depicts an oxygen saturation curve for myoglobin and hemoglobin.

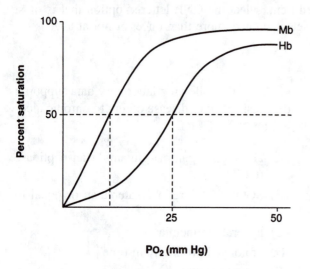

6. All of the following statements about the oxygen saturation curve depicted are true EXCEPT

(A) myoglobin has a higher oxygen affinity than hemoglobin

(B) myoglobin irreversibly binds a single molecule of oxygen

(C) hemoglobin exhibits cooperative binding of oxygen

(D) partial pressure of oxygen (P_{O_2}) needed to achieve half saturation of the binding sites (P_{50}) for myoglobin is approximately 10 mm Hg

(E) P_{O_2} needed to achieve P_{50} for hemoglobin is approximately 26 mm Hg

7. All of the following are true about 2,3-diphosphoglycerate EXCEPT

(A) it is the most abundant organic phosphate in the red blood cell

(B) the concentration of 2,3-diphosphoglycerate in red blood cells increases in response to chronic hypoxia

(C) it decreases the oxygen affinity of hemoglobin by binding to oxyhemoglobin

(D) it is synthesized from intermediates of glycolysis

(E) one molecule of 2,3-diphosphoglycerate binds to a pocket in the center of the deoxyhemoglobin tetramers formed by the two β-chains in hemoglobin

8. All of the following statements about digitalis are true EXCEPT

(A) it increases contractility of the cardiac muscle

(B) it inhibits Na^+/K^+ exchange by Na^+, K^+-ATPase

(C) severe digitalis toxicity can result in ventricular tachycardia

(D) hyperkalemia is a factor that predisposes to digitalis toxicity

9. All of the following statements about the inhaled general anesthetic isoflurane are true EXCEPT

(A) it does not induce cardiac arrhythmias

(B) it sensitizes the heart to the action of epinephrine

(C) it does not raise intracranial pressure

(D) it has a low rate of biotransformation

(E) it has low organ toxicity

10. All of the following statements about methotrexate are true EXCEPT

(A) it is structurally related to folic acid

(B) it acts as an antagonist of folic acid

(C) leucovorin rescues cells from methotrexate cytotoxicity by binding to methotrexate

(D) resistance to methotrexate is characteristic of nonproliferating cells

(E) it inhibits dihydrofolate reductase

11. All of the following increase the extent of sickling in sickle cell anemia by increasing the proportion of deoxygenated hemoglobin S (Hb S) EXCEPT

(A) decreased oxygen tension caused by high altitude or flying in a nonpressurized plane

(B) increased carbon dioxide concentration

(C) increased concentration of 2,3-diphosphoglycerate in erythrocytes

(D) increased pH

12. All of the following conditions increase erythrocyte sedimentation rate (ESR) EXCEPT

(A) inflammatory disorders

(B) anemia

(C) pregnancy

(D) congestive heart failure

(E) hypercholesterolemia

13. Asplenic patients are most prone to develop infections from all of the following organisms EXCEPT

(A) *Streptococcus pneumoniae*

(B) *Haemophilus influenzae*

(C) *Staphylococcus aureus*

(D) *Neisseria meningitidis*

(E) *Trichinella spiralis*

14. All of the following statements about classic galactosemia are true EXCEPT

(A) galactosemia is caused by a galactokinase deficiency

(B) it is an autosomal recessive disorder

(C) galactosemia causes the accumulation of galactose 1-phosphate and galactitol in nerve tissues, liver, and kidneys

(D) infants with this deficiency have severe vomiting and diarrhea

(E) therapy for galactosemia involves rapid diagnosis and removal of galactose from the diet

15. All of the following coenzymes are derived from vitamins EXCEPT

(A) coenzyme A (CoA-SH)

(B) pyridoxal phosphate

(C) thiamine pyrophosphate (TPP)

(D) coenzyme Q (CoQ)

16. All of the following laboratory findings are consistent with a diagnosis of pheochromocytoma EXCEPT

(A) elevated urinary vanillylmandelic acid

(B) elevated urinary free catecholamines

(C) elevated basal plasma catecholamine level

(D) elevated plasma catecholamine level following glucagon administration

(E) elevated plasma catecholamine level following clonidine administration

Questions 17–20

(A) Immunoglobulin D (IgD)
(B) IgA
(C) IgE
(D) IgG
(E) IgM

For each method of activating (fixing) complement listed, select the immunoglobulin most closely associated with that method.

17. Fixes complement efficiently via the C_H2 domain

18. Fixes complement via the C_H3 domain

19. Fixes complement via the alternative pathway only

20. Fixes complement most efficiently in lytic reactions

21. Each of the following commonly causes peripheral vertigo EXCEPT

(A) Meniere's disease
(B) vestibular neuronitis
(C) multiple sclerosis
(D) acoustic neuroma

22. All of the following statements about calcium oxalate kidney stones are correct EXCEPT

(A) they are the most common type of kidney stone in the United States
(B) they are radio-opaque
(C) in most cases, endoscopic therapy or lithotripsy is not performed until more than 1 month after onset of symptoms
(D) recurrence is rare after treatment of the initial incidence
(E) intravenous pyelography should be performed after the incident, even if the stone has passed

23. A patient who is receiving cyclophosphamide for her breast cancer begins to experience nausea, vomiting, weakness, and an inability to think clearly. No evidence of infection is found, but her serum sodium has dropped to 115 mEq/L (normal = 134–146 mEq/L). Although there are no signs of edema, a urinalysis reveals a urinary sodium level of 500 mEq/L. Which one of the following statements is most likely correct?

(A) Because the patient is hyponatremic, she must also be volume depleted
(B) Diuretics should not be given to this patient
(C) Administration of normal saline is the only form of treatment required
(D) No treatment is required, because this patient should recover rapidly on her own
(E) This case is consistent with a diagnosis of syndrome of inappropriate secretion of antidiuretic hormone (SIADH)

24. Which one of the following statements concerning the effects of diuretics on the kidney is correct?

(A) Diuretics that affect the proximal tubule are the most efficacious class of diuretics, because the majority of reabsorption occurs in the proximal tubules
(B) Loop diuretics may cause kidney stone formation, because of the reduction of the electrical potential that normally enhances the reabsorption of calcium
(C) Thiazide-type diuretics, which act in the distal tubule, can cause a metabolic acidosis
(D) Because only approximately 20% of sodium reabsorption occurs in the loop of Henle, loop diuretics are only suitable for cases of very mild edema
(E) Aldosterone antagonists act mainly in the proximal tubule
(F) Osmotic diuretics are frequently useful as oral agents in patients with severe edema

25. Which one of the following statements correctly describes the mechanism of action of mast cells in people with allergies?

(A) Fc receptors on the surface of mast cells bind to immunoglobulin E (IgE). When antigen cross-links the bound IgE antibodies, the mast cell is triggered to release its secretory granules that contain inflammatory mediators (e.g., leukotrienes and histamine).

(B) Mast cells are triggered by the release of cytokines during the allergic response. Interleukin-4 (IL-4) and IL-5 cause the mast cell to release secretory granules containing more IL-4 and IL-5 in a positive feedback loop.

(C) Receptors on the surface of mast cells can specifically bind to foreign antigen. Upon binding, mast cells begin to secrete and release inflammatory mediators.

(D) The IgD antibody binds to mast cells via Fab receptors. When antigen cross-links the bound antibodies, the mast cell is triggered to release its secretory granules, which contain inflammatory mediators such as leukotrienes and histamine.

(E) Mast cells phagocytose foreign antigen and process it for presentation to other mast cells. These cells will then begin secreting IL-8 and tumor necrosis factor (TNF)-α.

26. All of the following statements about insulin are true EXCEPT

(A) in the liver, insulin increases glycogenesis

(B) it is a polypeptide hormone made up of the A and B chain

(C) its action is anabolic, increasing the storage of glucose

(D) it facilitates the entry of glucose into red blood cells

(E) it is produced by β-cells of the pancreatic islets

(F) in the liver, insulin inhibits gluconeogenesis

27. A particular recessive trait (e.g., purple fingers) is found in 4.5% of a population, and the penetrance of the trait is 50% in the homozygous recessive state (0% in heterozygotes and dominant homozygotes). What is the percentage of the population that is heterozygous for the purple finger allele, assuming only two possible alleles (dominant and recessive), random mating, no selection bias for the trait, and no new mutations?

(A) 5.82%

(B) 9%

(C) 30%

(D) 42%

(E) 49%

28. A 62-year-old woman presents with symptoms of dyspnea that have gradually worsened over the past 5 years, but have recently become more severe coupled with the "cold" that she has had. The physician notices clubbing of the fingers and toes and hears inspiratory crackles. A chest radiograph shows a bilateral, basilar, reticulonodular infiltrate. A lung biopsy shows a mononuclear cell infiltrate and interstitial scarring with honeycombing. Which one of the following statements is true?

(A) The patient will likely respond well to steroids

(B) The disease that this patient has is often associated with connective tissue diseases

(C) The patient has bronchiolitis obliterans organizing pneumonia (BOOP)

(D) The abnormalities seen on the biopsy appear temporally homogeneous

(E) The infiltrate seen on the biopsy is diffuse rather than patchy

29. All of the following associations of hormones, site of production, and chemical structure are correct EXCEPT

(A) androgens—zona reticularis of adrenal cortex—steroid

(B) vasopressin—zona glomerulosa of adrenal cortex—steroid

(C) cortisol—zona fasiculata of adrenal cortex—steroid

(D) norepinephrine—adrenal medulla—catecholamine

(E) glucagon—α-cells of the pancreas—peptide

30. A patient who has had poorly controlled diabetes mellitus type 2 for 20 years presents to his physician with a large lesion on the bottom of his foot. All of the following statements could be true EXCEPT

(A) he has a sensory neuropathy that did not allow him to feel any pain from the ulcer

(B) he has a motor neuropathy in his foot that predisposed his foot to ulcers due to changing of the pressure points on his feet

(C) although neuropathies can in some cases cause a lack of sensation, in other cases neuropathies are a cause of severe pain

(D) the length of time that one has diabetes is the major risk factor for complications; thus, because this variable cannot be affected, nothing can be done to prevent their occurrence

(E) peripheral vascular insufficiency is another important factor in the development of foot ulcers in diabetic patients

Questions 31–33

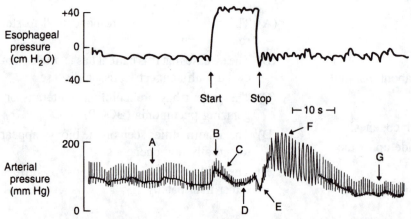

The esophageal and arterial pressure tracings depicted were made from a normal subject during a voluntary effort to exhale against significant resistance (the Valsalva maneuver), which is a useful test of cardiac function. Match the descriptions that follow with the labeled arterial pressure readings.

31. Loss of this vagally mediated change in arterial pressure is a useful diagnostic aid in assessing autonomic insufficiency.

32. Changes in arterial blood pressure and pulse pressure are caused by a decrease in venous return.

33. This area of the arterial blood pressure tracing is consistent with reflex tachycardia.

Questions 34–38

(A) Obsessive–compulsive
(B) Borderline
(C) Dependent
(D) Narcissistic
(E) Antisocial

Match each disease characteristic with the personality disorder that is most apt to be associated with it.

34. Associated with childhood conduct disorder

35. Overly rigid

36. Hypersensitive to criticism

37. Repetitive self-cutting

38. Perfectionistic

Questions 39–42

(A) Osteosarcoma
(B) Chondrosarcoma
(C) Ewing's sarcoma
(D) Giant cell tumor
(E) Osteoid osteoma
(F) Chondroblastoma

Based on the clinical information given, select the bone tumor that is most likely to occur in each patient.

39. Epiphyseal lesions in a patient younger than 20 years of age

40. Epiphyseal lesions in a patient older than 20 years of age

41. Metaphyseal lesions in a patient younger than 20 years of age

42. A diaphyseal lesion with concentric onion-skin layering in a patient younger than 20 years of age

43. A 46-year-old man with diabetes, who is taking an angiotensin-converting enzyme (ACE) inhibitor for his hypertension, recently reports having developed the symptoms of vomiting, increasing muscle weakness, and periods in which his heart rate seems "uncomfortably fast." An electrocardiogram shows the presence of peaked T waves. Which one of the following statements is most likely correct?

(A) The patient is hypolkalemic and should be given potassium chloride supplements
(B) The patient is hypokalemic and should be given a β-blocker
(C) The patient is hyperkalemic and should be given a β-blocker
(D) The patient is hyperkalemic and should be given intravenous calcium, followed by insulin and sodium polystyrene sulfonate
(E) The patient is hyperkalemic but does not require treatment other than insulin, if his glucose is uncontrolled, and he should continue the use of the angiotensin-converting enzyme (ACE) inhibitor

44. All of the following statements referring to renal tubule acidosis (RTA) are correct EXCEPT

(A) type I RTA is caused by a defect in H^+ secretion in the distal nephron

(B) type IV RTA is often associated with hypokalemia or hyperaldosteronism

(C) type II RTA is caused by a defect in H^+ secretion in the proximal tubule

(D) type IV RTA is frequently associated with diabetes

(E) type II RTA is usually associated with hypokalemia

45. An oliguric patient being treated for a gram-negative infection has a sudden increase in his blood urea nitrogen and creatinine ratio. Which one of the following statements would lead to the diagnosis of an acute interstitial nephritis rather than an acute tubular necrosis?

(A) The patient is taking gentamicin for a gram-negative infection

(B) The patient does not have proteinuria

(C) The patient's urine has dirty brown casts

(D) The patient was taking penicillin for a gram-negative infection and has developed a rash and arthralgia

(E) The patient had a computed tomography scan in which contrast material was used

46. Major histocompatibility complex class I (MHC-I) is an important protein facilitating the immune response. One of its functions is to

(A) present processed antigen to $CD4^+$ T lymphocytes

(B) bind to whole antigens in the antigen-presenting cell's environment for presentation to $CD8^+$ T lymphocytes

(C) regulate the natural killer cell's cytolytic activity

(D) bind to extracellular bacteria to enhance phagocytosis by neutrophils

(E) facilitate cell-to-cell contact between B lymphocytes to enhance antibody production

47. A 12-year-old patient who has an insatiable appetite, is short in stature, and is mildly retarded is diagnosed with Prader-Willi syndrome. Knowing that Prader-Willi syndrome involves an imprinted gene on chromosome 15, which one of the following genetic mechanisms could have caused this syndrome?

(A) Trisomy of chromosome 15

(B) Uniparental diploidy

(C) A deletion of a portion of the paternal chromosome 15

(D) Monosomy of chromosome 15

(E) Uniparental disomy of chromosome 2

48. All of the following scenarios are indications for prenatal diagnostic tests (e.g., amniocentesis, chorionic villus sampling) EXCEPT

(A) the father has a known chromosomal rearrangement

(B) the mother is 36 years old and has had three healthy children

(C) the father was affected with spina bifida, and the mother is a healthy 23-year-old

(D) the mother had a previous miscarriage for unknown reasons

(E) the mother had a previous child with Down syndrome

49. If a patient has a partial obstruction of an airway leading to a segment of one of his lungs, he will have a ventilation/perfusion mismatch. This scenario leads to an elevated level of the partial pressure of carbon dioxide (Pco_2) and a decreased level of the partial pressure of oxygen (Po_2). Which statement concerning the normal physiologic ability to compensate for such a defect is correct?

(A) The patient will be able to compensate for both the elevated Pco_2 and decreased Po_2

(B) The patient will be able to compensate for the decreased Po_2 but not the elevated Pco_2

(C) The patient will be able to compensate for the elevated Pco_2 but not the decreased Po_2

(D) The patient will not be able to compensate for either the elevated Pco_2 or the decreased Po_2

(E) Administration of supplemental oxygen would be helpful

50. A colleague is designing a clinical trial for a new drug that he has developed and asks how the study might be affected by patients' adherence to the trial regimen. Which one of the following statements is most accurate?

(A) Because the researcher is dealing with a serious disease, he does not need to worry about patient compliance; compliance is only a problem when patients do not believe that they need the therapy to get better

(B) He should limit his study group to men only, because men are more compliant than women

(C) The socioeconomic status of his patient group will not affect patient compliance, as long as the patients do not have to pay for the drug

(D) If there is poor compliance, the trial will overestimate the toxicity of the drug

(E) If the drug is given in the hospital, he does not need to worry because all of the patients will receive the entire regimen

51. All of the following statements concerning the classification of joints are correct EXCEPT

(A) the sutures of the skull are examples of synarthroses

(B) diarthroses allow for the widest range of motion

(C) amphiarthroses are hinge joints (e.g., the knee)

(D) diarthroses include both a synovium and a joint capsule

(E) diarthroses include both intracapsular and extracapsular ligaments

(F) the tendons that support diarthroses contain type I collagen

52. A patient has a transverse fracture of his left humerus. Which one of the following statements is correct?

(A) The fracture was likely due to compression, because bone is weaker in compression than in torsion or bending

(B) If a small gap needs to be filled in, a hard callous forms instead of cartilage

(C) Lamellar bone is formed and then is remodeled to cortical bone

(D) The presence of a physis on the radiograph indicates that the patient's skeleton is not fully mature

(E) If the fracture does not heal by 6 months, it is called a malunion

53. In evaluating a patient who has joint pain, which one of the following statements is characteristic of osteoarthritis but not rheumatoid arthritis?

(A) The joint pain is symmetrical

(B) The patient has morning stiffness that lasts for more than 1 hour

(C) The patient has ''swan neck'' deformities on his second and third fingers

(D) The patient has pain in the distal interphalangeal joints that is worse after activity and is relieved with rest

(E) Fluid removed from a painful joint has a low viscosity and a high white blood cell count

(F) The patient has swelling of the metacarpophalangeal joints

Questions 54–58

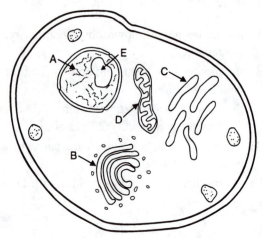

Match each description below with the appropriate organelle in the accompanying diagram.

54. It is involved in sorting and targeting proteins

55. It is the site of cleavage of introns from messenger RNA (mRNA)

56. It is the site of ribosomal RNA (rRNA) synthesis

57. It is the site of steroid synthesis

58. It is the main site of adenosine triphosphate (ATP) synthesis

Questions 59–63

(A) Albumin
(B) Transferrin
(C) Haptoglobin
(D) Transcobalamin
(E) None of the above

For each function, select the associated transport protein.

59. Iron transport

60. Vitamin B_{12} transport

61. Clot formation

62. Plasma osmotic pressure maintenance

63. Hemoglobin transport

64. A surgeon is considering performing a splenectomy on a 9-year-old girl for staging of her Hodgkin's disease. Which one of the following statements is correct concerning the effects of this procedure on the immune system?

(A) Because the patient has already had all of her immunizations, it is not important that the patient will no longer have a spleen; she will be no more susceptible to disease after the splenectomy

(B) The patient should have all of her immunizations repeated after the surgery

(C) *Staphylococcus aureus* is the organism that is of most concern following splenectomy

(D) The physician should be sure that the patient has already had (or receives before surgery) a *Haemophilus influenzae* B vaccination and a Pneumovax vaccination; in addition, prophylactic antibiotics should be prescribed for her after the surgery

(E) The patient will be highly susceptible to viral infections after the surgery

65. Which one of the following statements about abnormalities that may be present at birth is correct?

(A) A malformation is an abnormality that is caused by intrauterine compression

(B) A cleft lip is a common example of a deformation

(C) Dysplasias are abnormalities of cells and tissues rather than organs; therefore, they rarely are due to a genetic defect

(D) The presence of amniotic bands is an example of a disruption

(E) Associations have only one cause, whereas syndromes are thought to have multiple causes

66. A pregnant woman has myotonic dystrophy. Her mother also had a mild form of the disease. The patient's symptoms include distal muscle weakness and a ''hatchet-faced'' appearance. There is no history of the disorder on her father's side of the family. The patient has two healthy children. Her ultrasound shows that the fetus is a boy. Which one of the following statements is correct?

(A) The fetus is not at risk of having myotonic dystrophy because it affects only females

(B) The fetus has a lower risk of having myotonic dystrophy because the two previous infants did not have the disease

(C) The fetus has a higher risk of having myotonic dystrophy because the two previous infants did not have the disease

(D) If the fetus has myotonic dystrophy, it will likely be less severe than it is for his mother

(E) If the fetus has myotonic dystrophy, he has a high risk of being more severely affected than his mother

67. A patient with hypertension, hirsutism, a-menorrhea, acne, and an excess of truncal fat with peripheral muscle wasting is referred to an endocrinologist for evaluation. The patient has never taken any form of steroids. The patient has increased levels of cortisol, which are not suppressed by exogenous dexamethasone. The plasma adrenocorticotropic hormone (ACTH) levels are elevated and are not suppressed by dexamethasone. Which of the following disorders is the most likely diagnosis?

(A) Addison's disease
(B) Waterhouse-Friderichsen syndrome
(C) Cushing's syndrome caused by a pituitary tumor
(D) Cushing's syndrome caused by an adrenal tumor
(E) Cushing's syndrome caused by ectopic production of ACTH

68. A nondiabetic, 35-year-old patient has been experiencing postprandial hypoglycemia. Which one of the following statements is most likely correct?

(A) The patient has insulinoma
(B) The insulin and C-peptide levels are the same; therefore, the patient has factitious hypoglycemia
(C) Alimentary hypoglycemia is consistent with this scenario
(D) An oral glucose tolerance test is required to determine the etiology of hypoglycemia
(E) The patient's history of alcohol abuse is unimportant because alcohol causes hyperglycemia, not hypoglycemia
(F) Chronic hypoglycemia can be caused by the loss of as little as 20% of the liver mass, because there is only a small surplus in the liver's capacity for gluconeogenesis and glycogen storage

69. A 38-year-old man complains of pain in his right big toe and ankle. His toe and ankle are erythematous and swollen. The night before he had a large meal, including a steak and a "few" glasses of wine. In the middle of the night he awoke with severe pain. Which one of the following statements is correct?

(A) The patient has pseudogout rather than acute gouty arthritis
(B) That the patient ingested alcohol the previous night makes a diagnosis of acute gouty arthritis less likely because alcohol speeds the excretion of uric acid
(C) This patient will likely develop tophi in the next few weeks
(D) One would expect the synovial fluid to display needle-shaped negatively birefringent crystals under polarized light
(E) Treatment must be administered as soon as possible; otherwise, the patient's symptoms will continue indefinitely

70. All of the following statements about Paget's disease are true EXCEPT

(A) the bone of patients with Paget's disease has an increased thickness of the osteoid layer
(B) Paget's disease is also known as osteitis deformans
(C) Paget's disease is often asymptomatic
(D) the bone of patients with Paget's disease has cement lines that are arranged in a "mosaic" pattern
(E) in a histologic section of bone, osteoclasts with up to 100 nuclei may be seen

71. All of the following support an initial diagnosis of reactive arthritis (Reiter's syndrome) EXCEPT

(A) the patient has lower back pain
(B) the patient has increased pain with bed rest and inactivity
(C) the patient is positive for the histocompatibility antigen (HLA)-B27
(D) a positive gonococcal culture is obtained from the synovium
(E) the patient has an elevated erythrocyte sedimentation rate
(F) the patient has unilateral conjunctivitis

Questions 72–74

(A) T cell
(B) B cell
(C) Macrophage
(D) Natural killer (NK) cell
(E) Eosinophil
(F) Basophil
(G) Neutrophil
(H) Mast cell

For each cell characteristic or function described below, select the cell with which it is most closely associated.

72. Functions as helper in antibody response

73. Functions as suppressor cell

74. Phagocytizes and processes antigen in the immune response

Questions 75–77

(A) Piaget
(B) Freud
(C) Maslow
(D) Kohlberg
(E) Erikson

Match each of the following descriptions of developmental theory with the correct researcher.

75. Psychosexual development proceeds with different parts of the body serving as the focus of sexual gratification during different stages

76. Development of the ego takes place within a social context across the entire life cycle; each stage is characterized by a struggle that must be resolved before progressing to the next stage

77. Childhood thinking processes develop in stages, with most children passing through each stage in a sequential fashion; reasoning power in each stage is qualitatively different from the previous stage because new skills have been acquired

Questions 78–80

An acutely ill 3-year-old boy is brought to the emergency room. His breathing is extremely labored, and he is producing rust-colored sputum. A Gram stain of the sputum reveals numerous gram-positive cocci in random clusters. A diagnosis of staphylococcal pneumonia is made, and the child is hospitalized and placed on an intravenous methicillin. The mother reports that the child has experienced several such episodes previously that were successfully controlled with antibiotics. Further discussion of the child's medical history reveals that he had experienced a normal recovery from measles approximately 6 months earlier.

78. The most probable diagnosis, based on this history, is

(A) DiGeorge's syndrome
(B) Nezelof's syndrome
(C) Wiskott-Aldrich syndrome
(D) selective immunoglobulin deficiency

79. Leukocyte function studies are performed and indicate that phagocytosis, intracellular killing, and chemotactic responses are all within normal limits. These features rule out defects in non-specific resistance, a characteristic of all of the following disorders EXCEPT

(A) chronic granulomatous disease (CGD)
(B) lazy leukocyte syndrome
(C) Job's syndrome
(D) dysgammaglobulinemia

80. An immunoglobulin profile is ordered. The child has no detectable IgA or IgM in his serum. A small amount of IgG (30 mg/dl) is detected when the assay is repeated with low-level radial immunodiffusion plates. Based on this information, the most probable diagnosis is

(A) selective immunoglobulin deficiency
(B) common variable hypogammaglobulinemia
(C) Wiskott-Aldrich syndrome
(D) Bruton's hypogammaglobulinemia
(E) transient hypogammaglobulinemia of infancy

Questions 81–86

(A) Defective chloride ion channel regulation throughout the body
(B) Defective sodium channels in excitable tissues
(C) Defective androgen receptors in target tissues
(D) Defective 21-hydroxylase activity in steroid producing tissues
(E) Defective 17-β-hydroxysteroid dehydrogenase activity in steroid producing tissues
(F) Defective hydroxylation of proline residues in collagen
(G) Defective lysyl oxidase activity in fibroblasts
(H) Defective phenylalanine hydroxylase activity in the liver
(I) Defective cystathionine β-synthase activity in the liver
(J) Defective porphobilinogen deaminase activity in the liver

Match each of the following clinical or historical descriptions with the cellular or biochemical defect underlying the disease.

81. An 18-year-old man with moderately severe, diffuse abdominal pain has dark red urine and an increased heart rate. He is nauseated and says that he has been vomiting severely over the last several hours. Deep tendon reflexes are diminished, and he has a generalized muscular weakness. He admits to using barbiturates last night at a party, but says it was his first time.

82. A 2-month-old male infant in the neonatal intensive care unit with microcephaly and severe growth retardation has met few of the developmental milestones for his age. His mother vaguely remembers that she had dietary restrictions as a child.

83. A 3-week-old 46;X,X infant has moderate signs of virilization at birth including clitoral hypertrophy and partial fusion of the labioscrotal folds. Radiographic evaluation indicates normal internal female anatomy. She has been admitted to the neonatal intensive care unit for anorexia, vomiting, and hypotension.

84. A 7-year-old white girl is hospitalized with chronic pulmonary infections and malabsorption. Her development has been retarded secondary to her medical problems, which existed from birth.

85. The sternum of an 8-month-old female infant is sunken inward, and she has not stopped crying since her arrival in the emergency room 2 hours ago. Large ecchymoses are evident all over her body, but a careful examination reveals no signs of abuse. The mother, who is unemployed, and the infant live by themselves.

86. An 18-year-old woman with primary amenorrhea has normal breast development, and her body habitus is clearly female. Pubic hair is scanty but present, and she has no facial hair. Her clitoris and external genitalia are normal. A karyotype reveals that chromosomally she is 46; X,Y.

87. All of the following statements concerning mitochondrial DNA and proteins are true EXCEPT

(A) mitochondria use exactly the same genetic code that is used for nuclear genes

(B) the majority of proteins within a mitochondria are encoded by the nuclear DNA

(C) mitochondrial DNA has a higher mutation rate than nuclear DNA

(D) there may be genetic differences among the mitochondrial genomes within a single cell

(E) mitochondrial DNA is maternally inherited, and the genes lack introns

88. The parents of the boy, indicated with an arrow in the pedigree below, are seeking genetic counseling because of the genetic disease that the boy's father and several of his relatives have (shaded in pedigree). This disease causes severe symptoms beginning at about 10 years of age. Their youngest child is now 6 years old, and they would like to know what the chances are that this boy has the disease. The boy and several family members have been tested for a marker of the disease-causing locus that has a theta value of 0.01. The results are shown below the individuals in the pedigree. What should the family be told about the mode of inheritance and the likelihood that their son is affected?

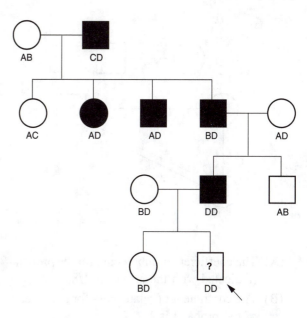

(A) Autosomal dominant, with a probability of 1 that the boy is affected

(B) Autosomal dominant, with a probability of 0.49 that the boy is affected

(C) Autosomal dominant, with a probability of 0.50 that the boy is affected

(D) Autosomal dominant, with a probability of 0.51 that the boy is affected

(E) Autosomal recessive, with a probability of 0.49 that the boy is affected

89. All of the following processes are matched with the correct direction EXCEPT

(A) DNA replication, leading strand—DNA is synthesized in a 5' to 3' direction
(B) DNA replication, lagging strand—DNA is read in a 3' to 5' direction
(C) transcription—DNA is read in a 5' to 3' direction
(D) translation—mRNA is read in a 5' to 3' direction
(E) translation—protein is synthesized from amino terminus to carboxy terminus

90. Using the pedigree below, which one of the following statements is true?

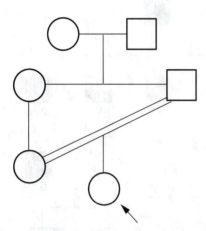

(A) The coefficient of inbreeding for the proband (indicated with the arrow) is 1/8
(B) The coefficient of relatedness for the parents of the proband is 1/2
(C) The coefficient of relatedness for the parents of the proband is 1/8
(D) The coefficient of inbreeding cannot be determined without knowledge of the proband's genotype
(E) If the proband is homozygous at a particular locus, it must be identity by descent
(F) The coefficient of inbreeding of the proband equals the coefficient of relatedness of her parents

91. Which one of the following statements about Graves disease is correct?

(A) Patients with Graves disease have symptoms due to the thyrotoxic effects
(B) Patients with Graves disease have high levels of thyroid-stimulating hormones (TSH)
(C) Although the thyroxine (T_4) index is elevated in patients with Graves disease, the tri-iodothyronine (T_3) is within normal limits
(D) A goiter is not usually seen in patients with Graves disease
(E) Graves disease occurs more commonly in women than in men
(F) Exophthalmos is a requirement for the diagnosis of Graves disease

92. A 49-year-old novelist who has been spending many hours at her computer complains of burning pain in her hands and numbness of her index and middle fingers. The pain is relieved by vigorously shaking her hands. All of the following statements are true EXCEPT

(A) the patient's symptoms are caused by compression of the median nerve
(B) the hand pain is caused by compression of the ulnar nerve as it passes through Guyon's canal
(C) a splint is helpful in reducing the symptoms
(D) the patient has carpal tunnel syndrome; if she does not receive treatment, she will develop an enlarged thenar eminence
(E) the patient has a positive Phalen test

93. All of the following are characteristic features of achondroplasia EXCEPT

(A) autosomal dominant inheritance
(B) normal intramembranous bone formation
(C) normal length of spine, short limbs
(D) increased lumbar lordosis
(E) metaphyseal flaring of long bones and bowing of legs
(F) mutation in the fibroblast growth factor receptor 3 gene
(G) mental retardation

94. A patient who recently had surgery involving his right hip area has a waddling gait. His pelvis tilts to the left when he lifts his left leg. All of the following statements are true EXCEPT

(A) the patient has a positive Trendelenburg sign
(B) the muscles that normally prevent a limp of this nature are the gluteus medius and the gluteus minimus
(C) the patient limp was caused by damage to the superior gluteal nerve during his surgery
(D) a dislocated hip would not cause a limp of this nature
(E) poliomyelitis may cause a limp of this nature

95. A 38-year-old woman is worried about developing osteoporosis. Her aunt recently had a hip fracture as a complication of osteoporosis. All of the following statements are correct concerning her fears EXCEPT

(A) cigarette smoking can increase one's risk of osteoporosis
(B) excessive alcohol use can increase one's risk of osteoporosis
(C) because one does not normally attain peak bone mass until 40 years of age, the patient should continue to get sufficient calcium and exercise
(D) after menopause, estrogen replacement therapy can reduce the amount of bone loss from that which is normally seen in postmenopausal women
(E) heredity plays an important role in determining one's peak bone mass

96. Which one of the following statements concerning smoking cessation is accurate?

(A) If a patient wants help, they will ask for it; otherwise, it is not useful to ask a patient about their smoking
(B) If a patient is going to succeed in quitting, it will likely be in his first attempt
(C) Most smokers have the desire to quit and have tried to quit at least once
(D) Both withdrawal symptoms and cravings for cigarettes last for several months after smoking cessation
(E) Pharmacologic treatment alone is as effective as any other method of smoking cessation
(F) A patient should never quit smoking "cold turkey," but rather reduce the number of cigarettes gradually

97. Which one of the following statements about eating disorders is correct?

(A) The difference between anorexia nervosa and bulimia nervosa is that bulimia nervosa involves purging behavior, and anorexia nervosa does not

(B) A patient may be diagnosed with bulimia nervosa, even if he or she is of normal weight

(C) A patient may be diagnosed with anorexia nervosa, even if he or she is of normal weight

(D) Although more often diagnosed in women, anorexia nervosa is equally common in men

(E) Eating disorders are acquired conditions that are brought about by societal pressures not genetic factors

Questions 98–100

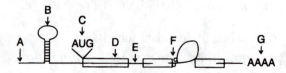

Using the diagrammatic representation of nucleic pre-messenger RNA, match the following descriptions with the correct lettered structure.

98. Site of translation initiation once the message has entered the cytoplasm

99. Site of autocatalytic activity of some RNA molecules; small nuclear ribonucleoproteins (snRNPs) can bind here

100. Site of specially modified base (N7-methyl-guanylate)

ANSWER KEY

1-D	21-C	41-A	61-E	81-J
2-D	22-D	42-C	62-A	82-H
3-C	23-E	43-D	63-C	83-D
4-C	24-B	44-B	64-D	84-A
5-B	25-A	45-D	65-D	85-F
6-B	26-D	46-C	66-E	86-C
7-C	27-D	47-C	67-F	87-A
8-D	28-B	48-D	68-C	88-C
9-B	29-B	49-C	69-D	89-C
10-C	30-D	50-C	70-A	90-A
11-D	31-F	51-C	71-D	91-E
12-D	32-C	52-D	72-A	92-D
13-E	33-D	53-D	73-A	93-G
14-A	34-E	54-B	74-C	94-D
15-D	35-A	55-A	75-B	95-C
16-E	36-D	56-E	76-E	96-C
17-D	37-B	57-C	77-A	97-B
18-E	38-A	58-D	78-D	98-C
19-B	39-F	59-B	79-D	99-F
20-E	40-D	60-D	80-D	100-A

ANSWERS AND EXPLANATIONS

1. The answer is D. *(Pathology; hypertension)*
Factors that indicate a poor prognosis in hypertension are male gender, persistent diastolic pressure greater than 115 mm Hg, hypercholesterolemia, diabetes mellitus, smoking, obesity, and evidence of end-organ damage. There is no dividing line between normal and high blood pressure; arbitrary levels have been established to define those who have increased risk of developing a morbid cardiovascular event. These definitions should consider not only the level of diastolic pressure but also systolic pressure, age, sex, and race. When hypertension is suspected, blood pressure should be measured at least twice on two separate examinations. In adults, a diastolic pressure of 115 mm Hg or greater is considered severe hypertension. A diastolic pressure of less than 90 mm Hg, with systolic pressure of 160 mm Hg or greater, is considered isolated systolic hypertension.

2. The answer is D. *(Biochemistry; ketones)*
Ketogenesis occurs when there is a high rate of fatty acid oxidation in the liver. Acetoacetate, β-hydroxybutyrate, and acetone are produced by this process. These substances are collectively known as ketone bodies. Higher than normal quantities of these substances in the blood or urine is a condition called ketosis. Ketone bodies are made in response to elevated levels of fatty acids in the liver, when the amount of acetyl CoA exceeds the oxidative capacity of the liver. Acetone is a breakdown product of acetoacetate that cannot be metabolized by the body. The liver cannot utilize ketone bodies because it lacks the enzyme necessary to convert acetoacetate into its acetoacetyl CoA form.

3. The answer is C. *(Behavioral science; pharmacology; alcohol withdrawal)*
Tremulousness, alcoholic hallucinosis, delirium tremens, and grand mal seizures are associated with alcohol withdrawal, and not petit mal seizures. Tremulousness occurs 8–12 hours after cessation of drinking. The patient manifests a tremor that is aggravated by inattention or agitation. Alcoholic hallucinosis usually occurs 12–24 hours after the cessation of drinking. The patient will experience auditory or visual hallucinations alternating with periods of lucidity. Grand mal seizures occur in 90% of cases between 6 and 48 hours after the cessation of drinking. Seizures are usually generalized and multiple. Delirium tremens usually occurs 3–4 days after the cessation of drinking. It manifests as confusion, hallucinations, tremors, and signs of autonomic hyperactivity.

4. The answer is C. *(Pathology; alcoholic liver disease)*
Elevation in gamma-glutamyl transpeptidase (GGT), serum glutamate oxaloacetate transaminase:serum glutamate pyruvate transaminase (SGOT:SGPT) ratio greater than or equal to 2:1, hypoalbuminemia, prolonged prothrombin time (PT), thrombocytopenia, low blood urea nitrogen (BUN), low glucose, and macrocytosis of red blood cells are laboratory data that support a diagnosis of liver disease owing to chronic alcohol abuse; hyperalbuminemia does not. Anemia may result from acute and chronic gastrointestinal blood loss, coexistent folic acid deficiency, and hypersplenism. Some patients may have leukopenia and thrombocytopenia resulting from hypersplenism or the inhibitory effect of alcohol on bone marrow. SGOT:SGPT ratio greater than 2 may result from the proportionally higher inhibition of SGPT synthesis by ethanol. Prolonged serum prothrombin time reflects reduced synthesis of clotting proteins, most notably vitamin K–dependent factors. Hypoalbuminemia reflects overall impairment in hepatic protein synthesis.

5. The answer is B. *(Pharmacology; antibiotics; erythromycin)*
Erythromycin binds reversibly to the 50s ribosomal subunit. It can interfere with the action of chloramphenicol, which also binds at this site. Gram-positive bacteria accumulate about 100 times more erythromycin than do gram-negative microorganisms. Erythromycin may be bactericidal or bacteriostatic, depending on the microorganism and the concentration of the drug, and can be used as a penicillin substitute. It is primarily

concentrated and excreted in an active form in the bile, and is contraindicated in patients with hepatic dysfunction.

6–7. The answers are: 6-B, 7-C. *(Biochemistry, hemoglobin)*

Myoglobin reversibly binds a single molecule of oxygen. The more tightly oxygen is bound, the lower the P_{50}. Therefore, the P_{50} of myoglobin is approximately 10 mm Hg, which is less than the P_{50} of hemoglobin, which is approximately 26 mm Hg. The oxygen dissociation curve for hemoglobin is sigmoidal, indicating that its subunits cooperate in binding oxygen. This cooperative binding results from the fact that the binding of one oxygen molecule at one heme increases the affinity of the remaining hemes for oxygen.

2,3-Diphosphoglycerate decreases the oxygen affinity of hemoglobin by binding to deoxyhemoglobin, but not to oxyhemoglobin. This preferential binding stabilizes the taut configuration of deoxyhemoglobin, thereby decreasing the oxygen affinity of hemoglobin. 1,3-Diphosphoglycerate, an intermediate of glycolysis, can be converted to 2,3-diphosphoglycerate by a mutase. 2,3-Diphosphoglycerate is hydrolyzed by a phosphatase to 3-phosphoglycerate, which is also an intermediate of glycolysis.

8. The answer is D. *(Pharmacology; digitalis)*

Hypokalemia, and not hyperkalemia, predisposes patients to digitalis toxicity. Hypercalcemia, hypernatremia, hypermagnesemia, and alkalosis also predispose to digitalis toxicity. Digitalis increases contractility of the cardiac muscle. This increased myocardial contraction leads to a decrease in diastolic volume, thus increasing the efficiency of contraction. The resulting improved circulation results in a decrease in sympathetic activity, which reduces peripheral resistance. All of this causes a reduction in heart rate. Digitalis inhibits Na^+/K^+ exchange by Na^+, K^+-ATPase. This causes an increase in intracellular sodium, which results in a decrease in Ca^{2+} exported from the cell and favors the import of Ca^{2+} into the cell by the Na^+/Ca^{2+} exchange mechanism. Severe digitalis toxicity can result in ventricular tachycardia.

9. The answer is B. *(Pharmacology; general anesthetics)*

Isoflurane is a halogenated anesthetic that does not sensitize the heart to the action of epinephrine. Inhaled gases are the mainstay of anesthesia and are used for the maintenance of anesthesia after the administration of an intravenous agent. A benefit of inhaled anesthetics over intravenous agents is that the depth of anesthesia can be rapidly altered by changing the concentration of the inhaled anesthetic. In addition, most of these agents are rapidly eliminated from the body and therefore do not tend to cause postoperative respiratory depression.

10. The answer is C. *(Pharmacology; methotrexate)*

Leucovorin (N^5-formyl-FH_4) rescues cells from methotrexate cytotoxicity by bypassing the blocked enzyme dihydrofolate reductase. It replenishes the folate pool by its conversion to N^5, N^{10}-methylene-FH_4, which bypasses the inhibited dihydrofolate reductase. Methotrexate is structurally related to folic acid, which enables it to inhibit dihydrofolate reductase. Resistance to methotrexate is characteristic of nonproliferating cells.

11. The answer is D. *(Physiology; sickle cell anemia)*

Increasing the blood pH of the patient shifts the oxygen saturation curve such that the proportion of deoxygenated hemoglobin S (Hb S) is decreased. Decreased oxygen tension, increased carbon dioxide concentration, and increased 2,3-diphosphoglycerate in erythrocytes all increase the proportion of Hb S in the deoxygenated state. Decreased oxygen tension increases the amount of deoxygenated Hb S. Increased 2,3-diphosphoglycerate shifts the oxygen curve to the right, causing the proportion of Hb S that is deoxygenated to increase. Elevated carbon dioxide levels increase the amount of carbon dioxide available to bind to Hb S, allowing Hb S to stabilize in its deoxygenated form.

12. The answer is D. *(Pathology; erythrocyte sedimentation rate)*
The erythrocyte sedimentation rate (ESR) is a nonspecific index of inflammation. Whether the ESR is normal, increased, or decreased depends on the sum of forces acting on the red blood cells. These include the downward force of gravity, the upward buoyant forces, and the bulk plasma flow. ESR can be increased by hypercholesterolemia, inflammatory disorders, anemia, and pregnancy. ESR is decreased by congestive heart failure.

13. The answer is E. *(Microbiology; asplenia)*
Patients who are asplenic because of anatomic absence or functional asplenia are prone to infection from encapsulated organisms such as *Streptococcus pneumoniae*, *Haemophilus influenzae*, *Staphylococcus aureus*, and *Neisseria meningitidis*. Pneumococci cause pneumonia, bacteremia, meningitis, and upper respiratory tract infections. *N. meningitidis* mainly causes menigitis and meningococcemia. *S. aureus* cause both invasive disorders, such as deep abscesses, carbuncles, and pyoderms, and toxigenic disorders, such as food poisoning, toxic epidermal necrolysis, and scaled skin syndrome. *H. influenzae* is a leading cause of meningitis in young children, an important cause of upper respiratory infection and sepsis in children, and causes pneumonia in adults. *Trichinella spiralis* is a nematode that causes trichinosis and is not commonly associated with infections in asplenic patients.

14. The answer is A. *(Biochemistry; carbohydrate metabolism)*
Galactosemia is caused by uridyl transferase deficiency, not a galactokinase deficiency. Galactokinase deficiency would cause galactosuria and causes galactitol accumulation if galactose is present in the diet.

15. The answer is D. *(Biochemistry; coenzymes)*
Coenzyme Q transfers hydrogen atoms and electrons in the mitochondrial oxidative phosphorylation system. Humans synthesize their own coenzyme Q. Coenzyme A is generated in the liver from pantothenic acid (a B vitamin) combining with adenosine triphosphate (ATP) and cysteine. Pyridoxal phosphate is converted from vitamin B_6. Thiamine pyrophosphate is an ester of thiamine (vitamin B_1).

16. The answer is E. *(Pathology; endocrinology; pheochromocytomas)*
Pheochromocytoma is a tumor derived from catecholamine-producing chromaffin cells. These cells release excessive catecholamines (i.e., epinephrine and norepinephrine) into the blood, causing a classical clinical triad of headaches, sweating, and palpitations. In addition, a plethora of other symptoms, including nausea, tremors, fatigue, chest or abdominal pain, dyspnea, and dizziness, may be noted. Physical findings that are consistent with the presence of a pheochromocytoma are hypertension (sustained or paroxysmal), tachycardia, tremor, lean body habitus, and Raynaud's phenomenon. Syncope is not generally associated with the presence of a pheochromocytoma. Diagnosis is based upon finding elevated catecholamines in the blood or urine. The urine may also contain catecholamine metabolites, such as metanephrines and vanillylmandelic acid.

Pharmacologic testing may be necessary to distinguish pheochromocytoma from essential hypertension. Administration of glucagon increases plasma catecholamine levels in patients with pheochromocytoma but not in patients with essential hypertension. Calcium-channel blockers are given to safeguard against the risk of severe hypertension following glucagon administration. Clonidine may also be administered to distinguish between a pheochromocytoma and essential hypertension. Clonidine suppresses serum catecholamine levels in patients with essential hypertension but has no effect in patients with a pheochromocytoma.

Pheochromocytomas characteristically present as benign, unilateral, intra-adrenal tumors in adults. However, it is important to remember that 10% of pheochromocytomas are bilateral, 10% are extra-adrenal (associated with sympathetic ganglia), 10% are malignant, and 10% are found in the pediatric population. Finally, 10% are familial and are associated with several syndomes, including MEN-IIA and IIB (also referred to as MEN-II and III, respectively), neurofibromatosis, and von Hippel-Lindau.

17–20. The answers are: 17-D, 18-E, 19-B, 20-E. *(Immunology; immunoglobulins)*
The complement system, which plays a major role in host defense and the inflammatory process, can be activated (fixed) via the classic or alternative pathways. Activation of the pathways may occur via antigen–antibody complexes or by aggregated immunoglobulins. IgG molecules (mainly the IgG1 and IgG3 subclasses) are capable of fixing complement. Activation of the classic pathway follows binding of complement to the C_H2 domain on the Fc fragment of IgG. Serum IgA fixes complement via the alternative pathway only. Activation of this pathway can be triggered immunologically primarily by IgA (and to a lesser degree by some IgG). IgM is the most efficient immunoglobulin at activating complement via the classic pathway. Only one molecule of IgM is required to react with complement. Activation of the classic pathway follows binding of complement to the C_H3 domain on the Fc fragment of IgM.

21. The answer is C. *(Neurology; vertigo)*
Patients with vestibular dizziness complain of vertigo, which is a sense of spinning or the turning of themselves or their environment. This sensation of motion, when none is present, is a hallucination. Vertigo can be central (a brain stem lesion) or peripheral (an ear lesion). Central vertigo is frequently accompanied by other signs of brain stem dysfunction (e.g., double vision, weakness or numbness of the face, and dysphagia). Peripheral vertigo is usually accompanied by tinnitus or hearing loss, but no other neurologic abnormalities. Multiple sclerosis is a disease associated with central nervous system lesions, not lesions of the ear, and it would cause central vertigo, not peripheral vertigo. Vestibular neuronitis, Meniere's disease, and acoustic neuroma are all associated with ear lesions, and the vertigo associated with these disorders would be considered peripheral vertigo.

22. The answer is D. *(Physiology; kidney stones)*
Calcium oxalate kidney stones are the most common form of kidney stone in the United States. Because they are calcified, they are apparent on radiograph. Patient's with these stones frequently present with hematuria or flank pain. Unless there are complications (e.g., complete obstruction, infection, severe hematuria, and intolerable pain that cannot be controlled by analgesics), endoscopic therapy or lithotripsy is usually delayed approximately 2 months. The reason for the delay is that 70% of calculi smaller than 5 mm will pass spontaneously (only 30% of those larger than 6 mm will pass spontaneously). Intravenous pyelography should be performed after the incident to confirm that the urinary tract has been cleared. More than 70% of patients will have recurrences; however, increased fluid intake may help to prevent recurrences.

23. The answer is E. *(Physiology; syndrome of inappropriate secretion of antidiuretic hormone)*
The syndrome of inappropriate secretion of antidiuretic hormone (SIADH) is characterized by a urine osmolality that is too concentrated relative to serum tonicity. In the case of hyponatremia, the urine should be maximally dilute to limit further sodium losses. Diagnosis also includes the exclusion of other causes of water retention (e.g., volume depletion and congestive heart failure). Total body sodium must also be normal. Although water restriction may be sufficient therapy for mild cases, symptoms of the central nervous system and a serum sodium level lower than 120 mEq/L require treatment with both saline and diuretics. Correction of the hyponatremia; however, must be done slowly to avoid causing brain damage.

24. The answer is B. *(Pharmacology; diuretics)*
The majority of reabsorption takes place in the proximal tubule, but diuretics that act in this segment are not very efficacious because their effects may be compensated for by increased reabsorption in the loop of Henle. Conversely, although only approximately 20% of sodium reabsorption occurs in the loop of Henle, drugs that act in this segment make up the most efficacious class of diuretics. Thus, loop diuretics are often used for rapid diuresis in severe cases of edema. Kidney stones are a possible side effect of loop diuretics, because they decrease the electrical potential that increases the reabsorption of calcium and magnesium.

Thus, the calcium concentration increases in the tubular lumen, and kidney stones may form. Loop diuretics and thiazide-type diuretics may cause a metabolic alkalosis, because of the increased proton secretion in the collecting duct. This excess secretion of hydrogen ions is caused by increased sodium delivery to the collecting duct. Aldosterone antagonists act in the collecting duct, and they may cause a metabolic acidosis because of the reduction in sodium reabsorption and proton secretion. Almost all osmotic diuretics are ineffective orally and are not efficacious for severe edema.

25. The answer is A. *(Immunology; mast cells and allergies)*
Upon first encounter between an allergic individual and the allergen, immunoglobulin E (IgE) antibodies are produced. These antibodies then bind to high-affinity Fc receptors on the surface of mast cells and basophils. The antigen-binding portion of the antibodies are unbound and can bind to allergens during the next encounter. When enough IgE coats the mast cell so that antibodies are close to one another, the allergen cross-links the adjacent IgE, triggering the release of granules containing inflammatory mediators (i.e., leuko-trienes, histamine, and serotonin).

26. The answer is D. *(Physiology; endocrine system)*
Insulin facilitates the entry of glucose into cells of all tissues except the brain, kidney tubules, intestinal mucosa, and red blood cells. Insulin is produced by the β-cells of the pancreatic islets. It is a polypeptide hormone made up of A and B chains, which are connected by disulfide bonds. The action of the hormone is anabolic, increasing glucose, fatty acid, and amino acid storage. Insulin increases glycogenesis in the liver by stimulating glucokinase and glycogen synthetase. It also inhibits gluconeogenesis in the liver by inhibiting phosphorylase.

27. The answer is D. *(Genetics; Hardy-Weinberg equilibrium)*
The Hardy-Weinberg equilibrium equation ($p^2 + 2pq + q^2 = 1$) includes random mating and no selection or mutations. If the penetrance of the trait is only 50%, then the percentage of people that are homozygous recessive is twice the percentage with the trait (4.5% $\times$ 2 = 9%). Thus, q may be calculated by taking the square root of 0.09 (= 0.3), and p may be determined by subtracting $1 - q$ (= 0.7). Thus, the percentage of heterozygotes in the population should be 2pq, or 2 $\times$ 0.3 $\times$ 0.7 = 0.42 = 42%.

28. The answer is B. *(Pathology; chronic interstitial lung disease)*
These symptoms are typical of usual interstitial pneumonia (UIP), also known as idiopathic pulmonary fibrosis. This disease responds to steroid therapy in only a relatively small percentage of cases. UIP is frequently associated with connective tissue diseases. It can be differentiated from bronchiolitis obliterans organizing pneumonia (BOOP) by the length of time during which the symptoms developed. BOOP generally develops over a period of less than a couple of months. Also, BOOP tends to have a ground-glass appearance on chest radiographs, rather than the reticular or reticulonodular appearance seen in UIP. UIP is characterized by a patchy and temporally heterogeneous pattern of injury on examination of the lung biopsy.

29. The answer is B. *(Biochemistry; hormone synthesis)*
Vasopressin and oxytocin are peptides that are synthesized in the hypothalamus and secreted from the posterior pituitary. The adrenal cortex synthesizes three types of steroid hormones including glucocorticoids (e.g., cortisol) in the zona fasiculata, mineralocorticoids (e.g., aldosterone) in the zona glomerulosa, and androgens in the zona reticularis. The adrenal medulla synthesizes catecholamines including norepinephrine. The pancreatic islet cells secrete the peptide hormones insulin (β-cells) and glucagon (α-cells), as well as other hormones.

30. The answer is D. *(Medicine; complications of diabetes mellitus)*
Although the incidence of foot ulcers and the need for amputations do increase with the duration of diabetes, the glucose level control also has a strong effect. A person who has had diabetes for 20 years is less likely to have complications if he has maintained control of his glucose levels. Other behavioral aspects (e.g., good hygiene and properly fitted shoes) can reduce the risk of foot ulcers and the need for amputations. The cause of foot ulcers in diabetic patients is often multifactorial. Motor neuropathies can cause atrophy of the foot muscles leading to abnormal pressure points. A sensory neuropathy can make diabetic patients unable to feel a cut or lesion on their foot, allowing it to progress without treatment. However, although diabetic neuropathies often cause a lack of sensation in the feet, they cause extremely severe pain in some individuals. Vascular insufficiency to the foot can reduce the ability of the immune system to effectively heal a lesion, as effector cells cannot easily reach the lesion and eliminate infection.

31–33. The answers are: 31-F, 32-C, 33-D. *(Physiology; Valsalva maneuver)*
The subject described in the question exhaled against a small leak, requiring the use of thoracic and abdominal muscles to maintain voluntarily an elevated esophageal (and intrathoracic) pressure of 40 cm H_2O. Transmission of applied pressure causes a rise in blood pressure (*B*) followed quickly by a decrease in arterial pressure and pulse pressure (*C*) as venous return is cut off. A reflex change during the maneuver prevents further decline in blood pressure with accompanying reflex tachycardia (*D*). When the strain ends, the blood pressure falls, and venous return is restored (*E*). In a normal subject, an overshoot in pressure followed by a vagally mediated bradycardia ensues (*F*).

34–38. The answers are: 34-E, 35-A, 36-D, 37-B, 38-A. *(Behavioral science; personality disorders)*
Antisocial behavior in an adult has roots in similar behavior as a child or teenager; such children are termed conduct-disordered. Obsessive–compulsive individuals are rigid, perfectionistic, overly organized, and have difficulty relaxing or having fun. Narcissistic individuals are self-centered with a grandiose sense of self, yet they have underlying poor self-esteem and become enraged when they perceive criticism, even if slight. Individuals with borderline personalities frequently cut themselves, even superficially, and often have multiple scars.

39–42. The answers are: 39-F, 40-D, 41-A, 42-C. *(Pathology; musculoskeletal tumors)*
A chondroblastoma is a benign tumor composed of small immature chondrocytes, each with a single nucleus, dispersed among benign-appearing, multinucleated giant cells and chondroid matrix. This tumor most often occurs within the epiphyseal region of long, tubular bones of individuals between the ages of 10 and 20 years. Males are affected twice as often as females.

A giant cell tumor is a benign, but locally invasive, lesion characterized by many multinucleated giant cells distributed in a stroma of neoplastic, smaller, mononucleated cells. Over 50% of these ''brown'' tumors develop in the distal femur or proximal tibia or fibula. The majority of individuals with this tumor are between 20 and 40 years of age. Females are affected slightly more often than males. The tumor frequently recurs many years after surgical removal.

An osteosarcoma is a malignant tumor that most often arises in the medullary cavity of the metaphyseal end of the long bones of the extremities. It is a tumor of mesenchymal cells in which there is deposition of osteoid or new bone. This tumor is most often seen in adolescent or young adult males. Deletions of the long arm of chromosome 13, which are associated with retinoblastoma, are hypothesized to be associated with osteosarcoma development. Radiographs of osteosarcomas often show Codman's triangle—an angle formed between the elevated periosteum and the plane of the outer surface of the cortical bone.

Ewing's sarcoma is a malignant neoplasm, most often seen in the pelvis and long tubular bones. It is characterized radiographically by ''onion-skin'' layering of the cortex and widening of the diaphyseal region. Ewing's sarcoma usually arises before the age of 20 years, and it appears twice as often in males as in females. This tumor is associated with translocation of portions of the long arms of chromosomes 11 and 22.

43. The answer is D. *(Physiology; potassium homeostasis)*
Although both cardiac and neuromuscular symptoms can be caused by either hypokalemia or hyperkalemia, the electrocardiogram patterns are distinct for each abnormality. Hyperkalemia is associated with peaked T waves, a wide QRS complex, a prolonged PR interval, absent P waves, and a sine wave pattern. Hypokalemia causes flattened T waves, U waves, and ST segment depression. Treatment of hyperkalemia should include rapid administration of intravenous calcium followed by insulin, albuterol, and sodium bicarbonate and then a potassium-binding agent (e.g., sodium polystyrene sulfonate). Treatment is emergent because cardiac arrest or arrythmias could occur. Angiotensin-converting enzyme (ACE) inhibitors and β-blockers should be avoided because these drugs, as well as diabetes, are potential causes of hyperkalemia. Treatment of hypokalemia is less urgent, but should include potassium replacement as well as a search for the underlying cause.

44. The answer is B. *(Physiology; renal tubule acidosis)*
The various types of renal tubule acidosis (RTA) are disorders that cause a normal anion gap, metabolic acidosis. Type I involves a disturbance of the proton pumps in the distal nephron. Type II involves defects in the proton secretion and bicarbonate reabsorption in the proximal nephron. Type II frequently has concomitant hypokalemia, and hypophosphatemia is commom. Type IV involves defects in both potassium and proton secretion in the distal nephron. It is associated with decreased ammonia production, hyperkalemia, and hypoaldosteronism. Diabetic nephropathy is a factor in more than half of the cases.

45. The answer is D. *(Physiology; acute renal failure)*
Acute renal failure may be caused by acute tubular necrosis, acute interstitial nephritis, and many other problems. Acute tubular necrosis is frequently incited by aminoglycoside antibiotics, including gentamicin, or by the use of contrast media for radiologic studies. Dirty brown casts are often present in the urine specimen. Patients with acute tubular necrosis do not have proteinuria, red blood cells, white blood cells, and white blood cell casts, but these cells are often seen in patients with acute interstitial nephritis. Acute interstitial nephritis is associated with penicillin, dilantin, infections, and radiation. A hypersensitivity response (e.g., fever, rash, and arthralgia) may occur with acute interstitial nephritis, but is not seen in patients with acute tubular necrosis.

46. The answer is C. *(Immunology; major histocompatibility complex class I)*
MHC-I is a protein present on almost all cells of the body. Its function is to sample the intracellular contents and present peptides that come from inside the cell. In the uninfected, noncancerous cell, MHC-I presents normal cell peptides, and there is no immune response. If the cell is infected by a virus, intracellular bacteria, or if it is cancerous, then the peptides presented by the MHC-I may be recognized as non-self by CD8$^+$ T lymphocytes. Some viruses are able to down-regulate the MHC-I expression and avoid detection. Natural killer cells, which are part of the innate immune system and are antigen nonspecific, are inhibited by the presence of MHC-I on the cell surface. Virally infected cells with low expression of MHC-I have an increased risk of being killed by natural killer cells.

47. The answer is C. *(Genetics; imprinting)*
Genomic imprinting is defined as a difference in the expression of genetic material depending on whether it is maternal or paternal in origin. Although the mechanisms for this process are not entirely understood, it is known to occur. Prader-Willi syndrome is an example of a disease that is caused by the lack of a paternally derived copy of a certain genetic sequence on chromosome 15. Angelman syndrome is caused by the lack of a maternal copy of a nearby sequence. Prader-Willi syndrome may be due to either deletion of the specific region of the paternally derived chromosome 15 or, less commonly, due to maternal uniparental disomy of chromosome 15. Although maternal monosomy 15 and maternal uniparental diploidy would lead to Prader-Willi syndrome (if only the region of chromosome 15 is considered), these conditions are not compatible

with life. Trisomy 15 is also not compatible with life beyond fetal stages, nor would it lead to the absence of a paternal chromosome 15 or Prader-Willi syndrome.

48. The answer is D. *(Genetics; prenatal diagnosis)*
Prenatal tests such as amniocentesis and chorionic villus sampling are diagnostic tests, not a screen for a normal fetus. It is necessary to have some idea of what could be wrong for a prenatal test to be worthwhile. For a woman who had a miscarriage of unknown cause, prenatal testing may not be helpful. Prenatal tests also involve risk; therefore, if there is a low probability of diagnosis, performing the test may be unwise. In the case of a previous child with a trisomy, neural tube defect, or metabolic disease (e.g., Tay-Sachs disease); a parent with a chromosomal rearrangement or neural tube defect; or a mother older than age 35 years (risk of Down syndrome increases exponentially with age), prenatal diagnostic testing is indicated. The ultimate decision on whether testing is done should be made by the patient.

49. The answer is C. *(Physiology; ventilation/perfusion mismatch)*
In a patient with a ventilation/perfusion (V/Q) mismatch, the level of the partial pressure of carbon dioxide (P_{CO_2}) will increase and the level of the partial pressure of oxygen (P_{O_2}) will decrease. The decrease in the P_{CO_2} will cause the patient to increase his rate of ventilation because of central chemoreceptors, enabling the patient to compensate for the elevated P_{CO_2} and keep this value within the normal range. However, the patient will not be able to compensate for the lowered P_{O_2}. The reason for this failure is that the vast majority of oxygen in the blood is carried by hemoglobin, and under normal conditions the hemoglobin is near saturation of its oxygen-carrying capacity. Thus, even with hyperventilation, an area of high V/Q cannot increase the amount of oxygen that it is carrying to compensate for an area of low V/Q. Increasing the concentration of oxygen of the inspired air would not be beneficial.

50. The answer is C. *(Behavioral medicine; patient compliance)*
Patient compliance should be a major concern of physicians because up to 50% of patients are poorly adherent to some aspect of their treatment regimen. Adherence is even a problem for patients with life-threatening illnesses (e.g., cancer and transplants). Neither sex, race, nor socioeconomic status is related to the level of compliance. However, cost and the complexity of the regimen do affect adherence. Patients are more compliant if they are involved in the planning of the regimen. Even in the hospital, patients do not always receive the prescribed dosages at the prescribed times; furthermore, they may refuse to take certain treatments when offered. In terms of research protocols, poor adherence decreases the apparent efficacy of the treatment, but it also underestimates the toxicity of the regimen. Thus, it is an important parameter to measure. It may be assessed by several methods, including pill counting, patient report or daily diary, and biochemical tests.

51. The answer is C. *(Anatomy; classification of joints)*
Synarthroses do not permit any motion because they are made up of a thin layer of fibrous tissue. The sutures of the skull are a good example of this type of joint. Amphiarthroses allow only a small degree of motion, as they are made up of flexible fibrocartilage. The intervertebral discs of the spine are examples of amphiarthroses. Diarthroses are synovial-lined joints. They include hinge joints (e.g., the knee), ball-and-socket joints, saddle joints, and plane joints. Diarthroses also have a capsule, intracapsular and extracapsular ligaments, and tendons that are composed largely of type I collagen.

52. The answer is D. *(Anatomy; bone fractures and healing)*
Bone is weakest in tension, somewhat stronger in torsion and bending, and strongest in compression. Tension failure also leads to transverse fractures. Once a stable clot is formed, cartilage begins to be laid down to stabilize the wound enough for bone to grow (i.e., decrease the strain). However, cartilage formation may not occur if the bone ends are apposed to each other and no motion is allowed. A hard callous forms, and

woven bone is laid down. Then the woven bone is replaced by lamellar bone. Cortical bone and trabecular bone are subtypes of lamellar bone. Presence of a physis on radiograph indicates that the skeleton is not fully mature; the physis disappears once growth is complete. A fracture that does not heal within 6 months is termed a nonunion; a malunion is a fracture that heals in an abnormal position.

53. The answer is D. *(Anatomy; rheumatoid arthritis versus osteoarthritis)*
Rheumatoid arthritis (RA) is characterized by symmetrical joint pain, morning stiffness lasting more than 60 minutes; sparing of the distal interphalangeal joints (DIP); involvement of the wrist, metacarpophalangeal joints (MCP), and proximal interphalangeal joints (PIP); and the presence of systemic symptoms. The pain in patients with RA is relatively constant and not relieved by rest. "Swan neck" deformities are just one example of the complications that can arise. Fluid removed from an RA joint has a low viscosity but a high white blood cell count because of the inflammation. Osteoarthritis is less commonly symmetrical, involves morning stiffness for 5 to 10 minutes, often involves the DIP joints, typically worsens with activity, and is relieved by rest. It does not cause the vast array of systemic symptoms that are seen in patients with RA. Swelling is uncommon, and the MCP are less frequently involved in patients with osteoarthritis. Fluid removed from a painful osteoarthritis joint will be viscous, but will have few white blood cells.

54–58. The answers are: 54-B, 55-A, 56-E, 57-C, 58-D. *(Cell biology; organelle structure and function)*
The Golgi complex (*B*) is composed of flattened membranous sacs and functions in protein glycosylation, membrane recycling, and sorting and targeting of proteins. Introns are regions of DNA that are transcribed but not translated. In the nucleus (*A*), introns are cleaved from primary RNA transcripts to produce mature messenger RNA (mRNA). Ribosomes are composed of ribosomal RNA (rRNA), which is synthesized in the nucleolus (*E*) of the cell by RNA polymerase I. Smooth endoplasmic reticulum (*C*) has various functions, including steroid synthesis; calcium homeostasis; and lipid, cholesterol, and drug metabolism. Adenosine triphosphate (ATP) is synthesized by glycolysis in the cytosol and by oxidative phosphorylation in the mitochondria (*D*).

59–63. The answers are: 59-B, 60-D, 61-E, 62-A, 63-C. *(Biochemistry; transport proteins)*
The functions of transport proteins can be divided into three general classes: the control of diffusion into the tissues; the highly specific recognition of molecules; and the removal of toxins. Transferrin helps in transporting iron to storage and utilization sites in the bone marrow. The damage that free iron can cause to tissues other than the marrow is prevented when it is bound by transferrin. Transcobalamin binds vitamin B_{12} and prevents it from degrading while it is being transported to storage and utilization sites in tissues with high cellular turnover rates. Albumin is the main plasma protein responsible for the maintenance of plasma osmotic pressure. Haptoglobin is a plasma protein that binds free hemoglobin in the blood and delivers it to the liver for recycling. The degree of intravascular hemolysis is determined by measuring the levels of depleted free forms of haptoglobin in the blood.

64. The answer is D. *(Immunology; splenectomy)*
Splenectomy does cause an increased susceptibility to infection, but the risks can be reduced if the proper precautions are taken. Encapsulated bacteria, especially *Streptococcus pneumoniae* and *Haemophilus influenzae,* present the greatest threat to patients without a spleen. If possible, vaccinations to both of these organisms should be given to the patient before surgery. Prophylactic antibiotics should be taken following splenectomy, particularly when dental work or other invasive procedures are to be performed. Certain aspects of the immune system will remain intact after splenectomy. Thus, it is not necessary to repeat immunizations after surgery. In addition, splenectomy does not significantly increase susceptibility to viral infections or infections by *Staphylococcus aureus*. In fact, adults who have already been exposed to many microorganisms are less affected by removal of the spleen than are children.

65. The answer is D. *(Genetics; abnormalities of morphogenesis)*
Malformations are due to intrinsic processes and include abnormalities (e.g., cleft lip). Dysplasias are also often due to genetic causes, but they involve abnormalities of cells or tissues rather than organs (e.g., phacomatoses). Deformations and disruptions are caused by extrinsic factors (e.g., compression and teratogens, respectively). Examples include clubfoot (deformation) and amniotic bands (disruption). A syndrome is a pattern of abnormalities with one cause, whereas an association does not have a single cause.

66. The answer is E. *(Genetics; myotonic dystrophy)*
Myotonic dystrophy is an autosomal dominant disorder that may cause myotonia, distal muscle weakness, and mental retardation. This disorder is an example of an expansion disorder. In an affected individual the causative gene contains a repeated sequence that is present in an abnormally high number. The severity of the disease often worsens in successive generations (genetic anticipation). With myotonic dystrophy, this possibility in passage from the mother than the father is much more common. In fact, a child born to a mother with the disease is at risk for neonatal complications including respiratory distress and "floppiness." Previous healthy siblings do not change the risk to the fetus. Because the mother has this autosomal dominant disease, each of her children, male or female, will have a 50% chance of getting the disease.

67. The answer is E. *(Physiology; Cushing's syndrome)*
Cushing's syndrome symptoms are hypertension, impaired glucose tolerance, truncal fat, hirsutism, osteoporosis, abdominal striae, and amennorrhea. The causes of Cushing's syndrome include pituitary tumors, adrenal tumors, ectopic adrenocorticotropic hormone (ACTH) expression, and exogenous glucocorticoid use. Each of these etiologies results in increased levels of glucocorticoids. High levels of dexamethasone, which can act like cortisol through feedback inhibition to block the release of ACTH, can suppress the ACTH and cortisol release in nearly all pituitary tumors that cause Cushing's syndrome. In Cushing's syndrome caused by an adrenal tumor, the ACTH is kept low by the feedback inhibition of high levels of cortisol; however, ectopic production of ACTH, which is most commonly seen in lung cancer, remains elevated. Addison's disease is characterized by low levels of glucocorticoids. Waterhouse-Friderichsen syndrome is also characterized by adrenocortical insufficiency, and it occurs in the setting of sepsis.

68. The answer is C. *(Physiology; hypoglycemia)*
Hypoglycemia can be caused by several mechanisms in nondiabetic patients. Because the hypoglycemia occurs postprandially, insulinoma is unlikely, as they typically cause fasting hypoglycemia. If someone is taking excess insulin that is causing their hypoglycemia (factitious hypoglycemia), the level of insulin will be higher than the level of C-peptide because C-peptide is not included in exogenous preparations of insulin. A reactive cause of hypoglycemia (including alimentary and idiopathic) causes postprandial symptoms. In alimentary hypoglycemia, rapid gastric emptying (as a result of surgery or other factors) causes an excess of insulin secretion with meals. Alcohol, pentamidine, and several other drugs may also cause hypoglycemia. Liver damage can also be a cause of hypoglycemia; however, more than 80% of the liver mass must be dysfunctional before the rate of hepatic glucose production is reduced. An oral glucose tolerance test is not required for patients with hypoglycemia and may confuse the issue because the results are not consistent for patients in this setting.

69. The answer is D. *(Anatomy; acute gouty arthritis)*
Painful and swollen big toe and ankle, after consuming alcohol, are common symptoms of acute gouty arthritis. The metatarsophalangeal joint of the first toe is the joint that is most often affected, whereas the ankle is also frequently involved. This differs somewhat from pseudogout, which is a calcium pyrophosphate dihydrate deposition disease. Pseudogout commonly affects the knee; otherwise, pseudogout is similar to

gout symptomatically. Acute gouty arthritis is caused by the accumulation of monosodium urate crystals, a by-product of purine catabolism. These crystals can be seen under polarized light as negatively birefringent crystals that are bright yellow. Alcohol ingestion and dietary excess of purines can precipitate an attack. Alcohol accelerates the degradation of adenosine triphosphate. Although chronic gout and tophi may develop in this patient, it usually takes about 10 years after the initial symptoms for tophi to develop. In addition, the initial acute attacks are self-limited, and the symptoms resolve in 3–10 days without treatment.

70. The answer is A. *(Pathology; Paget's disease)*
Paget's disease, also known as osteitis deformans, is often asymptomatic, but it may cause deformity, pain, and other complications (e.g., pathologic fractures and, occasionally, sarcomas). It is a disease of disordered bone formation, not bone mineralization. Thus, the irregular cement lines that are formed in abnormal bone metabolism form a "mosaic" pattern. Large osteoclasts with up to 100 nuclei may also be present, demonstrating the abnormal bone remodeling. Because the mineralization of the bone is relatively unaffected in patients with Paget's disease, there is not an increased thickness of the osteoid layer as is seen in patients with osteomalacia.

71. The answer is D. *(Immunology; reactive arthritis)*
Reactive arthritis, also known as Reiter's syndrome, occurs in genetically susceptible individuals after an infection. The presence of the human leukocyte antigen (HLA)-B27 seems to play a role in the pathogenesis, but is not required for diagnosis of the disease. Symptoms may include lower back and joint pain that is commonly asymmetric and in the lower extremities. The back pain may radiate to the legs and worsens with inactivity. Conjunctivitis, or even uveitis, may occur unilaterally or bilaterally. Keratoderma blenorrhagica may be seen on the skin, and cardiac complications can occur. The syndrome is usually precipitated by a urogenital or gastrointestinal infection. The erythrocyte sedimenation rate is sometimes elevated, but this is a nonspecific result. A postive gonococcal culture from the synovium or blood indicates that the arthritis is most likely caused by a systemic gonococcal infection rather than reactive arthritis. The inflamed joints in patients with reactive arthritis should be sterile. However, finding gonococcal infection in the urethra is not as definitive, and the patient may still have reactive arthritis. This distinction is important as there are different treatments for the two diseases.

72–74. The answers are: 72-A, 73-A, 74-C. *(Cell biology; cell characteristics and function)*
The T cell—specifically the helper T (Th) cell—can help with the B-cell proliferation and differentiation to an antibody-secreting plasma cell that occurs in the antibody response. If antigen on an accessory cell (e.g., a macrophage) interacts with its homologous receptor on a T-cell surface, this will trigger lymphokine release from the Th cell, as well as proliferation and differentiation of the B cell, if both the cells are identical at the class II major histocompatibility complex (MHC). The Th cells that participate in B-cell maturation also show this MHC restriction.

There are several functional subsets of T cells. Cytotoxic T (Tc) cells cause lysis of antigen-bearing target cells (virally infected cells, tumor cells, transplanted allogeneic cells). Besides being important in B-cell maturation, Th cells also function in Tc-cell development. The suppressor T (Ts) cell has an opposing function: It serves to down-regulate (depress) the immune response. Ts cells suppress directly, or via suppressor factors, the function of other immunologically active cells (e.g., Th cells). Ts cells and Tc cells bear the CD8 membrane antigen but not the CD4; therefore they are $CD8^+$, $CD4^-$, and are easily distinguished from Th cells, which are $CD8^-$, $CD4^+$.

Macrophages and the dendritic cells of the spleen and the Langerhans cells of the skin are responsible for the initial processing of an antigen as it enters the spleen or lymph nodes. The processed antigen is complexed with class II MHC molecules in the cytoplasm and is presented to the lymphocytes on the membrane of the antigen-presenting cell. Peripheral blood neutrophils are phagocytic, as are the macrophages, but do not process antigen effectively.

75–77. The answers are: 75-B, 76-E, 77-A. *(Behavioral science; developmental theories)*
A broad range of thinking has contributed to our understanding of personal, moral, and cognitive development. Freud is best known for his classic description of the "superego" conscience and its battle of the immoral, irreverent, and aggressive "id." The unconscious battle results in the "ego," which is the outward manifestation of both components of our subconscious personality. According to Freud's theory, the development of the ego is a progression through a series of phases, during which different parts of the body serve as the focus of an individual's sexual gratification.

Erikson elaborated on Freud's thinking but maintained a similar structure. He emphasized the development of individuals as being a series of crises within a societal context. For example, an infant interacts with its mother and learns either to trust or distrust the world. In each stage a decision is made (i.e., to trust or to mistrust), and subsequent development is influenced by the outcome of earlier crises.

The French psychologist Piaget studied young children throughout their development. He asked them to explain commonplace events (e.g., what happens to the sun when it sets) and created a series of simple experiments to let them demonstrate their mode of reasoning. What he found was that most children in fact do proceed through a standard set of phases using qualitatively different intellectual tools at each stage.

Maslow was interested in "self-actualization" and motivation. What he described was the classic pyramid of goals for which people universally strive. In general, people cannot have altruistic goals and motives until their more basic needs are met. They do not seek companionship, for example, until they have sufficient food; nor will they look for intellectual stimulation until shelter has been found.

Kohlberg was primarily interested in moral development, and he described a series of stages through which people progress as they shape their behavior. Fear of punishment initially promotes children to obey their parents. Later, behaviors are based on "what others will think." Ultimately, some people achieve a moral character in which the needs of others are considered equal to their own when they make decisions.

78–80. The answers are: 78-D, 79-D, 80-D. *(Immunology; Bruton's hypogammaglobulinemia)*
Normal recovery from viral diseases suggests an intact thymus-dependent immune system, thus eliminating DiGeorge, Nezelof's, and Wiskott-Aldrich syndromes, all of which feature variable or total deficits in T-cell immunity. Selective immunoglobulin deficiency is a possible diagnosis because of its characteristic of normal T-cell function.

Dysgammaglobulinemia is a selective immunoglobulin deficiency, in which one or more, but not all, immunoglobulins show a decrease in serum levels; nonspecific immunity is normal in this disorder. Normal leukocytic function would not be characteristic of chronic granulomatous disease (CGD) [impaired intracellular killing], Job's syndrome (faulty chemotactic response), or the lazy leukocyte syndrome (defective chemotactic response and abnormal inflammatory response).

The patient has Bruton's hypogammaglobulinemia. The presence of a small amount of IgG is consistent with this diagnosis. Common variable hypogammaglobulinemia resembles Bruton's disease, except that symptoms first appear in patients 20 to 30 years of age. Selective immunoglobulin deficiency is characterized by a decrease in serum levels of one or more immunoglobulin class; in selective IgA deficiency, the most common form, there is little serum IgA but normal or increased levels of IgG and IgM. Wiskott-Aldrich syndrome features low IgM levels, elevated IgA and IgE, but normal IgG levels. Transient hypogammaglobulinemia of infancy is self-correcting by age 30 months, and thus would be an unlikely diagnosis by age 3 years.

81–86. The answers are: 81-J, 82-H, 83-D, 84-A, 85-F, 86-C. *(Biochemistry; biochemical basis of disease)*
The diagnosis of acute intermittent porphyria is rarely made before puberty, but the description given is classic. The disease is transmitted in an autosomal dominant fashion, but it has a variable degree of heterozygous expression. Generally, hemoglobin synthesis by the erythrocytes is normal, but the liver's ability to

synthesize heme is impaired. Most attacks are brought on by the introduction of a drug that is metabolized through the cytochrome P_{450} oxidase system. Diffuse abdominal pain, dark red urine, increased heart rate, nausea, and vomiting reflect a buildup of γ-aminolevulinic acid and porphobilinogen, which are the precursors of porphyrin synthesis. Because there is not a serum buildup of preformed porphyrin rings, the cutaneous photosensitivity seen in erythrogenic porphyrias does not occur. The abdominal pain and vomiting are thought to be related to an autonomic neuropathy induced by the deranged metabolism. The other neuropathies described are mild in the spectrum; more striking presentations might include paraplegias, delirium, and seizures.

The description of maternal phenylketonuria has become all too common. Women who were diagnosed and treated in childhood may have forgotten their disease because effective control is important only until growth and sexual development are complete. The disease reappears strikingly when they bear children. The extremely high maternal levels of phenylalanine and alternative phenylalanine metabolites diffuse across the placenta to the fetus. Effects on the fetus include retarded myelination, impaired synthesis of catecholamines, and reduced transport of other amino acids (thus reducing their availability for protein synthesis). Mental retardation in these children is almost uniform; congenital heart defects and microcephaly occur in many. Now that treated women are able to live and function as normal adults, it is critical to identify and treat them during pregnancy to prevent this alarming outcome. If a mother is effectively managed with dietary modifications during pregnancy, the fetus is not subjected to the toxic effects of the mother's disease. Generally, the infant is heterozygous for the disorder and will have normal phenylalanine metabolism and normal development after birth.

The 21-hydroxylase deficiency is inherited in an autosomal recessive fashion and is the most common cause of congenital adrenal hyperplasia (CAH). CAH occurs in both males and females with a spectrum of severity that roughly corresponds to the underlying defect in the steroid synthesis pathway. The earlier and more complete the defect, the less able the body is to compensate. In this case, normal female anatomy has developed because of a lack of müllerian inhibiting substance, whose expression is Y-chromosome dependent. However, estrogen-dependent development (e.g., urogenital sinus differentiation) is ambiguous, and in some cases can be strikingly male, resulting in misassignment of sex. As many as two thirds of these children inherit a defect severe enough that the body is unable to compensate despite adrenal hyperplasia. In this subset of children, secretion of cortisol and aldosterone are impaired enough to produce salt-wasting, volume depletion, anorexia, and vomiting within the first few weeks of life. In the remaining cases, the hyperplasia is sufficient to compensate for the synthetic defect, and the adrenal glands produce enough glucocorticoids and mineralocorticoids so that the signs of salt-wasting are not seen. Ambiguous genitalia or virilization is common to both the salt-wasting and the non–salt-wasting cases.

Cystic fibrosis is the most common autosomal recessive disease among white children. The malabsorption is a result of diminished secretion of digestive enzymes by both the exocrine pancreas and the liver. The chronic pulmonary infections (usually *Pseudomonas aeruginosa*) are generally the earliest manifestations and often the cause of death. Dysregulation of chloride channels results in viscous secretions from all exocrine organs, and diagnosis is made following a chloride sweat test. Better antibiotics, supplemental enzyme therapy, and earlier intervention can extend the average lifespan into the third decade, but the diagnosis still carries a grim prognosis.

Vitamin C deficiency (i.e., scurvy) is now a disease largely confined to the urban poor and elderly edentulous persons, both of whom are susceptible to a variety of malnourishment syndromes. The underlying biochemical defect of vitamin C deficiency involves the impairment of the hydroxylation of proline residues; ascorbic acid is required to maintain the enzyme in its reduced (active) form. Capillary fragility, poor wound healing, and abnormal joint and bone development result because the stability of the collagen triple helix is largely dependent on the hydroxyproline content. Bleeding into the periosteum of long bones can cause painful swellings, which are probably the source of the infant's incessant crying. All of the processes are reversible if the hemorrhage and resulting inflammation in the bones do not remain unchecked for long.

The complete testicular feminization syndrome is the third most common cause of primary amenorrhea. Prepubertal inguinal hernia would be the only other reason for otherwise normal phenotypic females to present. The vagina is often short and blind-ending in these women, and all internal genitalia are absent except for normal but undescended testes. Physical growth and bone age are normal, although late epiphyseal closure frequently results in rather tall women. As with all cryptorchidism, the major long-term complication is the development of testicular tumors. The physician can generally elicit a family history of a disorder of sexual development. The defective androgen receptor is a typical member of the steroid hormone receptor superfamily with DNA-binding properties; it is encoded on the long arm of the X chromosome. Testosterone levels are high as a result of lack of feedback inhibition on luteinizing hormone (LH), and estradiol levels are intermediate between normal females and normal males. However, because the normal expression of female characteristics is dependent on an estrogen–androgen balance, these androgen-insensitive, genotypic men tend to have a greater degree of feminization than do normal women (who are sensitive to the low levels of testosterone that they have).

Defective sodium channels, which do not inactivate like their normal voltage-gated sodium channel counterparts, are implicated in the pathophysiology of periodic paralysis, a relatively rare disorder of muscle tissue.

Defective 17-β-hydroxysteroid dehydrogenase in the testis results in a lack of virilization in 46;X,Y males (male pseudohermaphroditism), without any symptoms of congenital adrenal hyperplasia. Because this enzyme is only important for the final step in testosterone synthesis, there are no glucocorticoid or mineralocorticoid deficiencies. The lack of complete male development in male pseudohermaphroditism is different from the seemingly normal female development seen in testicular feminization syndrome.

Defective oxidation of lysyl residues in collagen is the underlying problem in the most common variant (type VI) of Ehlers-Danlos syndrome.

Defective cystathionine β-synthase activity is the most common cause of homocystinuria, a defect in the metabolism of sulfur-containing amino acids (i.e., methionine, cysteine).

87. The answer is A. *(Genetics; mitochondrial DNA and proteins)*
Although the genetic code that is used in mitochondria is very similar to that used in the nucleus, there are a few differences. Because four codons are read differently, it is important that mitochondria produce their own set of transfer RNAs (tRNAs). Mitochondrial DNA includes a higher mutation rate than nuclear DNA, a maternal inheritance pattern, a lack of introns, and a single promoter for each strand. Because there are several mitochondria per cell, there may be differences among the genomes of these mitochondria, a situation called heteroplasmy. As for the protein make-up of mitochondria, most of the proteins are encoded by nuclear genes; although, there are several structural proteins that are encoded within the mitochondria. These intricate relationships pose questions related to evolution and diseases related to mitochondria DNA.

88. The answer is C. *(Genetics; pedigree analysis)*
The mode of inheritance is autosomal dominant. It does not skip generations, and it can be passed from a father to a son or a daughter. The marker that was used is uninformative in this case because it cannot be determined which of the father's alleles was given to the son. The fact that there is a recombination frequency of 1% (theta value = 0.01) does not affect the probabilities in this case. The son has inherited either the mutant allele of the gene or the normal allele, but it is not known which one. Thus, the probability that he is affected remains the same as before the testing at 0.50.

89. The answer is C. *(Genetics; direction of cellular processes)*
DNA replication of both the leading and lagging strand occurs in a 5′ to 3′ direction reading the template strand in a 3′ to 5′ direction. However, the lagging strand must be synthesized in pieces called Okazaki fragments. The messenger RNA (mRNA) is synthesized (transcription) in a 5′ to 3′ direction; this process is achieved by reading the DNA in a 3′ to 5′ direction. Translation includes the reading of a mRNA strand in a 5′ to 3′ direction to produce protein in an N-terminus to C-terminus direction.

90. The answer is A. *(Genetics; inbreeding)*
There are several methods to determine the coefficients of inbreeding and relatedness from the pedigree. First, determine the coefficient of relatedness of the proband's parent; this term is used to describe the probability that two people share an allele with identity by descent (IBD). Because a brother and sister have half of their alleles in common, a niece and uncle (as are the parents in this case) would share 1/4 of their alleles IBD because the niece would have half of her mother's alleles IBD. Then the coefficient of inbreeding can be calculated, because it is equal to half of the coefficient of relatedness of the parents. The genotypes are not required for these calculations. If a person is homozygous at a locus, it is not necessarily IBD; it could be identity by state, meaning that the same allele was inherited from two different sources and not a common ancestor.

91. The answer is E. *(Physiology; Graves disease)*
Graves disease is an autoimmune disorder that may include hyperthyroidism, goiter, pretibial myxedema, and infiltrative ophthalmopathy. Goiter is the most common manifestation. Exophthalmos occurs less frequently and is not required for the diagnosis. The symptoms are caused by both the hyperthyroidism (thyrotoxicosis) and the immune system abnormalities. The thyroxine (T_4) index and triiodothyronine (T_3) level are characteristically increased, whereas the levels of thyroid-stimulating hormone (TSH) are below normal. Graves disease is similar to other thyroid diseases in that it is approximately eight times more common in women than in men.

92. The answer is D. *(Anatomy; carpal tunnel syndrome)*
Carpal tunnel syndrome involves the compression of the median nerve as it passes through the carpel tunnel. Symptoms are pain, tingling, and numbness. Weakness of the thumb and thenar muscle atrophy may also occur. Phalen's test, which involves holding the back of one's hands together with wrists flexed, may cause numbness in the index and middle fingers, as well as the radial half of the fourth finger. Tinel's sign may also be positive. A splint may be sufficient therapy in mild cases; corticosteroids or surgery may be required in severe cases. Entrapment of the ulnar nerve in Guyon's canal can cause hand pain in a way that is analogous to carpal tunnel syndrome. This syndrome may be differentiated from carpal tunnel syndrome, because it affects the hypothenar muscles as well as the fourth and fifth fingers.

93. The answer is G. *(Genetics; achondroplasia)*
Achondroplasia is the most common form of short-limb dwarfism. It is caused by a mutation leading to a single amino acid change in the fibroblast growth factor receptor 3. This condition has an autosomal dominant mode of inheritance. It affects endochondral ossification but not intramembranous bone formation. The phenotype includes short limbs with metaphyseal flaring and bowing of the legs. The length of the spine is not usually affected, but there is an increased lumbar lordosis. Intelligence is typically normal. Other characteristic features are a saddle nose; trident hand; and compression of the spinal cord, which often occurs at the narrowed foramen magnum.

94. The answer is D. *(Anatomy; Trendelenburg sign)*
The abnormal gait can be called either a positive Trendelenburg sign or a gluteus medius limp. The gluteus medius (and to a certain extent, the gluteus minimus) normally functions to prevent such a limp. It pulls against its origin to keep the pelvis from tilting toward the opposite side when the opposite leg is off the ground. Thus, a defect on the right side causes the pelvis to tilt toward the unaffected, left side when walking. A limp of this nature may be caused by a weak gluteus medius, damage to the superior gluteal nerve, a dislocated hip, poliomyelitis, or a deformity of the femoral neck.

95. The answer is C. *(Pathology; osteoporosis)*
Osteoporosis is a disease of decreased bone mass, which can often lead to pathologic fractures. An individual usually reaches peak bone mass at about 30 years of age, at which point loss of bone mass begins. Adequate

calcium intake and exercise are important in reaching an optimal peak bone mass. Genetic factors also play a large role. Both men and women lose bone mass as they age, but women have a period of accelerated bone loss after menopause. This accelerated loss may be prevented by estrogen replacement therapy, but not by calcium supplements alone. Smoking and alcohol use can increase the rate of bone loss. Once excessive bone loss has occurred, treatments include calcium, vitamin D, estrogen, calcitonin, and biphosphonates.

96. The answer is C. *(Behavioral medicine; smoking cessation)*
The majority of smokers wish to quit, and most have tried. Most are unsuccessful in their first attempt; however, many people eventually succeed in quitting long term. On average, it takes approximately three attempts to quit. It is critical to ask about a patient's smoking habits, because many people who want to quit and who want help will not mention it unless asked. Although cravings may last for a long time, withdrawal symptoms normally abate within 2 weeks. Pharmacologic treatment may be useful, particularly in patients who experience withdrawal symptoms, but behavioral counseling is still required to give the person the best chance of succeeding. Quitting "cold turkey" is effective in comparison to a gradual reduction. In fact, a person who is "cutting down" may be smoking a fewer number of cigarettes, but inhaling more deeply and more frequently, thereby providing the same amount of nicotine.

97. The answer is B. *(Behavioral medicine; eating disorders)*
A diagnosis of bulimia nervosa does not require that the person be below a normal body weight, but it does involve binge eating and compensatory behaviors. The compensatory behaviors may include purging by self-induced vomiting, laxative abuse, and other behavior (e.g., fasting and excessive exercise). A diagnosis of anorexia nervosa is only made when a person is 85% or less than their ideal body weight and has unrealistic concerns about gaining weight. They may or may not engage in binging and purging. Anorexia nervosa and bulimia nervosa are more common in women than in men, usually with an onset in late adolescence or early adulthood. Although social factors play a role in the development of eating disorders, genetic factors are also important, as concordance rates are higher in monozygotic than dizygotic twins.

98–100. The answers are: 98-C, 99-F, 100-A. *(Biochemistry; structure of messenger RNA)*
The AUG sequence (C) codes for methionine; in eukaryotes, the first AUG following the methylguanylate cap is the site of translation initiation. The 5′ N7-methylguanylate cap is a post-translational modification that involves an unusual high-energy phosphate bond. This cap seems to enhance translation by interacting with the ribosome. It also stabilizes the message against the action of phosphatases and nucleases.

A stem–loop (or hairpin) structure (B) is, so far, the only important secondary structure described for the linear, single-stranded RNA. These stem–loops are created by sequences that are rich in standard Watson-Crick base-pairing ability. They can be found in introns and exons, at the beginning of the message, in the middle, or at the end. Their importance has been demonstrated in prokaryotes (e.g., attenuation, tryptophan operon) as well as in eukaryotes (e.g., the half-life of transferrin).

Exons (D) are the blocks of nucleotide sequence that code for amino acids in the protein. The intervening sequences, or introns (E) do not code for amino acids. Although their role is not fully understood, it is clear that in some cases they can regulate termination of translation as well as the half-life of the message.

The elucidation of the splicing process by which introns are removed and adjacent exons attached marked a major milestone in molecular genetics. Some messages have the capability to splice themselves independent of protein interaction (e.g., autocatalytic activity of RNA). In other messages, the activity of the small nuclear ribonucleoproteins (snRNPs) [F] is essential for exon splicing. The drawing illustrates the lariat intermediate, which is important in both types of splicing.

The 3′ polyadenylate (poly-A) tail (G) is a post-transcriptional modification; adenosine nucleotides are not formally coded in the gene. However, it is clear that genomic sequences indicate the length of the poly-A tail, and many researchers believe that the poly-A tail performs additional functions other than regulation of message half-life.

NMS Review for the USMLE Step 1 Answer Sheet

TEST 1

1 A B C D E F G H I J
2 A B C D E F G H I J
3 A B C D E F G H I J
4 A B C D E F G H I J
5 A B C D E F G H I J
6 A B C D E F G H I J
7 A B C D E F G H I J
8 A B C D E F G H I J
9 A B C D E F G H I J
10 A B C D E F G H I J

11 A B C D E F G H I J
12 A B C D E F G H I J
13 A B C D E F G H I J
14 A B C D E F G H I J
15 A B C D E F G H I J
16 A B C D E F G H I J
17 A B C D E F G H I J
18 A B C D E F G H I J
19 A B C D E F G H I J
20 A B C D E F G H I J

21 A B C D E F G H I J
22 A B C D E F G H I J
23 A B C D E F G H I J
24 A B C D E F G H I J
25 A B C D E F G H I J
26 A B C D E F G H I J
27 A B C D E F G H I J
28 A B C D E F G H I J
29 A B C D E F G H I J
30 A B C D E F G H I J

31 A B C D E F G H I J
32 A B C D E F G H I J
33 A B C D E F G H I J
34 A B C D E F G H I J
35 A B C D E F G H I J
36 A B C D E F G H I J
37 A B C D E F G H I J
38 A B C D E F G H I J
39 A B C D E F G H I J
40 A B C D E F G H I J

41 A B C D E F G H I J
42 A B C D E F G H I J
43 A B C D E F G H I J
44 A B C D E F G H I J
45 A B C D E F G H I J
46 A B C D E F G H I J
47 A B C D E F G H I J
48 A B C D E F G H I J
49 A B C D E F G H I J
50 A B C D E F G H I J

51 A B C D E F G H I J
52 A B C D E F G H I J
53 A B C D E F G H I J
54 A B C D E F G H I J
55 A B C D E F G H I J
56 A B C D E F G H I J
57 A B C D E F G H I J
58 A B C D E F G H I J
59 A B C D E F G H I J
60 A B C D E F G H I J

61 A B C D E F G H I J
62 A B C D E F G H I J
63 A B C D E F G H I J
64 A B C D E F G H I J
65 A B C D E F G H I J
66 A B C D E F G H I J
67 A B C D E F G H I J
68 A B C D E F G H I J
69 A B C D E F G H I J
70 A B C D E F G H I J

71 A B C D E F G H I J
72 A B C D E F G H I J
73 A B C D E F G H I J
74 A B C D E F G H I J
75 A B C D E F G H I J
76 A B C D E F G H I J
77 A B C D E F G H I J
78 A B C D E F G H I J
79 A B C D E F G H I J
80 A B C D E F G H I J

81 A B C D E F G H I J
82 A B C D E F G H I J
83 A B C D E F G H I J
84 A B C D E F G H I J
85 A B C D E F G H I J
86 A B C D E F G H I J
87 A B C D E F G H I J
88 A B C D E F G H I J
89 A B C D E F G H I J
90 A B C D E F G H I J

91 A B C D E F G H I J
92 A B C D E F G H I J
93 A B C D E F G H I J
94 A B C D E F G H I J
95 A B C D E F G H I J
96 A B C D E F G H I J
97 A B C D E F G H I J
98 A B C D E F G H I J
99 A B C D E F G H I J
100 A B C D E F G H I J

101 A B C D E F G H I J
102 A B C D E F G H I J
103 A B C D E F G H I J
104 A B C D E F G H I J
105 A B C D E F G H I J
106 A B C D E F G H I J
107 A B C D E F G H I J
108 A B C D E F G H I J
109 A B C D E F G H I J
110 A B C D E F G H I J

111 A B C D E F G H I J
112 A B C D E F G H I J
113 A B C D E F G H I J
114 A B C D E F G H I J
115 A B C D E F G H I J
116 A B C D E F G H I J
117 A B C D E F G H I J
118 A B C D E F G H I J
119 A B C D E F G H I J
120 A B C D E F G H I J

121 A B C D E F G H I J
122 A B C D E F G H I J
123 A B C D E F G H I J
124 A B C D E F G H I J
125 A B C D E F G H I J
126 A B C D E F G H I J
127 A B C D E F G H I J
127 A B C D E F G H I J
129 A B C D E F G H I J
130 A B C D E F G H I J

131 A B C D E F G H I J
132 A B C D E F G H I J
133 A B C D E F G H I J
134 A B C D E F G H I J
135 A B C D E F G H I J
136 A B C D E F G H I J
137 A B C D E F G H I J
138 A B C D E F G H I J
139 A B C D E F G H I J
140 A B C D E F G H I J

141 A B C D E F G H I J
142 A B C D E F G H I J
143 A B C D E F G H I J
144 A B C D E F G H I J
145 A B C D E F G H I J
146 A B C D E F G H I J
147 A B C D E F G H I J
148 A B C D E F G H I J
149 A B C D E F G H I J
150 A B C D E F G H I J

151 A B C D E F G H I J
152 A B C D E F G H I J
153 A B C D E F G H I J
154 A B C D E F G H I J
155 A B C D E F G H I J
156 A B C D E F G H I J
157 A B C D E F G H I J
158 A B C D E F G H I J
159 A B C D E F G H I J
160 A B C D E F G H I J

161 A B C D E F G H I J
162 A B C D E F G H I J
163 A B C D E F G H I J
164 A B C D E F G H I J
165 A B C D E F G H I J
166 A B C D E F G H I J
167 A B C D E F G H I J
168 A B C D E F G H I J
169 A B C D E F G H I J
170 A B C D E F G H I J

171 A B C D E F G H I J
172 A B C D E F G H I J
173 A B C D E F G H I J
174 A B C D E F G H I J
175 A B C D E F G H I J
176 A B C D E F G H I J
177 A B C D E F G H I J
178 A B C D E F G H I J
179 A B C D E F G H I J
180 A B C D E F G H I J

TEST 2

1 A B C D E F G H I J
2 A B C D E F G H I J
3 A B C D E F G H I J
4 A B C D E F G H I J
5 A B C D E F G H I J
6 A B C D E F G H I J
7 A B C D E F G H I J
8 A B C D E F G H I J
9 A B C D E F G H I J
10 A B C D E F G H I J

11 A B C D E F G H I J
12 A B C D E F G H I J
13 A B C D E F G H I J
14 A B C D E F G H I J
15 A B C D E F G H I J
16 A B C D E F G H I J
17 A B C D E F G H I J
18 A B C D E F G H I J
19 A B C D E F G H I J
20 A B C D E F G H I J

21 A B C D E F G H I J
22 A B C D E F G H I J
23 A B C D E F G H I J
24 A B C D E F G H I J
25 A B C D E F G H I J
26 A B C D E F G H I J
27 A B C D E F G H I J
28 A B C D E F G H I J
29 A B C D E F G H I J
30 A B C D E F G H I J

31 A B C D E F G H I J
32 A B C D E F G H I J
33 A B C D E F G H I J
34 A B C D E F G H I J
35 A B C D E F G H I J
36 A B C D E F G H I J
37 A B C D E F G H I J
38 A B C D E F G H I J
39 A B C D E F G H I J
40 A B C D E F G H I J

41 A B C D E F G H I J
42 A B C D E F G H I J
43 A B C D E F G H I J
44 A B C D E F G H I J
45 A B C D E F G H I J
46 A B C D E F G H I J
47 A B C D E F G H I J
48 A B C D E F G H I J
49 A B C D E F G H I J
50 A B C D E F G H I J

51 A B C D E F G H I J
52 A B C D E F G H I J
53 A B C D E F G H I J
54 A B C D E F G H I J
55 A B C D E F G H I J
56 A B C D E F G H I J
57 A B C D E F G H I J
58 A B C D E F G H I J
59 A B C D E F G H I J
60 A B C D E F G H I J

61 A B C D E F G H I J
62 A B C D E F G H I J
63 A B C D E F G H I J
64 A B C D E F G H I J
65 A B C D E F G H I J
66 A B C D E F G H I J

67 A B C D E F G H I J	131 A B C D E F G H I J	11 A B C D E F G H I J	76 A B C D E F G H I J
68 A B C D E F G H I J	132 A B C D E F G H I J	12 A B C D E F G H I J	77 A B C D E F G H I J
69 A B C D E F G H I J	133 A B C D E F G H I J	13 A B C D E F G H I J	78 A B C D E F G H I J
70 A B C D E F G H I J	134 A B C D E F G H I J	14 A B C D E F G H I J	79 A B C D E F G H I J
71 A B C D E F G H I J	135 A B C D E F G H I J	15 A B C D E F G H I J	80 A B C D E F G H I J
72 A B C D E F G H I J	136 A B C D E F G H I J	16 A B C D E F G H I J	81 A B C D E F G H I J
73 A B C D E F G H I J	137 A B C D E F G H I J	17 A B C D E F G H I J	82 A B C D E F G H I J
74 A B C D E F G H I J	138 A B C D E F G H I J	18 A B C D E F G H I J	83 A B C D E F G H I J
75 A B C D E F G H I J	139 A B C D E F G H I J	19 A B C D E F G H I J	84 A B C D E F G H I J
76 A B C D E F G H I J	140 A B C D E F G H I J	20 A B C D E F G H I J	85 A B C D E F G H I J
77 A B C D E F G H I J			86 A B C D E F G H I J
78 A B C D E F G H I J	141 A B C D E F G H I J	21 A B C D E F G H I J	87 A B C D E F G H I J
79 A B C D E F G H I J	142 A B C D E F G H I J	22 A B C D E F G H I J	88 A B C D E F G H I J
80 A B C D E F G H I J	143 A B C D E F G H I J	23 A B C D E F G H I J	89 A B C D E F G H I J
	144 A B C D E F G H I J	24 A B C D E F G H I J	90 A B C D E F G H I J
81 A B C D E F G H I J	145 A B C D E F G H I J	25 A B C D E F G H I J	
82 A B C D E F G H I J	146 A B C D E F G H I J	26 A B C D E F G H I J	91 A B C D E F G H I J
83 A B C D E F G H I J	147 A B C D E F G H I J	27 A B C D E F G H I J	92 A B C D E F G H I J
84 A B C D E F G H I J	148 A B C D E F G H I J	28 A B C D E F G H I J	93 A B C D E F G H I J
85 A B C D E F G H I J	149 A B C D E F G H I J	29 A B C D E F G H I J	94 A B C D E F G H I J
86 A B C D E F G H I J	150 A B C D E F G H I J	30 A B C D E F G H I J	95 A B C D E F G H I J
87 A B C D E F G H I J			96 A B C D E F G H I J
88 A B C D E F G H I J	151 A B C D E F G H I J	31 A B C D E F G H I J	97 A B C D E F G H I J
89 A B C D E F G H I J	152 A B C D E F G H I J	32 A B C D E F G H I J	98 A B C D E F G H I J
90 A B C D E F G H I J	153 A B C D E F G H I J	33 A B C D E F G H I J	99 A B C D E F G H I J
	154 A B C D E F G H I J	34 A B C D E F G H I J	100 A B C D E F G H I J
91 A B C D E F G H I J	155 A B C D E F G H I J	35 A B C D E F G H I J	
92 A B C D E F G H I J	156 A B C D E F G H I J	36 A B C D E F G H I J	101 A B C D E F G H I J
93 A B C D E F G H I J	157 A B C D E F G H I J	37 A B C D E F G H I J	102 A B C D E F G H I J
94 A B C D E F G H I J	158 A B C D E F G H I J	38 A B C D E F G H I J	103 A B C D E F G H I J
95 A B C D E F G H I J	159 A B C D E F G H I J	39 A B C D E F G H I J	104 A B C D E F G H I J
96 A B C D E F G H I J	160 A B C D E F G H I J	40 A B C D E F G H I J	105 A B C D E F G H I J
97 A B C D E F G H I J			106 A B C D E F G H I J
98 A B C D E F G H I J	161 A B C D E F G H I J	41 A B C D E F G H I J	107 A B C D E F G H I J
99 A B C D E F G H I J	162 A B C D E F G H I J	42 A B C D E F G H I J	108 A B C D E F G H I J
100 A B C D E F G H I J	163 A B C D E F G H I J	43 A B C D E F G H I J	109 A B C D E F G H I J
	164 A B C D E F G H I J	44 A B C D E F G H I J	110 A B C D E F G H I J
101 A B C D E F G H I J	165 A B C D E F G H I J	45 A B C D E F G H I J	
102 A B C D E F G H I J	166 A B C D E F G H I J	46 A B C D E F G H I J	111 A B C D E F G H I J
103 A B C D E F G H I J	167 A B C D E F G H I J	47 A B C D E F G H I J	112 A B C D E F G H I J
104 A B C D E F G H I J	168 A B C D E F G H I J	48 A B C D E F G H I J	113 A B C D E F G H I J
105 A B C D E F G H I J	169 A B C D E F G H I J	49 A B C D E F G H I J	114 A B C D E F G H I J
106 A B C D E F G H I J	170 A B C D E F G H I J	50 A B C D E F G H I J	115 A B C D E F G H I J
107 A B C D E F G H I J			116 A B C D E F G H I J
108 A B C D E F G H I J	171 A B C D E F G H I J	51 A B C D E F G H I J	117 A B C D E F G H I J
109 A B C D E F G H I J	172 A B C D E F G H I J	52 A B C D E F G H I J	118 A B C D E F G H I J
110 A B C D E F G H I J	173 A B C D E F G H I J	53 A B C D E F G H I J	119 A B C D E F G H I J
	174 A B C D E F G H I J	54 A B C D E F G H I J	120 A B C D E F G H I J
111 A B C D E F G H I J	175 A B C D E F G H I J	55 A B C D E F G H I J	
112 A B C D E F G H I J	176 A B C D E F G H I J	56 A B C D E F G H I J	121 A B C D E F G H I J
113 A B C D E F G H I J	177 A B C D E F G H I J	57 A B C D E F G H I J	122 A B C D E F G H I J
114 A B C D E F G H I J	178 A B C D E F G H I J	58 A B C D E F G H I J	123 A B C D E F G H I J
115 A B C D E F G H I J	179 A B C D E F G H I J	59 A B C D E F G H I J	124 A B C D E F G H I J
116 A B C D E F G H I J	180 A B C D E F G H I J	60 A B C D E F G H I J	125 A B C D E F G H I J
117 A B C D E F G H I J			126 A B C D E F G H I J
118 A B C D E F G H I J		61 A B C D E F G H I J	127 A B C D E F G H I J
119 A B C D E F G H I J		62 A B C D E F G H I J	127 A B C D E F G H I J
120 A B C D E F G H I J	TEST 3	63 A B C D E F G H I J	129 A B C D E F G H I J
		64 A B C D E F G H I J	130 A B C D E F G H I J
121 A B C D E F G H I J	1 A B C D E F G H I J	65 A B C D E F G H I J	
122 A B C D E F G H I J	2 A B C D E F G H I J	66 A B C D E F G H I J	131 A B C D E F G H I J
123 A B C D E F G H I J	3 A B C D E F G H I J	67 A B C D E F G H I J	132 A B C D E F G H I J
124 A B C D E F G H I J	4 A B C D E F G H I J	68 A B C D E F G H I J	133 A B C D E F G H I J
125 A B C D E F G H I J	5 A B C D E F G H I J	69 A B C D E F G H I J	134 A B C D E F G H I J
126 A B C D E F G H I J	6 A B C D E F G H I J	70 A B C D E F G H I J	135 A B C D E F G H I J
127 A (B C D E F G H I J	7 A B C D E F G H I J		136 A B C D E F G H I J
127 A B C D E F G H I J	8 A B C D E F G H I J	71 A B C D E F G H I J	137 A B C D E F G H I J
129 A B C D E F G H I J	9 A B C D E F G H I J	72 A B C D E F G H I J	138 A B C D E F G H I J
130 A B C D E F G H I J	10 A B C D E F G H I J	73 A B C D E F G H I J	139 A B C D E F G H I J
		74 A B C D E F G H I J	140 A B C D E F G H I J
		75 A B C D E F G H I J	141 A B C D E F G H I J

142 A B C D E F G H I J	24 A B C D E F G H I J	89 A B C D E F G H I J	153 A B C D E F G H I J
143 A B C D E F G H I J	25 A B C D E F G H I J	90 A B C D E F G H I J	154 A B C D E F G H I J
144 A B C D E F G H I J	26 A B C D E F G H I J		155 A B C D E F G H I J
145 A B C D E F G H I J	27 A B C D E F G H I J	91 A B C D E F G H I J	156 A B C D E F G H I J
146 A B C D E F G H I J	28 A B C D E F G H I J	92 A B C D E F G H I J	157 A B C D E F G H I J
147 A B C D E F G H I J	29 A B C D E F G H I J	93 A B C D E F G H I J	158 A B C D E F G H I J
148 A B C D E F G H I J	30 A B C D E F G H I J	94 A B C D E F G H I J	159 A B C D E F G H I J
149 A B C D E F G H I J		95 A B C D E F G H I J	160 A B C D E F G H I J
150 A B C D E F G H I J	31 A B C D E F G H I J	96 A B C D E F G H I J	
	32 A B C D E F G H I J	97 A B C D E F G H I J	161 A B C D E F G H I J
151 A B C D E F G H I J	33 A B C D E F G H I J	98 A B C D E F G H I J	162 A B C D E F G H I J
152 A B C D E F G H I J	34 A B C D E F G H I J	99 A B C D E F G H I J	163 A B C D E F G H I J
153 A B C D E F G H I J	35 A B C D E F G H I J	100 A B C D E F G H I J	164 A B C D E F G H I J
154 A B C D E F G H I J	36 A B C D E F G H I J		165 A B C D E F G H I J
155 A B C D E F G H I J	37 A B C D E F G H I J	101 A B C D E F G H I J	166 A B C D E F G H I J
156 A B C D E F G H I J	38 A B C D E F G H I J	102 A B C D E F G H I J	167 A B C D E F G H I J
157 A B C D E F G H I J	39 A B C D E F G H I J	103 A B C D E F G H I J	168 A B C D E F G H I J
158 A B C D E F G H I J	40 A B C D E F G H I J	104 A B C D E F G H I J	169 A B C D E F G H I J
159 A B C D E F G H I J		105 A B C D E F G H I J	170 A B C D E F G H I J
160 A B C D E F G H I J	41 A B C D E F G H I J	106 A B C D E F G H I J	
	42 A B C D E F G H I J	107 A B C D E F G H I J	171 A B C D E F G H I J
161 A B C D E F G H I J	43 A B C D E F G H I J	108 A B C D E F G H I J	172 A B C D E F G H I J
162 A B C D E F G H I J	44 A B C D E F G H I J	109 A B C D E F G H I J	173 A B C D E F G H I J
163 A B C D E F G H I J	45 A B C D E F G H I J	110 A B C D E F G H I J	174 A B C D E F G H I J
164 A B C D E F G H I J	46 A B C D E F G H I J		175 A B C D E F G H I J
165 A B C D E F G H I J	47 A B C D E F G H I J	111 A B C D E F G H I J	176 A B C D E F G H I J
166 A B C D E F G H I J	48 A B C D E F G H I J	112 A B C D E F G H I J	177 A B C D E F G H I J
167 A B C D E F G H I J	49 A B C D E F G H I J	113 A B C D E F G H I J	178 A B C D E F G H I J
168 A B C D E F G H I J	50 A B C D E F G H I J	114 A B C D E F G H I J	179 A B C D E F G H I J
169 A B C D E F G H I J		115 A B C D E F G H I J	180 A B C D E F G H I J
170 A B C D E F G H I J	51 A B C D E F G H I J	116 A B C D E F G H I J	
	52 A B C D E F G H I J	117 A B C D E F G H I J	
171 A B C D E F G H I J	53 A B C D E F G H I J	118 A B C D E F G H I J	TEST 5
172 A B C D E F G H I J	54 A B C D E F G H I J	119 A B C D E F G H I J	
173 A B C D E F G H I J	55 A B C D E F G H I J	120 A B C D E F G H I J	1 A B C D E F G H I J
174 A B C D E F G H I J	56 A B C D E F G H I J		2 A B C D E F G H I J
175 A B C D E F G H I J	57 A B C D E F G H I J	121 A B C D E F G H I J	3 A B C D E F G H I J
176 A B C D E F G H I J	58 A B C D E F G H I J	122 A B C D E F G H I J	4 A B C D E F G H I J
177 A B C D E F G H I J	59 A B C D E F G H I J	123 A B C D E F G H I J	5 A B C D E F G H I J
178 A B C D E F G H I J	60 A B C D E F G H I J	124 A B C D E F G H I J	6 A B C D E F G H I J
179 A B C D E F G H I J		125 A B C D E F G H I J	7 A B C D E F G H I J
180 A B C D E F G H I J	61 A B C D E F G H I J	126 A B C D E F G H I J	8 A B C D E F G H I J
	62 A B C D E F G H I J	127 A B C D E F G H I J	9 A B C D E F G H I J
	63 A B C D E F G H I J	127 A B C D E F G H I J	10 A B C D E F G H I J
TEST 4	64 A B C D E F G H I J	129 A B C D E F G H I J	
	65 A B C D E F G H I J	130 A B C D E F G H I J	11 A B C D E F G H I J
1 A B C D E F G H I J	66 A B C D E F G H I J		12 A B C D E F G H I J
2 A B C D E F G H I J	67 A B C D E F G H I J	131 A B C D E F G H I J	13 A B C D E F G H I J
3 A B C D E F G H I J	68 A B C D E F G H I J	132 A B C D E F G H I J	14 A B C D E F G H I J
4 A B C D E F G H I J	69 A B C D E F G H I J	133 A B C D E F G H I J	15 A B C D E F G H I J
5 A B C D E F G H I J	70 A B C D E F G H I J	134 A B C D E F G H I J	16 A B C D E F G H I J
6 A B C D E F G H I J		135 A B C D E F G H I J	17 A B C D E F G H I J
7 A B C D E F G H I J	71 A B C D E F G H I J	136 A B C D E F G H I J	18 A B C D E F G H I J
8 A B C D E F G H I J	72 A B C D E F G H I J	137 A B C D E F G H I J	19 A B C D E F G H I J
9 A B C D E F G H I J	73 A B C D E F G H I J	138 A B C D E F G H I J	20 A B C D E F G H I J
10 A B C D E F G H I J	74 A B C D E F G H I J	139 A B C D E F G H I J	
	75 A B C D E F G H I J	140 A B C D E F G H I J	21 A B C D E F G H I J
11 A B C D E F G H I J	76 A B C D E F G H I J		22 A B C D E F G H I J
12 A B C D E F G H I J	77 A B C D E F G H I J	141 A B C D E F G H I J	23 A B C D E F G H I J
13 A B C D E F G H I J	78 A B C D E F G H I J	142 A B C D E F G H I J	24 A B C D E F G H I J
14 A B C D E F G H I J	79 A B C D E F G H I J	143 A B C D E F G H I J	25 A B C D E F G H I J
15 A B C D E F G H I J	80 A B C D E F G H I J	144 A B C D E F G H I J	26 A B C D E F G H I J
16 A B C D E F G H I J		145 A B C D E F G H I J	27 A B C D E F G H I J
17 A B C D E F G H I J	81 A B C D E F G H I J	146 A B C D E F G H I J	28 A B C D E F G H I J
18 A B C D E F G H I J	82 A B C D E F G H I J	147 A B C D E F G H I J	29 A B C D E F G H I J
19 A B C D E F G H I J	83 A B C D E F G H I J	148 A B C D E F G H I J	30 A B C D E F G H I J
20 A B C D E F G H I J	84 A B C D E F G H I J	149 A B C D E F G H I J	31 A B C D E F G H I J
	85 A B C D E F G H I J	150 A B C D E F G H I J	32 A B C D E F G H I J
21 A B C D E F G H I J	86 A B C D E F G H I J		33 A B C D E F G H I J
22 A B C D E F G H I J	87 A B C D E F G H I J	151 A B C D E F G H I J	34 A B C D E F G H I J
23 A B C D E F G H I J	88 A B C D E F G H I J	152 A B C D E F G H I J	35 A B C D E F G H I J

36 A B C D E F G H I J
37 A B C D E F G H I J
38 A B C D E F G H I J
39 A B C D E F G H I J
40 A B C D E F G H I J

41 A B C D E F G H I J
42 A B C D E F G H I J
43 A B C D E F G H I J
44 A B C D E F G H I J
45 A B C D E F G H I J
46 A B C D E F G H I J
47 A B C D E F G H I J
48 A B C D E F G H I J
49 A B C D E F G H I J
50 A B C D E F G H I J

51 A B C D E F G H I J
52 A B C D E F G H I J
53 A B C D E F G H I J
54 A B C D E F G H I J
55 A B C D E F G H I J
56 A B C D E F G H I J
57 A B C D E F G H I J
58 A B C D E F G H I J
59 A B C D E F G H I J
60 A B C D E F G H I J

61 A B C D E F G H I J
62 A B C D E F G H I J
63 A B C D E F G H I J
64 A B C D E F G H I J
65 A B C D E F G H I J
66 A B C D E F G H I J
67 A B C D E F G H I J
68 A B C D E F G H I J
69 A B C D E F G H I J
70 A B C D E F G H I J

71 A B C D E F G H I J
72 A B C D E F G H I J
73 A B C D E F G H I J
74 A B C D E F G H I J
75 A B C D E F G H I J
76 A B C D E F G H I J
77 A B C D E F G H I J
78 A B C D E F G H I J
79 A B C D E F G H I J
80 A B C D E F G H I J

81 A B C D E F G H I J
82 A B C D E F G H I J
83 A B C D E F G H I J
84 A B C D E F G H I J
85 A B C D E F G H I J
86 A B C D E F G H I J
87 A B C D E F G H I J
88 A B C D E F G H I J
89 A B C D E F G H I J
90 A B C D E F G H I J

91 A B C D E F G H I J
92 A B C D E F G H I J
93 A B C D E F G H I J
94 A B C D E F G H I J
95 A B C D E F G H I J
96 A B C D E F G H I J
97 A B C D E F G H I J

98 A B C D E F G H I J
99 A B C D E F G H I J
100 A B C D E F G H I J

101 A B C D E F G H I J
102 A B C D E F G H I J
103 A B C D E F G H I J
104 A B C D E F G H I J
105 A B C D E F G H I J
106 A B C D E F G H I J
107 A B C D E F G H I J
108 A B C D E F G H I J
109 A B C D E F G H I J
110 A B C D E F G H I J

111 A B C D E F G H I J
112 A B C D E F G H I J
113 A B C D E F G H I J
114 A B C D E F G H I J
115 A B C D E F G H I J
116 A B C D E F G H I J
117 A B C D E F G H I J
118 A B C D E F G H I J
119 A B C D E F G H I J
120 A B C D E F G H I J

121 A B C D E F G H I J
122 A B C D E F G H I J
123 A B C D E F G H I J
124 A B C D E F G H I J
125 A B C D E F G H I J
126 A B C D E F G H I J
127 A B C D E F G H I J
127 A B C D E F G H I J
129 A B C D E F G H I J
130 A B C D E F G H I J

131 A B C D E F G H I J
132 A B C D E F G H I J
133 A B C D E F G H I J
134 A B C D E F G H I J
135 A B C D E F G H I J
136 A B C D E F G H I J
137 A B C D E F G H I J
138 A B C D E F G H I J
139 A B C D E F G H I J
140 A B C D E F G H I J

141 A B C D E F G H I J
142 A B C D E F G H I J
143 A B C D E F G H I J
144 A B C D E F G H I J
145 A B C D E F G H I J
146 A B C D E F G H I J
147 A B C D E F G H I J
148 A B C D E F G H I J
149 A B C D E F G H I J
150 A B C D E F G H I J

151 A B C D E F G H I J
152 A B C D E F G H I J
153 A B C D E F G H I J
154 A B C D E F G H I J
155 A B C D E F G H I J
156 A B C D E F G H I J
157 A B C D E F G H I J
158 A B C D E F G H I J

159 A B C D E F G H I J
160 A B C D E F G H I J

161 A B C D E F G H I J
162 A B C D E F G H I J
163 A B C D E F G H I J
164 A B C D E F G H I J
165 A B C D E F G H I J
166 A B C D E F G H I J
167 A B C D E F G H I J
168 A B C D E F G H I J
169 A B C D E F G H I J
170 A B C D E F G H I J

171 A B C D E F G H I J
172 A B C D E F G H I J
173 A B C D E F G H I J
174 A B C D E F G H I J
175 A B C D E F G H I J
176 A B C D E F G H I J
177 A B C D E F G H I J
178 A B C D E F G H I J
179 A B C D E F G H I J
180 A B C D E F G H I J

TEST6

1 A B C D E F G H I J
2 A B C D E F G H I J
3 A B C D E F G H I J
4 A B C D E F G H I J
5 A B C D E F G H I J
6 A B C D E F G H I J
7 A B C D E F G H I J
8 A B C D E F G H I J
9 A B C D E F G H I J
10 A B C D E F G H I J

11 A B C D E F G H I J
12 A B C D E F G H I J
13 A B C D E F G H I J
14 A B C D E F G H I J
15 A B C D E F G H I J
16 A B C D E F G H I J
17 A B C D E F G H I J
18 A B C D E F G H I J
19 A B C D E F G H I J
20 A B C D E F G H I J

21 A B C D E F G H I J
22 A B C D E F G H I J
23 A B C D E F G H I J
24 A B C D E F G H I J
25 A B C D E F G H I J
26 A B C D E F G H I J
27 A B C D E F G H I J
28 A B C D E F G H I J
29 A B C D E F G H I J
30 A B C D E F G H I J

31 A B C D E F G H I J
32 A B C D E F G H I J
33 A B C D E F G H I J
34 A B C D E F G H I J
35 A B C D E F G H I J
36 A B C D E F G H I J
37 A B C D E F G H I J
38 A B C D E F G H I J

39 A B C D E F G H I J
40 A B C D E F G H I J

41 A B C D E F G H I J
42 A B C D E F G H I J
43 A B C D E F G H I J
44 A B C D E F G H I J
45 A B C D E F G H I J
46 A B C D E F G H I J
47 A B C D E F G H I J
48 A B C D E F G H I J
49 A B C D E F G H I J
50 A B C D E F G H I J

51 A B C D E F G H I J
52 A B C D E F G H I J
53 A B C D E F G H I J
54 A B C D E F G H I J
55 A B C D E F G H I J
56 A B C D E F G H I J
57 A B C D E F G H I J
58 A B C D E F G H I J
59 A B C D E F G H I J
60 A B C D E F G H I J

61 A B C D E F G H I J
62 A B C D E F G H I J
63 A B C D E F G H I J
64 A B C D E F G H I J
65 A B C D E F G H I J
66 A B C D E F G H I J
67 A B C D E F G H I J
68 A B C D E F G H I J
69 A B C D E F G H I J
70 A B C D E F G H I J

71 A B C D E F G H I J
72 A B C D E F G H I J
73 A B C D E F G H I J
74 A B C D E F G H I J
75 A B C D E F G H I J
76 A B C D E F G H I J
77 A B C D E F G H I J
78 A B C D E F G H I J
79 A B C D E F G H I J
80 A B C D E F G H I J

81 A B C D E F G H I J
82 A B C D E F G H I J
83 A B C D E F G H I J
84 A B C D E F G H I J
85 A B C D E F G H I J
86 A B C D E F G H I J
87 A B C D E F G H I J
88 A B C D E F G H I J
89 A B C D E F G H I J
90 A B C D E F G H I J

91 A B C D E F G H I J
92 A B C D E F G H I J
93 A B C D E F G H I J
94 A B C D E F G H I J
95 A B C D E F G H I J
96 A B C D E F G H I J
97 A B C D E F G H I J
98 A B C D E F G H I J
99 A B C D E F G H I J
100 A B C D E F G H I J